Qualitative Methods in Psychology

SECOND EDITION

LIVERPOOL JMU LIBRARY

3 1111 01397 8729

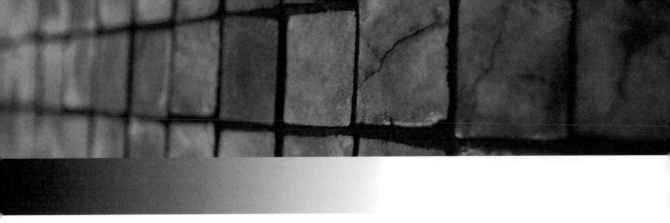

Qualitative Methods in Psychology

A research guide

SECOND EDITION

Peter Banister, Geoff Bunn, Erica Burman, John Daniels, Paul Duckett, Dan Goodley, Rebecca Lawthom, Ian Parker, Katherine Runswick-Cole, Judith Sixsmith, Sophie Smailes, Carol Tindall and Pauline Whelan

Manchester Metropolitan University

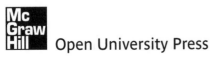

Open University Press

Open University Press
McGraw-Hill Education
McGraw-Hill House
Shoppenhangers Road
Maidenhead
Berkshire
England
SL6 2QL

email: enquiries@openup.co.uk
world wide web: www.openup.co.uk

and Two Penn Plaza, New York, NY 10121-2289, USA

First edition published 1994, this edition published 2011

Copyright © Peter Banister, Geoff Bunn, Erica Burman, John Daniels, Paul Duckett,
Dan Goodley, Rebecca Lawthom, Ian Parker, Katherine Runswick-Cole, Judith Sixsmith,
Sophie Smailes, Carol Tindall and Pauline Whelan 2011

All rights reserved. Except for the quotation of short passages for the purposes of criticism
and review, no part of this publication may be reproduced, stored in a retrieval system, or
transmitted, in any form or by any means, electronic, mechanical, photocopying, recording
or otherwise, without the prior written permission of the publisher or a licence from the
Copyright Licensing Agency Limited. Details of such licences (for reprographic reproduction)
may be obtained from the Copyright Licensing Agency Ltd of Saffron House, 6-10 Kirby Street,
London, EC1N 8TS.

A catalogue record of this book is available from the British Library

ISBN-13: 978-0-33-524305-1(pb)
ISBN-10: 0335241352 (pb)
e-ISBN: 9780335243068

Library of Congress Cataloging-in-Publication Data
CIP data applied for

Typeset by Graphicraft Limited, Hong Kong
Printed in the UK by Bell and Bain Ltd, Glasgow

Fictitious names of companies, products, people, characters and/or data that may be used
herein (in case studies or in examples) are not intended to represent any real individual,
company, product or event.

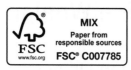

Contents

Preface   *vii*

Part I   Orientations   *1*
1 Phenomenology   *3*
2 Action research   *22*
3 Positionalities   *38*

Part II   Methodologies   *61*
 4 Observation   *63*
 5 Ethnography   *75*
 6 Interviewing   *88*
 7 The repertory grid and its possibilities   *100*
 8 Psychosocial analysis   *116*
 9 Narrative inquiry   *129*
10 Historical analyses   *143*

Part III   Representations   *163*
11 Future directions for qualitative research   *165*
12 New and emerging forms of representation   *179*
13 Writing up   *194*
14 ~~Problems~~ in/of qualitative research   *208*

    Glossary   *223*
    Index   *227*

Preface

This book, although headlined as the second edition of *Qualitative Methods in Psychology: A Research Guide*, is in many ways (though not entirely) a fundamentally different book. The original edition was published in 1994 arising out of a module on qualitative methods run on the MSc Psychology here at Manchester Metropolitan University. This MSc degree was originally a joint run degree in Psychology involving modules from a variety of local institutions, including the University of Manchester, Manchester Polytechnic, Salford University and Bolton Institute. It was felt that most psychology degrees made some attempt at covering quantitative methods, but that there was little coverage at the undergraduate level re. qualitative methods. Thus, providing a module for our joint MSc students was felt to be useful in helping them to develop a 'tool-kit' for research and to develop their critical appreciation of different methods within psychology. It was also felt to be useful for supporting bids to research funding councils for increasing taught postgraduate input for postgraduate students.

The module proved to be very successful, and there was a growing realisation that there were not many books available for students who wished to find out more about qualitative methods. The then five staff who produced the module thus suggested that a jointly written text arising from our experience of teaching the students would be useful for the academic community. Thus, the aim from the outset was to provide an introductory text to the area of qualitative research, intended for advanced undergraduate and postgraduate students. Its emphasis was very much on *methods* within psychology, and it assumed some basic knowledge of the discipline. We therefore expect the reader to have a preliminary acquaintance with the approach of psychology and more conventional methods, including some familiarity with the philosophy of psychological research, the research process, research methods and quantitative approaches. Thus the book was not aimed at introductory psychology students, but is a resource for academics and professionals who use psychological methods in their work. The book provided an understanding of the assumptions underlying such research methods, presenting them as both a *critique* and a *complement* to quantitative approaches, and was also presented as a practical guide to carrying out such research, along with the basis for a critical evaluation of it.

The book was later adopted as a set text for the Open University final year module in Social Psychology, and is still utilised in the current presentation of this module. In the interim years there have been a number of major changes which have also impacted on this area, emphasising the importance of qualitative methods for psychology students. There has been the publication by the Quality Assurance Agency (2007) of a benchmark for psychology undergraduate education. In Section 4.8 where research methods in psychology are specifically mentioned, there is a subheading that stresses the coverage of 'quantitative and qualitative methods' (p. 5), and p. 6 emphasises that the subject-specific skills include the ability to 'analyse data using both quantitative and qualitative methods'. In addition, the British Psychological Society (2010) in their curriculum for the graduate basis for chartered membership includes as an essential the ability to analyse data using both quantitative and qualitative methods. Thus qualitative methods in the last 16 or so years have now become much more accepted as part of mainstream psychology.

We continue to provide our module, but it too has altered over time to much more reflect the sharing of experiences by staff who are actively using qualitative methods in their own research. There are now many more postgraduate research students who are actively choosing to use qualitative methods to investigate their research questions. New methods have arisen in the intervening years, and these are included in this new edition. Nonetheless, for many of our postgraduate taught students there is still some reluctance to explore new ways of looking at psychological issues using qualitative methods. This book to some extent is intended to help them to open up their eyes to the potential of this approach and to serve as an adjunct to their current studies. We want to encourage them, as new researchers, to go beyond positivism and to do psychology in a way that is useful and relevant. A common thread throughout the book is an emphasis on reflexivity, not only concerning the research process and its outcomes, but also in terms of acknowledging and using your own position as a researcher.

Thus, there is still an emphasis on how to carry out research in this area, but also there is an attempt to broaden out the area to get the students to engage further with important concepts such as epistemology, positionality, subjectivity, politics and standpoints.

The contributors

All the co-authors have carried out research using qualitative methods and are committed to this general approach. Brief biographical notes are as follows.

Peter Banister is the Head of Department of Psychology at Manchester Metropolitan University, where he teaches qualitative methods, social psychology and forensic psychology.

Geoff Bunn is a Senior Lecturer in Psychology at Manchester Metropolitan University with specialist interests in conceptual and historical issues in psychology.

Erica Burman is Professor of Psychology and Women's Studies in Manchester Metropolitan University where she codirects the Discourse Unit and teaches and supervises critical, feminist and discursive work.

John Daniels is a Senior Lecturer for the Exercise and Sport Science Department at Manchester Metropolitan University. His research interests are in community interventions that seek to increase physical activity levels and participation in sport.

Paul Duckett is a critical community psychologist at Manchester Metropolitan University who works in the fields of disability, mental health and unemployment.

Dan Goodley is Professor of Psychology and Disability Studies at Manchester Metropolitan University who has published and researched widely in these areas.

Rebecca Lawthom is Reader in Community Practice at Manchester Metropolitan University, where she specialises in community psychology and feminist research.

Ian Parker is Professor of Psychology in the Discourse Unit at Manchester Metropolitan University (www.discourseunit.com).

Katherine Runswick-Cole is a Research Fellow in Disability Studies and Psychology at Manchester Metropolitan University.

Judith Sixsmith is Professor of Adult Social Care at Manchester Metropolitan University. Her research interests are in health, social care and community psychology where she works with people marginalised within social systems, often applying action research frameworks in real-world contexts.

Sophie Smailes is a Senior Lecturer in Social Change at Manchester Metropolitan University with interests in qualitative research, feminist methodologies and psychotherapy.

Carol Tindall has recently retired from Manchester Metropolitan University. She has extensive teaching and research interests in counselling and psychotherapy, specialising in exploring both the individual experiences of distress and how these experiences are sociopolitically framed.

Pauline Whelan is a doctoral student at the Centre for Research into Higher Education, Carnegie Research Institute, Leeds Metropolitan University.

This is not an edited collection of articles. All authors have circulated copies of their drafts to all members of the team, and there has been agreement across the team as to the final format of each chapter. This does not mean that this is a coherent seamless text. Just as there are contrasts and conflicts (as well as continuities) between the assumptions underlying quantitative and qualitative research, so there are tensions and differences in approach between the various qualitative methods and researchers. Such divisions are inevitable, given the nature of research. Indeed, some of these researchers would not accept the designation 'method' at all, seeing this as partaking in the scientist division between experience, theory and action.

We recognise that readers may want to use this book as an aid to carrying out research using a particular methodological technique from within qualitative methods, and may thus just look at the appropriate chapter. However, we think that a few words here about the book in general may well encourage you to read a little more than just one particular chapter.

The book starts off with three chapters that provide, under the general title of Orientations, some broad considerations about qualitative research. The next seven chapters, under the general heading of Methodologies, concentrate on what we consider to be currently the major different research approaches within psychology practised under the general heading of 'qualitative methods': observation, ethnography, interviewing, the repertory grid, psychosocial analysis, narrative enquiry and historical analyses. These chapters to some extent follow a common format and include a brief résumé of the specific area, its historical development, a description of the method as applied to a particular research example, a review of the advantages of the approach and a discussion of problems with the method. The final section of the book is on 'Representations', and suggests to some extent future direction for the area, and also includes a chapter on the writing up of qualitative research, with an emphasis on reflexivity, ethics, the role of values and the relationship between psychology and social change.

Thanks are due to Emma Turley for reading and commenting on an earlier version of Chapter 1 and to Professor Carolyn Kagan for reading and commenting on an earlier version of Chapter 7. Thanks also to the Econmic and Social Research Council funded project "Does Every Child Matter Post Blair? The interconnections of disabled childhoods". http://post.blairposterow.com/pages/home, which Dan Goodley and Katherine Runswick-Cole draw on in their chapters.

Our collective thanks are due to our students, who have helped us to refine our thoughts, and to appreciate the problems faced by those who are intending to start research using the exciting and challenging approaches of qualitative methods.

References

British Psychological Society (2010) *Accreditation through Partnership Handbook: Guidance for Undergraduate and Conversion Psychology Programmes.* Leicester: British Psychological Society.

Quality Assurance Agency (2007) *Subject Benchmark Statement Psychology.* London: Quality Assurance Agency for Higher Education.

PART I

Orientations

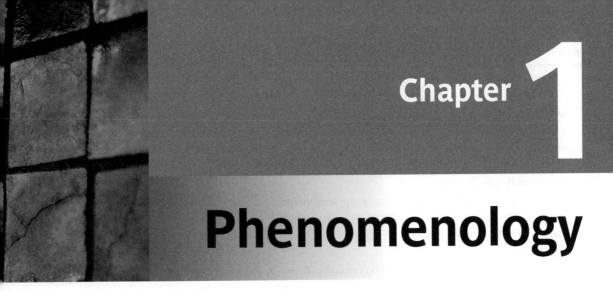

Chapter 1

Phenomenology

Rebecca Lawthom and Carol Tindall

Introduction

This chapter is situated in a section of text called Orientations and rather like guiders or orienteers we want to point you towards some markers and direction in phenomenology. We orient this work as interested practitioners and facilitators of qualitative research. One of us (CT) writes very much from a feminist phenomenological perspective and this articulation is clearly present both here and in Chapter 7 on the repertory grid. The other (RL) does not work from an explicit phenomenological perspective but works with interpretation and construction more broadly in qualitative work. In mapping and orienting, we will use examples throughout to situate and explain the terms. Of course experience belongs to us all, so use your experience to ground the terms for you.

Below, as an example of an account of experience, is Roxy Freeman's (2009) wonderfully rich and evocative first person narrative of change and of the phenomena of living within the built environment, which appeared in *The Guardian* under the title 'My Gypsy Childhood'. This offers you a flavour of the type of data that phenomenologists are interested in:

> My siblings and I were born into this lifestyle, but we weren't taught to carve clothes pegs and sell lucky heather. We were brought up with strict morals, values and guidelines. We don't look or act particularly different to anybody else. We just had a different path, and weren't brought up living in a house.
>
> After completing my access course (thanks to a wonderful tutor, I got distinctions in all the units), I did a degree with the Open University, and that meant completely changing my way of life. Last November, at the age of 30, I moved to Brighton to study at Brighton Journalist Works. I live here with my boyfriend in a flat, which is bizarre and alien to me. My family are, admittedly, no longer truly nomadic, and my parents support my decision to transform my life, but I have never lived within bricks and mortar before, and I feel completely out of touch with nature now.

I can't see or feel the change from one season to the next, I crave greenery, and I constantly wrestle with the emotion of feeling trapped. I spend half my life opening doors and windows, trying to get rid of the airless, claustrophobic feeling that comes with being inside. I get woken up by bin lorries, the rush-hour traffic and my neighbours shouting, instead of birdsong and the wind in the trees. I can't sense when it's going to rain because I can no longer smell it in the air, and when it does rain I can't hear it landing on the roof.

I live near the sea because it gives me some sense of openness and freedom, but I don't think I will ever feel truly settled here – or anywhere else. My instinct is to travel, and when you have grown up waking to different scenery every day, it's easy to feel trapped. But to reach my dream, I have to put down roots.

(Roxy Freeman. Reprinted with permission from *The Guardian*, Monday, 7 September 2009)

Phenomenology is all about lived experience, the richness and texture of experience which is understood through rich engagement with another person's 'lifeworld'. You may be familiar with the term phenomenology or phenomenological inquiry and this is not surprising. It has been utilised widely within the social sciences and is often used to refer to a research perspective, which is distinct from and in opposition to positivist forms of inquiry (Bogdan and Taylor 1979). Whilst we can locate phenomenology broadly within the interpretivist paradigm (Burrell and Morgan 1979; Holstein and Gubruim 1994), there is a sense of confusion between phenomenology as a paradigm and phenomenological inquiry as a stance or approach to conducting research (Patton 1990). In this chapter, we articulate some clear aims around phenomenology which both position phenomenology more broadly and explore the approach as a way of doing research. Space precludes in-depth coverage of analysis but we aim to paint a journey which captures the elements of the approach, signposting you on to further reading (if interested). In subsequent chapters you are introduced to different axes within which to understand qualitative approaches (action and structure). In this chapter, we turn to phenomenology which embraces subjectivity and also engages with interpretation and structure. However, the key pivot or essence of this understanding is around the primacy of subjective experience – so here, how the individual interprets the world and structure around them. Phenomenology is an approach which explicitly focuses on sense making and subjectivity where a person's world is therefore one of personal meanings.

Orientations

Everybody comes to qualitative methods from somewhere – often students and ourselves included happen upon it after induction into more dominant ways of knowing, i.e. positivist forms of knowledge. In this sense, it is a relational concept – we are considering it, in relation to other more privileged ways of doing 'science'. It seems useful to locate what we know about phenomenology both as a paradigm or philosophy and as a method. Understanding how phenomenology fits into the discipline of psychology generally and how it fits into debates around methods can allow us to see knowledge as situated. This term, situated knowledge, locates knowledge in time and place, within cultures and bodies, rather than as a free floating entity. In order to situate phenomenology it is useful to define it (whatever it is).

However, defining phenomenology is no easy task as the landscape of phenomenology is fissured and fragmented. Here, in this chapter, we offer an overview of the current scene, and include a wide range of examples rather than detailing the variety of phenomenologists' positioning. Indeed, as Caelli (2000) points out, it is possible to identify 18 different forms of phenomenology. There are shared features between these different schools, but also some distinct differences. The dynamic tension between phenomenologists – evident initially when existentialists such as Heidegger, Sartre and Merleau-Ponty challenged Husserl's (1859–1938) descriptive stance – is still apparent in phenomenology today (see, for example, Giorgi 2010). The divisions and tensions that began with Husserl and Heidegger are still evident today as Giorgi's descriptive stance (2010) contrasts with a more methodologically driven interpretative phenomenological stance advocated by Smith (2010). It is an evolving approach, although knowing something of the historic and cultural grounding of perspectives, theories and methods enables us to have a better understanding of their purpose and value. Whilst Husserl is seen as the 'founding father' of the philosophy. Others such as Heidegger developed it from being philosophically oriented to a methodological research approach. Phenomenology is a rich and complex philosophy which has been taken into psychology and other social sciences. From this, it has variously developed as an approach and research method resulting in different emphases and some confusion, which makes it a tricky area to map effectively.

That said, there are commonalities: all privilege the experiential subjective world of the individual, what many phenomenologists call the 'lifeworld'; that is, how things seem to the perceiver, how the phenomena (the appearance of things) are experienced and understood by the person having the experience, as it is through experiencing our world that we come to know it. This was a radical challenge to earlier dualist thinking where mind and body were thought of as separate entities. Later, in the 1960s, phenomenologists keen to resist the determinist and antihumanist tendencies of behaviourism and psychoanalysis joined forces and together with humanists such as Rogers emphasised the need to understand how people experience themselves, others and the contexts within which they are embedded, from their own viewpoint. So the primacy of experience, as filtered through the perceiver, is key to phenomenology's alternative understandings of people. Roxy's account (given above) captures her current lifeworld as not being able to smell or hear the rain, distinct from her childhood immersed in nature.

Some phenomenologists, when aiming to understand lived experience follow Husserl's focus on description (Ashworth 2003a, 2003b; Giorgi 2010), whilst others follow the existentialists (Packer and Addison 1989; Van Manen 1990; King 2004) and favour a more interpretive approach. Giorgi (2010) argues that the phenomenological method is richly descriptive and encompasses three interlocking steps: (a) the phenomenological reduction; (b) description; and (c) search for essences. Alongside this framework, a plethora of variations flourishes which pays differential emphasis to the lifeworld and ability to bracket off. In addition, there are phenomenological methods such as interpretative phenomenological analysis (IPA, Smith *et al.* 2009). You may well have heard of this, as it is probably the most popular method of phenomenological analysis and is a particular branch of interpretive analysis. This approach, with its distinctive analytical frame, has gained much ground within psychological research in the UK. We see this as an analytical development of phenomenology which can be fruitfully explored elsewhere. All phenomenologists, whatever their differences, aim to explore how the world is humanly experienced by gaining first-person accounts of the quality and texture of individual experience (Spinelli 2003), with the goal of using the accounts to elucidate the nature of the phenomena. However, given that 'psychologists . . . have turned their attention to particular areas of experience and have sought to draw out the human meanings of these areas using empirical material such as interviews and observation' (King *et al.* 2008: 81), it may be more accurate now in the twenty-first century to talk about phenomenologically based psychology.

Mapping

The landscape of qualitative research is rich and complex and it is useful to map where phenomenology fits into the wider picture. Burrell and Morgan's paradigmatic model (1979) proposed that particular lens or ways of viewing the social world are related to methods and knowledge (Figure 1.1).

The initial premise of Burrell and Morgan's work was to relate theories of organisation to their wider context. Their map, whilst originally developed around organisational theory, raises broader questions around nature and science. Questioning fundamental assumptions around ontology, epistemology, human nature and methodology, the model proposed pivots around two meta-theoretical assumptions about the nature of the society and the nature of social science. The debate (they choose) around the nature of social science is objectivity versus subjectivity. The society debate lies around regulation versus radical change. Given these two broad axes: the subjective–objective spectrum of social science and the regulatory–radical change spectrum of society, Burrell and Morgan conceive of four paradigms. The term paradigm itself is problematic, but they use it to mean the commonality of perspective which binds theoretical work together. Thus, the paradigms (here) are defined by the meta-theoretical assumptions

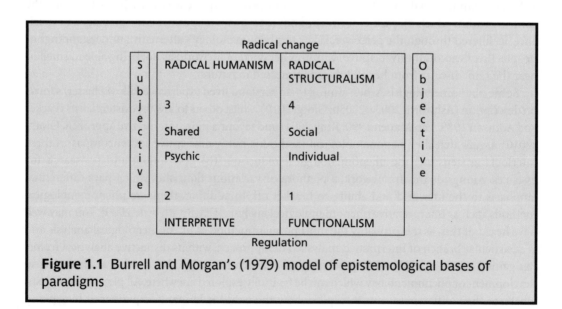

Figure 1.1 Burrell and Morgan's (1979) model of epistemological bases of paradigms

about the theorising and *modus operandi* of the theorists who work under this problematic. Each set identifies a separate social scientific reality. Of the four paradigms, we are interested in the interpretive paradigm which is allied with social theories that see the social world as stable (versus radical change) and privileges subjectivity – individual interpretation rather than an objective view. This paradigm seeks to explain the stability of behaviour from the individual's viewpoint. Researchers in this paradigm try to observe ongoing processes to better understand individual behaviour and the spiritual nature of the world – in essence then, phenomenologists.

In terms of locating this approach in contemporary maps of qualitative research, a commonly utilised model is that given by Guba and Lincoln (2005). They identify five main paradigms of contemporary qualitative research: positivism, postpositivism, critical theories, constructivism, and participatory/cooperative paradigms. Each of the paradigms listed by Guba and Lincoln is characterised by axiomatic differences in axiology (the value of the research), intended action of research, control of research process/outcomes, relationship to foundations of truth and knowledge, validity, textual representation and voice of the researcher/participants, and commensurability with other paradigms. Rather than try to position phenomenology within one of these paradigms, we aim to unpack what these distinctions mean for the phenomenologist.

Defining and mapping phenomenology as an approach

Bogdan and Taylor (1975) noticed early the potential for qualitative methods. Through them we learn about people we would not otherwise know: 'We hear them speak about themselves and their experiences and, though we do not accept their perspectives as truth, develop an empathy which allows us to see the world from their points of view' (p. 9). The distinctiveness of phenomenological research specifically is that it offers the ability to explore the diversity and variability of human experience in all its complexity from first-person accounts, with the intention to gain new understandings of how the world is experienced from those actually experiencing the phenomena of interest. Willig, who was interested in exploring 'the meaning and significance of an embodied experience' (2007: 209), demonstrates how using Colaizzi's descriptive method to explore the experience of taking part in extreme sport allowed 'genuinely new and surprising insights to emerge from participants' accounts of their subjective experience' (2007: 217).

There are common features within the broad and complex school that is phenomenology and which distinguish it from other approaches. First, from a phenomenological viewpoint, the world of subjects and objects cannot be separated from our experience of it. Whilst we may locate ourselves (as humans) distinct from objects in our world, these objects present themselves to us and we experience them as something. The appearance of this object is dependent upon intentionality – the perceiver's location, context, angle and mental orientation (e.g. desires, wishes, judgements, emotions, aims and purposes).

Michalko (1999) writes as a blind disability theorist and demonstrates the vitality of phenomenological theory. He notes that sighted people tend to dislike mundane tasks such as dusting – they are visually reminded that objects need dusting. There is a need to dust and many objects gather dust. However, few like doing it and see it as a chore or may pay others to do it.

For Michalko the act of dusting is intrinsically tied to the stuff that needs dusting. Stuff that needs dusting can be found everywhere and for a blind person presents an opportunity to connect with the material. The feeling at home experience afforded to a sighted person is of being surrounded visually by artifacts (clean or in need of dusting). One knows one is at home through being surrounded with familiar stuff. It is probable that the artefacts (stuff) that one has in one's home contain souvenirs and mementos from holiday, personal and familial photos, cards, gifts from others. For most people, however, the primary mode of coming into contact with their stuff is through seeing – an equivalent to touch with the eyes. For Michalko, this recognition comes through touching where the meaning of the object is embedded in the act of touching and knowing. The practice of touching here connects the person and the object in knowing and belonging. Dusting here is a practice of understanding and connecting with what may be termed the lifeworld.

Another clear demonstration of how intentionality shapes understanding and experience comes from Willig's (2008) review of Langdridge's (2007) text. She was enthusiastic about the book that she was already making use of and indeed recommending to students and thus initially keen to write the review. However, once her aim and purpose became that of a critic rather than a teacher, she 'read' the book quite differently. Reflecting on this shift she claims 'intentionality made all the difference! After all, it is not really possible to review the "book" itself (as object); instead, the "review" arises from, and tells us about, the relationship between the reviewer and the book' (2008: 429). This relationality between the subject/perceiver/toucher and the object is a very different feature of phenomenological theory.

Second, no other perspective in psychology focuses on people's lived experience as phenomenology does. The aim is to gain an understanding of the participants' lived experiences in their own terms, to focus on the uniqueness of experience from the point of view of those who live it. 'Phenomenology takes accounts at face value in that it treats them as an expression of experience itself' (Willig 2007: 210). Sometimes universal features or essences of the lived experience are sought (see Woodgate 2006). Other times, followers of Husserl seek the common features or essence of the phenomenon, rather than the experience (see Wade 2006). In the literature there is considerable variance and lack of clarification of the term lived experience. The intention is – via exposure to the participants' accounts of experience, mediated by the research process and the researcher – to gain a deep and useful understanding of the phenomena of interest.

Michalko (1999), in recounting his relationship with Smokie his guide dog, developed the notion of the two in one (together as one, yet distinct, species, both in some ways alienated from society):

> Smokie decides how we will get where we are going in the midst of human society. His judgement takes me and my blindness into account. He is not going anywhere: we are. He bases his judgement of the best way to a destination not on what is best for him or for me, but what is best for us. Smokie has also turned my blindness into an occasion for me. With Smokie I see a world which has never been seen by a sighted person. Alone together, Smokie and I decide what is best for us in a sighted human world, a world with which we are familiar but from which we are estranged.
>
> (Michalko 1999: 106)

Here, the essence of the lived experience is communicated as sensory uniqueness of being a blind person and a sighted guide dog, together as two-in-one. The livedness of this experience is unique to the writer and his construal of it is central to making sense of it. We may empathise with this construal and imagine this experience but it belongs to the writer.

Another distinctive and much contested feature of phenomenology is the setting aside of researcher reality, theoretical and other meaning-giving structures, often referred to as an 'attitude of openness' or 'empathy' throughout the research process in order to allow the participants' lived reality to emerge. This setting aside, epoche (bracketing) or phenomenological reduction is never completely achievable, in our view, and it is here, in the level of openness and interpretation that is acceptable and involved in practice that much of the variance and tensions within the perspective arise (more of this later). Various schools of phenomenology approach the possibility of epoche and reduction rather differently.

Individual subjectivity or lived experience is understood by many phenomenologists as the lifeworld that we are all immersed in which is highly personal, and it is this individuality that is key. However, all lifeworlds are understood as including some common features such as embodiment, spatiality, intersubjectivity, temporality and selfhood (Ashworth 2003b). Some general definitions of these terms may help:

- *Embodiment*. It is through our bodies, our felt sense, or the subjective meanings of the lived experience of the body that we communicate with and come to know and understand our world.

- *Spatiality*. Our space includes other people, a variety of natural and cultural objects and of course cultural institutions. Toombs highlights how lived space impacts on the quality of experience: 'the subjective feeling of space is intimately related both to one's bodily capacities and the design of the surrounding world' (2001: 249). More specifically, Van Manen suggests that it is 'the nature of lived space that renders that particular experience its quality of meaning' (1997: 102).

- *Intersubjectivity*. It is through intersubjective experience, connection with others, that we gain an understanding of the social world. Individual subjectivity is formed in an ongoing process of exchange and interaction with others (Grunwald and Thiersch 2009: 5). Although the focus is on individual experience of intersubjectivity, we recognise that collective forms of subjectivity such as ethnicity, culture and religion also impact on how relations with others are played out and experienced.

- *Temporality*. An awareness of the finiteness of life, of lived time and time left to live. Self project refers to the ways in which we engage in ongoing projects that change and transform the self. Finlay and Molano-Fisher (2008) show the changing lifeworld of a woman following a cochlear impact and how this shift impacts upon her notions of self.

Example

A worked example here will help unpack what temporality, spatiality and other terms mean. Temporality and spatiality are prominent features of Roxy's narrative which appears at the beginning of this chapter. First, temporality, there is a real sense of time past – we 'weren't brought up living in a house' – being part of time present, of her earlier experiencing being absorbed by her and shaping her current experiencing – 'I crave greenery – I spend half my life opening doors and windows, trying to get rid of the airless, claustrophobic feeling that comes with being inside' – and the sense of heightened awareness of what seem to be experienced as intrusive noises – 'I get woken up by bin lorries, the rush-hour traffic and my neighbours shouting', rather than the more familiar, natural (and no doubt gentler) noises of her childhood – 'of birdsong and the wind in the trees'.

In terms of spatiality she writes of feeling trapped within her flat, of trying to gain the space she had as a child by living near the sea 'because it gives me some sense of openness and freedom'. The whole piece paints a textured picture of something that many of us take for granted, living in a built environment, being for Roxy 'bizarre and alien'. Finally she claims that 'my instinct is to travel', but recognises that 'to reach my dream, I have to put down roots'. Her self project requires that she locates herself within the built environment and all that that means to her.

Locating the phenomenological approach in terms of ontology, epistemology, methodology and positionality

Willig (2008) proposes that asking questions about methodology allows us to identify the epistemological and ontological roots. If we take each question in turn this may help us entangle this approach.

First, what kind of knowledge does the methodology aim to produce? For phenomenology, knowledge is messy in that it is neither realist (assuming there is some direct access to reality) nor relativist (assuming that all knowledge is constructed). Phenomenology occupies a position somewhere in between these approaches which takes on board that knowledge/experience is always at some level constructed and interpreted although it is for the person 'real'. The epistemological position of interpretive phenomenology then is one of 'critical realism' (Willig 1999) that maintains a central focus on the ways in which people make meaning of their experience, whilst being aware of the influences that broader social structures have on those meanings. Descriptive phenomenology after Husserl is more realist. The aim is to 'give voice' to participants. However, their 'voice' is always mediated through the research process and the researchers' understandings. Researchers play an active role in analysis, in identifying and presenting themes and patterns. Themes do not naturally emerge from the data (Taylor and Ussher 2001), thus interpretation is to some degree an inevitable feature of the findings. Descriptive phenomenologists would not see their analysis as mediated through the research process because, in a purist research process, engagement with the epoche and the phenomenological reduction would prevent this, allowing them to see the world 'in its appearing'. For a recent account of these distinctions, see Finlay (2009) which debates differing construals of phenomenological practice.

An example helps shed light on this voice-giving, although here it is the writer who is constructing a phenomenology of blindness. A leading disability theorist (Michalko) writes about blindness and sightedness (from an insider perspective) using phenomenological lens. Michalko (1999) argues that the experience of being disabled is of course a real phenomenon which has real effects living in a dominant sighted world. However, the construction of blindness as an impairment occurs both for him and the wider society which positions him often as a person in need of being handled, 'helped' to cross the road or offered money if standing alone. The knowledge about being blind for Michalko is both a product of his actual experience and his knowledge of how it is viewed and treated in a wider sense. In this account he is both researcher/theorist and participant. For Michalko, and for us, guide dogs are inexorably tied to blindness. We cannot see guide dogs without interpreting the need for them, i.e. blindness:

'Excuse me.'
'Me? Are you talking to me?'
'Yep. Is that one of those blind dogs?'
'Jeez, I hope not.'

(Michalko 1999: 41)

Here the dog in harness, leading, brings the observer to query the status of the dog. Of course the dog is not blind but the observer reads the cues and uses familiar constructions of blindness and guide dogs to wrongly label the dog as blind. The kinds of knowledge produced by phenomenological approaches are either first person accounts, co-constructed accounts between researcher and the researched, or accounts around first-person experience but analysed by researchers.

Second, what kinds of assumptions does the methodology make about the world? This question is about ontology – what is there to know and what is the nature of the thing we are trying to know? Taking on board the idea that experience is primary, this approach focuses on the consciousness of experience. The Greek word *phainomenon* means 'how things appear' and here reality is important for the person who is having the experience. For the phenomenologist the *lived* experience from the view of those who live it is central, although there is acceptance that people can be in the same setting and experience this differently. These individual realities are understood as multiple, subtle constructions which are both socially and experientially based, as well as local and specific in nature (Guba and Lincoln 1994; Denzin and Lincoln 2000). A further assumption is that these individual subjectivies or realities are often understood as lifeworlds (see above).

An example here of the utilty of the lifeworld comes from Thome *et al.* (2004) who explored the meaning of living with cancer in old age for ten participants aged 75 plus, using Van Manen's (2001) phenomenological method. The four essential themes of the lived experience identified within the accounts of these ten participants were understood in terms of lifeworld features. The researchers revealed how the lived body (embodiment) was disturbed by fatigue, loss of bodily capacity and bodily discomfort. That participants' available lived space (spatiality) was much reduced and that their illness had brought with it 'a sudden awareness of the finiteness of life . . . leading to a reorientation in present time' (2004: 5) (temporality). Finally, intersubjectivity was evident in their renewed closeness with family and friends which seemed to give new meaning to the illness and gave participants strength. These insights of experience gained from those actually living with cancer provided new understandings to health care professionals about how best to meet with, be with and support people in their 'disintegrated life situation' (Thome *et al.* 2004: 1). A very different study by Roxberg *et al.* (2009) of survivors' accounts of the tsunami catastrophe demonstrates that the participants experienced a heightened awareness of time as embedded and lived now (temporality) when the tsunami cut through their taken-for-granted view of the world and caused disruption and turmoil. According to the authors 'the theoretical and methodological framework made it possible to some extent to reveal the invisible threads between the world of the victims and the world of the tsunami catastrophe' (2009: 26). The tsunami seemed to survivors to be 'timeless' with features of motion, both of the waves and the disorder felt, of stillness, characterised by endless waiting and shifts in perspective from focusing on helping themselves and others to a complete lack of understanding of what had happened, compounded by the lack of information. The nature of the knowledge in phenomenological lens is brought to life through features highlighted above, such as temporality and intersubjectivity.

Third, how does the methodology conceptualise the role of the researcher in the research process? In traditional phenomenological practice the idea of the researcher is one where the participant's lifeworld is understood through bracketing off or epoche. This requires the researcher to set aside assumptions, judgements and prior interpretations before immersing oneself fully in the data. This positionality is not without critics and certain forms of analysis such as IPA do not advocate this. A creative piece of research by King *et al.* (2008) allows us to see the importance of positionality, of how different positioning within phenomenology and different uses of bracketing or phenomenological reduction together with underlying assumptions affect findings. Five phenomenologist researchers analysed a single detailed narrative of the experience of mistrust within an organisational setting. The only agreement was that the analysis should be descriptive, that is, not offering explanation or cause. Between them they produced a consensual analysis with many links to lifeworld features, which is exactly what is expected. However, what is interesting for us here is that they 'demonstrate how different approaches can usefully draw out different meanings' (p. 96). King and Smith, who both position themselves as interpretive phenomenologists, focus on Kath's use of metaphor, supported by symbolism as this was seen by them as most striking, in order to reveal her experiences of organisational mistrust, essentially that she experienced colleagues within her institutional context as both a 'small and silly nest of chickens' and simultaneously as a 'dangerous and malevolent nest of vipers'. Butt and Langdridge, on the other hand, distance themselves from the realist notion that the interview narrative produced came 'from within the research participant' (p. 92). Instead, working with it as a narrative jointly produced during the process of the interview they each explore the 'rhetorical structure of the mistrust narrative'. In their connected individual commentaries they highlight Kath's resistance to being positioned as client within the interview and suggest that this may be due to Kath's need to take responsibility for her actions. They also track Kath's changing tone through the narrative from relatively neutral to one that becomes more 'brave and battling' in response to the interviewer's construction of Kath's situation. Finally, Finlay, who positions herself as an existential-hermeneutic phenomenologist and who was the only one to meet Kath and work with her face to face, focuses on embodied intersubjectivity. Finlay also understands the narrative as co-constructed within the process yet accepts that it also reflects Kath's meanings, which positions Finlay somewhere between realism and relativism.

However, she reveals how her felt sense or embodied empathic reaction to Kath's evolving story facilitated her understanding. She argues that her sense of closing down, reducing to a paler version of herself, mirrored Kath's own felt sense as she recounted her experiences: 'The crucial question is to what extent was I reflecting Kath's response or was it my own self creation?' (p. 96). One narrative with a variety of phenomenological readings produced rich yet inevitably partial understandings of Kath's lifeworld. The authors, while acknowledging shortcomings, claim to have glimpsed and represented something of Kath's meanings around her experience of organisational mistrust.

The definitions of reflexivity within qualitative research are necessarily rich, although phenomenology, with its emphasis on experience, forefronts how the researcher can and should position oneself in relation to the data.

Phenomenology as method

Whilst tenets of phenomenology have filtered into many qualitative approaches, we here outline what is distinctive in gathering data and analysing it. Much of the published work on phenomenology seems to feature issues related to health and illness or disruption. This is interesting as it begs the question as to why? Is it difference that excites and hence work privileges that which is not normal to us (ill health, disability, 'abnormality', crisis)? Alternatively, is it shifts in experience – the changing status of a medical condition, the ageing process, being in the midst of a crisis – which remind us to feel and think differently?

Details of methodological decisions that are driven by philosophical assumptions are often not clearly articulated in research papers, which promotes the unhelpful notion of the free floating method. This idea that methods stand alone and can be applied to data is critiqued as technicist and value free (Hughes 1997; Parker 2007). Philosophical grounding and the rationales for decisions made through the process of the research need to be made transparent. This enables readers to have an understanding of how the findings have been produced and how the study might be evaluated.

When gathering data, all phenomenologists aim to gain the richest possible account of subjective experience from the participant in order to enable the depth and complexities of experience to be revealed and thus ultimately strengthen the authenticity of findings. To achieve this, researchers adopt an attitude of openness throughout the research. Finlay maintains that an 'open phenomenological attitude . . . enables me to be curious and ready to be surprised' (King *et al.* 2008: 100). The most popular data collection method is the one-to-one, in-depth interview, based around few open-ended questions or topics, although any first-hand accounts may be used. For example, Roxberg *et al.* (2009) used Swedish television footage of survivors talking of their experiences of the 2004 tsunami as it took place in Thailand, which had the advantage of immediacy, of participants being in the world of the tsunami experience as they spoke, and the disadvantage of lack of engagement between researchers and participants. Initially researcher attitude of openness needs to be empathic, meeting and being with the participants in a noncensorial manner in order to gain access to the participants' reality as understood by them. It is a matter of encouraging participants to tell their story of experience in as much detail as they wish and are able to. This attitude is succinctly expressed by King *et al.* (2008: 84): 'The interviewer, Linda, aimed to be a non judgmental, sensitive listener and to promote natural, spontaneous conversation.'

Descriptive approaches tend to use participants' written descriptions of one concrete experience rather than interviews, whereas the interpretive approach favours interviews. Descriptive and interpretive methods differ most strikingly in the way that the data are both gathered and treated. Having highlighted the importance of the philosophical base of the approach, we will follow good practice and outline the background philosophy of descriptive and interpretive traditions before directing you to some good examples of recent research which illustrate some of the different phenomenological positions.

First, the descriptive tradition after Husserl: the focus here is to reveal the lived experience of those being studied, without any researcher interpretation. To achieve this lack of bias the researcher must achieve the Husserlian concept of transcendental subjectivity via use of epoche. Husserl (1983) called for epoches, or abstentions from any influences that might bias description. These include bracketing off personal and professional presumptions and the theoretical frameworks of science to access the phenomena as they are experienced by participants, rather than as the phenomena might be understood professionally or through a particular scientific framework. Willig (2007) provides a clear example of articulating her presuppositions about phenomenology and the embodied experience of taking part in extreme sport in the early stages of her study.

Descriptive phenomenologists are interested in the essential features of lived experience, that is, the commonalities within accounts of experience of the phenomena. Such essences are taken as objective and true descriptions of the phenomenon, which stems from the realist ontology of this school of phenomenology and Husserl's enthusiasm to ensure that all research in this tradition is scientifically rigorous. Importantly, Husserl considered people as free agents responsible for shaping their environment and culture, rather than understanding the environment and culture as influencing the person. This concept he called radical autonomy (Husserl 1970).

If you are interested in descriptive phenomenology we suggest reading any or all of the following very different examples: Wertz (2005) who explores the use of this method in the field of counselling psychology and thus provides a helpful overview; Bargdill (2000) who makes use of Giorgi's approach to investigate the experience of life boredom; Mastain (2006) who aims to reveal the structure and meaning of the lived experience of spontaneous altruism.

Second, the interpretive tradition, after Heidegger, which is not so much interested in description of phenomena but in making explicit the meanings within participants' accounts of everyday experiences, specifically the links between participants and their lifeworld, which are sometimes expressed as metaphors. As Lopez and Willis make clear: 'It is not the pure content of human subjectivity that is the focus of a hermeneutic inquiry but, rather, what the individual's narratives imply about what he or she experiences every day' (2004: 729).

In contrast to the descriptive tradition there is an assumption of 'situated freedom' (Leonard 1999), of choices being limited and variously influenced by the web of social structures and access to resources that people live within. Such structures are understood as having a profound effect on individual experience.

Researcher presuppositions, including knowledge of the relevant literature, that are bracketed off within the descriptive tradition are seen here, in the interpretive tradition, as a resource, a guide to the research process and the transformation of data. Through an ongoing process of reflexivity, researcher understanding in all its guises (personal and professional suppositions as well as theoretical frameworks) is critically engaged with throughout and how each impacts and shapes the decision making and eventual understanding gained is made transparent. It is not unusual within this tradition to make use of a theoretical frame to provide a lens for the research.

Intersubjectivity between researcher and participant is also recognised as key to generating data and thus influencing findings. The meanings within participant transcripts are understood as produced by the topic of the research and the interconnection of researcher and participant. Thus interpretation at a number of levels is acknowledged as inherent in data production. Ricouer (1970) emphasised that the interpretive work is always with the intent of 'bringing out' the meaning of experience' (cited in King *et al.* 2008: 82). Findings, recognised as interpretative, must nevertheless be firmly grounded in participant narratives and be coherent within the parameters of the study. However, it is also acknowledged that findings are inevitably partial and that other readings are always possible. This positions the interpretive tradition as relativist rather than realist.

The examples of work we would direct you to if interested in interpretive phenomenology include: King *et al.* (2002) who explore how people adjust to living with diabetic renal disease; Thome *et al.*'s (2004) work using Van Manen's method to reveal what living with cancer in old age means to participants; Katz *et al.*'s (2010) US-based study aiming to understand the experiences of Native American nurses working within their tribal communities with the intention of improving the retention of such professionals.

Critical hermeneutics, a particular branch of the broad school that is phenomenology favoured by critical theorists such as feminists and Marxists, explores how participants' lives, often those of marginalised groups, are structured by dominant ideologies. The purpose here is to look beneath the accounts of experience, to explore and surface how the invisible threads of power and socially accepted thinking impact on the life chances and often diminish the experiences of specific groups. In traditional formulations of phenomenology it is the researcher whose experiences are studied although accounts from others are more commonly found in contemporary research. Critical hermeneutics allows a critical reading of subjective experience in interpreting the wider social world.

Analytical approaches prioritise the process of treating the data, although Smith *et al.* (2009: 1) argue that 'interpretative phenomenological analysis' is 'committed to the examination of how people make sense of their own life experiences'. This approach accepts that researchers' views and interactions with participants will influence the data and the subsequent interpretation of the account. The systematic process towards analysis is well covered elsewhere (Flowers *et al.* 1997; Smith *et al.* 2009) and utilises a form of annotating issues and then labelling themes. The analysis then becomes structured around clusters and themes representing participants' meanings.

Good and varied examples of IPA that you may want to read include: Johnson *et al.*'s (2004) exploration of how women in the later stages of pregnancy and early stages of motherhood experience their changing body; Flowers *et al.*'s (2000) study, looking at how gay men understand and manage their HIV risk; Rhodes and Smith's (2010) analysis of what depression actually feels like for their 46-year-old participant.

Evaluation

IPA is at least one qualitative approach that does derive from psychological traditions. Critics argue that in seeing the world through others this approach lacks a focus on the wider social context and hence politics. But there is an argument that personal phenomenological accounts are in themselves political. Mohanty notes that 'the point is not just "to record" one's history of struggle, or consciousness, but how they are recorded; the way we read, receive and disseminate such imaginative records is immensely significant' (1991: 34). So we may question whether personal narratives simply privilege the personal over the political, or whether they can displace the opposition between public and private by rewriting personal experience as part of a common struggle, whilst contributing to the collective memory that sustains political community.

In the current forever busy but ailing capitalist climate of the UK in the twenty-first century, driven by the need to achieve targets and meet satisfactory outcome measures, commonly called the 'audit culture', people's lived experience is often overlooked or erased as unimportant by policymakers and researchers alike. However, it is just this – our sense of being in the world, our subjectivity – which is the core concern of phenomenology. Rather than personal experiences being silenced or ignored, they are positioned centre stage by phenomenologists and accepted as rich veins of understanding that are ideally used to inform practice. Many psychologically based practices, traditionally informed solely by more superficial outside-in understandings such as those imposed by 'experts' and/or professionals, often fail users. If you are interested in this aspect do read Bentall's (2010) text detailing the many failings of psychiatry, which conventionally ignores the voice of its patients/consumers. Bentall applauds the rise of an increasingly vocal consumer movement within psychiatric practice and highlights the Hearing Voices Network as one such organisation. He suggests that when consumers' understandings are recognised as important 'perhaps then we really would see services that people in distress would want to make use of' (2010: 287).

Phenomenology with subjectivity as its core has the potential to be accepting of difference as difference and not as deficit or deviance, and thus connects with a social justice agenda. Shifting the power base as phenomenology does to the participant and their narrative of lived experience allows individuals or groups to position themselves and have their own story told, rather than to be positioned as pathological or deviant by the stories told of them by professionals or researchers through various structural or theoretical frameworks. The target-driven audit culture frames this common practice; it is a necessary element of being professional and maintaining standards. We do not wish to demonise professionals whom we recognise are mostly concerned to respect their clients/patients/users and do the best for them. However, it is necessary to point out that the political and social structures within which we all work require that we as practitioners conform. See Bentall (2010) for an example of the structural power of companies to frame understandings of mental health in ways that support the companies and feed capitalism with vast financial profit, whilst often failing to actually meet the needs of the individuals in distress. Langdridge and Butt's (2004) work provides another example of how those electing to be involved in sadomasochism have traditionally been pathologised, positioned as deviant, whereas more recent phenomenologically based research has focused on 'the individual life stories of people engaging in these practices and the struggle "SMers" may have to realise their identities' (Langdridge 2009: 1).

New directions

Phenomenologists have in recent years responded to the critique that they tend to neglect how language and politics structure people's subjective experience, which in turn limits understandings and change to the individual rather than recognising that structural understandings and change can often be more useful. To counter this critique and in the spirit of progress reflecting current trends in social psychology, some authors (Langdridge 2007; Smith *et al.* 2009) have been discussing combining phenomenological approaches with various forms of discourse analysis to add a critical aspect to phenomenological understandings. Smith *et al.* (2009) explore in some detail how IPA and Foucauldian discourse analysis (FDA) may usefully be combined to provide a deeper analysis, which potentially paves the way for social change:

> While IPA studies provide a detailed experiential account of the person's involvement in the context, FDA offers a critical analysis of the structure of the context itself and thus touches on the resources available to the individual in making sense of their experience.
>
> (Smith *et al.* 2009: 196)

There are relatively few studies making use of IPA and FDA as yet, but one example of this combination is 'Does My Bump Look Big In This?' (Johnson *et al.* 2004). The combined analysis suggests that the women are positioned by others and themselves in complex and varied ways within the discursive possibilities of mothers-to-be within our culture, and that these positions influence their experiencing in ways more likely to be limiting than empowering as their pregnant state transgresses the idealised female body discourse. What is needed is structural change, specifically the availability of other cultural representations of women which allow them to understand themselves differently and do not pathologise them, pregnant or otherwise.

Rather than combining approaches Langdridge (2007) has developed a more radical phenomenological approach grounded in the phenomenological tradition of maintaining a focus on storytelling and respecting the narrative of lived experience, yet also making explicit the role of the political. His critical narrative analysis (CNA) recognises that as narratives can be interrogated via hermeneutic empathy to reveal individual meanings, so too can they be critically interrogated in terms of how power impacts on and is revealed within the narratives. Langdridge (2007) is keen to point out that the purpose of taking the axes of power is not to overrule personal understandings, such as is the aim of the hermeneutics of suspicion, by uncovering buried truths or causal explanations, but rather the purpose is to open up possibilities for new ways of living. Langdridge suggests that such developments are necessary if social psychology is 'to meet the needs of people, communities and societies . . . in these fast changing late modern times' (2008: 139).

Newer directions for phenomenology

Whilst phenomenology has long-standing historical roots, it is also continually evolving. For example, Ahmed (2006) demonstrates how queer studies can put phenomenology to productive use. Focusing on the 'orientation' aspect of 'sexual orientation' and the 'orient' in 'orientalism', Ahmed examines what it means for bodies to be situated in space and time. Bodies take shape as they move through the world directing themselves toward or away from objects and others. Being 'orientated' means feeling at home, knowing where one stands, or having certain objects within reach. Orientations affect what is proximate to the body or what can be reached. A queer phenomenology, Ahmed contends, reveals how social relations are arranged spatially, how queerness disrupts and reorders these relations by not following the accepted paths, and how a politics of disorientation puts other objects within reach, those that might at first glance seem awry. Ahmed proposes that a queer phenomenology might investigate not only how the concept of orientation is informed by phenomenology but also the orientation of phenomenology itself.

Theorists have also turned to race studies and Lee (2008) articulates how phenomenology sheds light on race. Phenomenology elucidates this difficult situation where race continues as a key social indicator by addressing an important but glaring chasm – a lived experiential understanding of race. Experience eludes analysis because the ephemeral structure of experience counters theory's systematising tendencies. Descriptions of experience range from the too specific to the too broadly sweeping to be useful for analysis. Despite such difficulties, a lived sense of race aims to portray this immediate, everyday experience of race. This is precisely the aim of existential phenomenologists' work on race. Frantz Fanon, Jean-Paul Sartre and scholars in this tradition, working on race, have illustrated the experience of living as racialised subjects in the aftermath of colonialism. An exploration of a lived understanding of race through phenomenology provides insights about the workings of racism.

Chapter summary

Opening up the world of experience through phenomenological lens offers possibility for engagement and resonance. As Behar (1996, cited in Bochner 2001: 143) argued with reference to anthropology, research which 'doesn't break your heart just isn't worth doing anymore'. The richness of phenomenological work and the diversity within should not dissuade. Wertz (2005: 175) noted that 'phenomenology is a low-hovering, in-dwelling, meditative philosophy that glories in the concreteness of person-world relations and accords lived experience, with all its indeterminancy and ambiguity, primacy over the known'. Not knowing or uncertainty may well be the future for much of science, representing a shift in scientists celebrating uncertainty (Jha 2011). What phenomenology affords within qualitative research is primacy of lived experience, even if the approach itself is less certain or knowing about how best to access and represent this. Being comfortable with uncertainty is undoubtedly worthy of further phenomenological inquiry.

In this chapter we have given you only a glimpse of the phenomenological tradition. The chapter has mapped key theorists and used examples to showcase the kind of approach a phenomenological lens sheds light on. In phenomenology, subjective experience is key so there is an assumption that understanding comes from being.

References

Ahmed, S. (2006) *Queer Phenomenology: Orientations, Objects, Others*. Durham, NC: Duke University Press.

Ashworth, P. (2003a) 'The phenomenology of the lifeworld and social psychology'. *Social Psychological Review*, **5**(1), 18–34.

Ashworth, P. (2003b) 'An approach to phenomenological psychology: the contingencies of the lifeworld'. *Journal of Phenomenological Psychology*, **34**(2), 145–56.

Bargdill, R. (2000) 'The study of boredom'. *Journal of Phenomenological Psychology*, **31**(2), 188–219.

Behar, R. (1996) *The Vulnerable Observer: Anthropology that Breaks Your Heart*. Boston, MA: Beacon Press.

Bentall, R. P. (2010) *Doctoring the Mind: Why Psychiatric Treatments Fail*. London: Penguin.

Bochner, A. P. (2001) 'Narrative's virtues'. *Qualitative Inquiry*, **7**(2), 131–57.

Bogdan, R. and Taylor, S. (1975) *Introduction to Qualitative Research Methods*. New York: Wiley.

Burrell, G. and Morgan, G. (1979) *Sociological Paradigms and Organisational Analysis: Elements of the Sociology of Corporate Life*. London: Heinemann.

Caelli, K. (2000) 'The changing face of phenomenological research: traditional and American phenomenology in nursing'. *Qualitative Health Research*, **10**(3), 366–77.

Denzin, N. K. and Lincoln, Y. S. (2000) 'Paradigms and perspectives in transition', in N. Denzin and Y. S. Lincoln (eds) *Handbook of Qualitative Research*, 2nd edn. Thousand Oaks, CA: Sage.

Finlay, L. (2009) 'Debating phenomenological research methods'. *Phenomenology and Practice*, **3**(1), 6–25.

Finlay, L. and Molano-Fisher, P. (2008) '"Transforming" self and world: a phenomenological study of a changing lifeworld following a cochlear implant'. *Medicine, Health Care and Philosophy*, **11**(3), 255–67.

Flowers, P., Duncan, B. and Frankis, J. (2000) 'Community, responsibility and culpability: HIV risk-management amongst Scottish gay men'. *Journal of Community and Applied Psychology*, **10**, 285–300.

Flowers, P., Sheeran, P., Beail, N. and Smith, J. A. (1997) 'The role of psychosocial factors in HIV risk reduction among gay and bisexual men: A quantitative review'. *Psychology and Health*, **12**, 197–230.

Giorgi, A. (2010) 'Phenomenology and the practice of science'. *Existential Analysis*, **21**(1), 3–22.

Grunwald, K. and Thiersch, H. (2009) 'The concept of the "lifeworld orientation" for social work and social care'. *Journal of Social World Practice*, **23**(2), 131–46.

Guba, E. and Lincoln, Y. (1994) 'Competing paradigms in qualitative research', in N. Denzin and Y. Lincoln (eds) *Handbook of Qualitative Research*, Thousand Oaks, CA: Sage.

Guba, E. G. and Lincoln, Y. S. (2005) 'Paradigmatic controversies, contradictions, and emerging influences', in N. K. Denzin and Y. S. Lincoln (eds), *The Sage Handbook of Qualitative Research*, 3rd edn. London: Sage.

Holstein, J. A. and Gubrium, J. F. (1994) 'Phenomenology, ethnomethodology, and interpretive practice', in N. K. Denzin and Y. S. Lincoln (eds) *Handbook of Qualitative Research*. Thousand Oaks, CA: Sage.

Hughes, C. (1997) 'Mystifying through coalescence: the underlying politics of methodological choices', in K. Watson, C. Modgil and S. Modgil (eds) *Educational Dilemmas: Debate and Diversity, Quality in Education*. London: Cassell.

Husserl, E. (1970) *Logical Investigation*. New York: Humanities Press.

Jha, A. (2011) 'Learn to love uncertainty and failure, say leading thinkers'. Accessed January 15, 2011. www.guardian.co.uk.

Johnson, S., Burrows, A. and Williamson, I. (2004) '"Does my bump look big in this?": the meaning of bodily changes for first-time mothers -to-be'. *Journal of Health Psychology*, **9**, 361–74.

Katz, J., O'Neal, G., Stricklow, C. and Doutrich, D. (2010) 'Retention of Native American nurses working in their own communities'. *Journal of Transcultural Nursing*, **21**(4), 393–401.

King, N. (2004) 'Using interviews in qualitative research', in C. Cassell and G. Symon (eds) *Essential Guide to Qualitative Methods in Organizational Research*. London: Sage.

King, N., Carroll, C., Newton, P. and Dornan, T. (2002) '"You can't cure it so you have to endure it": the experience of adaptation to diabetic renal disease'. *Qualitative Health Research*, **12**(3), 329–46.

King, N., Finlay, L., Ashworth, P., Smith, J. A., Langdridge, D. and Butt, T. (2008) '"Can't really trust that, so what can I trust?": a polyvocal qualitative analysis of the psychology of mistrust'. *Qualitative Research in Psychology*, **5**, 80–102.

Langdridge, D. (2007) *Phenomenological Psychology: Theory, Research and Method*. Harlow: Pearson.

Langdridge, D. (2009) 'Relating through difference: a critical narrative analysis', in L. Finlay and K. Evans (eds) *Relational Centred Research for Psychotherapists: Exploring Meanings and Experience*. Chichester: Wiley-Blackwell.

Langdridge, D. and Butt, T. (2004) 'A hermeneutic phenomenological investigation of the construction of sadomasochistic identities'. *Sexualities*, **7**(1), 31–53.

Lee, E. S. (2008) 'A phenomenology for Homi Bhabha's postcolonial metropolitan subject'. *Southern Journal of Philosophy*, **46**, 537–57.

Leonard, V. W. (1999) 'A Heideggerian phenomenological perspective on the concept of the person', in E. C. Polifroni and M. Welch (eds) *Perspectives on Philosophy of Science in Nursing: An Historical and Contemporary Anthology*. Philadelphia: Lippincott.

Lopez, K. and Willis, D. (2004) 'Descriptive versus interpretive phenomenology: their contributions to nursing knowledge'. *Qualitative Health Research*, **14**(5), 726–34.

Mastain, L. (2006) 'The lived experience of spontaneous altruism: a phenomenological study'. *Journal of Phenomenological Psychology*, **37**(1), 25–52.

Michalko, R. (1999) *The Two in One: Walking with Smokie, Walking with Blindness*. Philadelphia, PA: Temple University Press.

Michalko, R. (2010) 'Touch and belonging'. Paper presented at Normalcy Conference, Manchester, May.

Mohanty, C. (1991) 'Cartographies of struggle: Third World women and the politics of feminism', in C. Mohanty, A. Russo and T. Lourdes (eds) *Third World Women and the Politics of Feminism*. Bloomington, IN: Indiana University Press.

Packer, M. and Addison, R. (eds) (1989) *Entering the Circle: Hermeneutic Investigation in Psychology*. Albany, NY: State University of New York Press.

Parker, I. (2007) *Revolution in Psychology: Alienation to Emancipation*. London: Pluto Press.

Patton, M. Q. (1990) *Qualitative Evaluation and Research Methods*, 2nd edn. Newbury Park, CA: Sage.

Rhodes, J. and Smith, J. A. (2010) '"The top of my head came off": an interpretative phenomenological analysis of the experience of depression'. *Counselling Psychology Quarterly*, 23(4), 399–409.

Ricouer, P. (1970) *Freud and Philosophy: An Essay on Interpretation*. New Haven, CT: Yale University Press.

Roxberg, A., Dahlberg, K., Stolt, C.-M. and Fridlund, B. (2009) 'In the midst of the unthinkable: A phenomenological lifeworld approach to the experiences of suffering and relieved suffering during the tsunami catastrophe, 2004'. *International Journal of Qualitative Studies on Health and Well-being*, 4, 17–27.

Smith, J. A. (2010) 'Interpretative phenomenological analysis: a reply to Amedeo Giorgi'. *Existential Analysis*, 21(2), 186–91.

Smith, J. A., Flowers, P. and Larkin, M. (2009) *Interpretative Phenomenological Analysis: Theory, Method and Research*. London: Sage.

Spinelli, E. (2003) 'The existential–phenomenological paradigm', in R. Woolfe, W. Dryden and S. Strawbridge (eds) *The Handbook of Counselling Psychology*, 2nd edn. London: Sage.

Taylor, G. W. and Ussher, J. M. (2001) 'Making sense of S&M: a discourse analytic account'. *Sexualities*, 4, 293–313.

Thome, B., Esbensen, B. A., Dykes, A. K. and Hallberg, I. R. (2004) 'The meaning of having to live with cancer in old age'. *European Journal of Cancer Care*, 13(5), 399–408.

Toombs, S. K. (2001) *Handbook of Phenomenology and Medicine*. Dordrecht: Kluwer.

Van Manen, M. (1990) *Researching Lived Experience*. Albany, NY: State University of New York Press.

Van Manen, M. (1997) 'From meaning to method'. *Qualitative Health Research*, 7, 345–96.

Wade, J. (2006) '"Crying alone with my child": parenting a school aged child diagnosed with bipolar disorder'. *Issues in Mental Health Nursing*, 27(8), 885–903.

Wertz, F. J. (2005) 'Phenomenological research methods for counseling psychology'. *Journal of Counseling Psychology*, 52(2), 167–77.

Willig, C. (2007) 'Reflections on the use of a phenomenological method'. *Qualitative Research in Psychology*, 4(3), 209–25.

Willig, C. (2008) 'Book review of *Phenomenological Psychology: Theory, Research and Method* by Darren Langdridge (2007)'. *Existential Analysis: Journal of the Society for Existential Analysis*, 19(2), 429–32.

Woodgate, R. L. (2006) 'Living in a world without closure: reality for parents who have experienced the death of a child'. *Journal of Palliative Care*, 22(2), 75–82.

Chapter **2**

Action research

Judith Sixsmith and John Daniels

Introduction

In this chapter, action research (AR) is described and the principles and practices of action research are overviewed with attention to issues of epistemology, positionality, subjectivity, politics, quality and ethics. The value of action research in the context of policy is discussed and correspondences between evaluation research and action research are examined.

What is action research?

Action research is an approach to improving social practice by changing it and evaluating the impact of change (Bradbury and Reason 1993; Bargal 2008). In contrast to many other ways of doing research, AR is done by taking *action* (i.e. not simply by observing or measuring what already exists in the world) and attempting to understand the impact of that *action* within a *research* process. The emphasis on action differentiates AR from mainstream scientific approaches often used in psychology since intervention in a problem area is essential. The emphasis on research differentiates AR from community development or change management since research to understand the context and processes of change are critical elements. Taken together action+research (Dick and Swepson 1997) at once attempts to institute 'learning by doing', or taking action to solve practical problems while simultaneously furthering goals in social science. Being based in the world of practice, AR is an applied approach in which the complexity of real-world settings replaces the experimental psychologists' laboratory.

This is an important point as one founding father of AR Kurt Lewin (1946) pointed out: the complexity of human problems do not often lend themselves to the simplistic reductionist approach of traditional scientific enquiry, rather social problems need to be addressed within the holistic complexity of their psychosocial, cultural, environmental, political and historical contexts. Lewin described action research as 'comparative research on the conditions and effects of various forms of social action and research leading to social action' that uses 'a spiral of steps, each of which is composed of a circle of planning, action, and fact-finding about the result of the action' (1946: 34).

Lewin felt that tangible solutions to real-world problems needed to be based on a thorough understanding of the 'facts' of the situation (this is often where scientific enquiry ends), followed by planning and action to address the problem (i.e. some form of targeted intervention or process of dialogue), reflection on what happened as a result of the action and why, followed by further enquiry and perhaps adjustments to the intervention and so on. Lewin's cyclical process still constitutes the foundations of AR today.

However, more radical approaches developed in the 1970s and beyond, particularly aimed at people who were experiencing marginalisation and oppression and felt alienated from the processes of research and change which affected their lives. Radical approaches place import-ance on 'co-learning' and 'critical reflection' or reflexivity (Freire 1970; Fals-Borda 1987) and are framed with an implicit emancipatory focus to identify and question traditional power bases and challenge the status quo. The emancipatory process is most commonly achieved via reflexive and dialogical approaches of progressive problem solving led by marginalised people working in collaboration with others (often but not always researchers) in organised, thoughtful team-work or as part of a 'community of practice'.[1] For example, prefigurative action research (PreAR; Kagan and Burton 2000) examines the motivations and practices of those in power such that their positions are understood and power relations intrinsic to those positions are scrutinised. It is in this sense, that, once again, AR departs from traditional forms of scientific inquiry since it takes on an explicitly political orientation; one which adopts a position prioritising social justice and the fight against oppression (Kagan and Burton 2000) by relocating sources of control within and without the research process, as Barnes (2001: 5) notes in relation to critical disability studies:

> Above all the emancipatory research agenda warrants the transformation of the material and social relations of research production. In short, this means that disabled people and their organisations, rather than professional academics and researchers, should have control of the research process. Also, that this control should include both funding and the research agenda.

To be effective, PreAR does not simply work with people facing oppressive practices in their lives, but also engages with those in power within the change process and is strengthened when all acknowledge the need for change. Issues of social justice and challenges to oppression are priorities in the design, implementation and evaluation of PreAR:

> [Prefigurative action research] . . . is characterised by: an analysis of both the structural and ideological dimensions of oppression; an emphasis on creating and sustaining examples of alternative forms of social relations that provide a vision of a just society; the participation of less powerful people;

---

[1] A community of practice (CoP) is a group of people who share an interest, hobby, and/or profession (Lave and Wenger 1991). CoPs can evolve naturally out of common interests held by group members or can be created specifically with the aim of gaining or creating knowledge in a particular area or domain. Members learn from each other by sharing information and experiences with the group and can expand their horizons in terms of personal and professional development. CoPs are not restricted to real-world, real-time settings; they can exist in the virtual online world of the Internet.

multiple cycles of reflection, doing and knowing; simultaneous attention to both agency and structure in emancipatory practice.

(Kagan and Burton 2000: 73)

The radical forms of AR developed in the 1970s paved the way for participatory versions of AR whereby mutual enquiry is aimed at social change (Minkler 2000) and the empowerment of all stakeholders within the AR process is prioritised. In contrast to a top-down and more elitist version of scientific enquiry where independent and objective researchers are positioned to hold relevant knowledge and expertise and control the enquiry process, participatory action research (PAR) equally values the experiential knowledge of stakeholders such as community members or organisational staff (i.e. the people who experience the focal problem). This means stakeholders bring their experiential knowledge and local skills to the table to work together *with* researchers on a *jointly* identified problem, subsequent intervention and assessment of what works. In addition, researchers are positioned as *integrally involved in* the practice of AR and not simply in charge of it. Their subjectivity[2] is both acknowledged and helps to shape the AR process. No longer is research framed as a search for 'facts' which taken together reveal a greater, knowable and single 'truth', rather AR takes a pragmatic perspective to reveal what works and why. In fact, AR encourages an embracing of subjectivity as the basis from which inquiry progresses since we cannot escape from our immersion in the world around us (Ladkin 2005). We are always in the world which we apprehend through our own perceptions and construct our realities accordingly. This does not mean that we are lost in subjectivity, an inescapable internal place that we look out from, rather we recognise that multiple, socially constructed realities exist pointing to recurrent patterns in the world which are knowable in an everyday rather than a scientific sense. We affect the world by being in it, who we are, our values, beliefs and attitudes are intrinsic to shaping our research, just as they are intrinsic to shaping the actions we imagine and conduct. Moreover, our gender, our age, our ethnicity and social class intersect to position us in ways which enable us to see certain aspects of the world but not others. At once, they enable and curtail our understanding of what is important, what is valuable and what is possible. Action researchers, by working within the confines of their subjectivities, 'understand that how something is known will have an impact on how one relates to it' (Ladkin 2005: 114). In other words, how we try to address a problem will depend on our relation to it, how we perceive it and what we want to achieve.

Not surprisingly, different forms of action research or participatory action research have emerged over the years and there is no standardised way, and certainly no single set of rules, that govern how best to do (P)AR. Dick (2009) has examined the themes and trends in AR over recent years and lists action research approaches under the following headings: action learning; community-based participatory research; youth work; educational action research; appreciative inquiry; and action science. This variety of approaches stands testament to the crossover between AR and other literatures which value the application and democratisation of knowledge and practice (Smith *et al.* 2010). This may indicate that the design of AR is being conceptualised to

---

[2] After Ladkin (2005) subjectivity refers to a way of knowing located in the person's own perspective, created through their experiences, expectations and perceptions.

fit the situation rather than being applied in a prescriptive way (like following a recipe). The intention in this chapter is not to attempt to describe these very many different forms, but rather to overview their guiding principles, highlighting the epistemological underpinnings of (P)AR, exploring issues of social positioning and discussing the value of (P)AR with respect to practical, quality and ethical standpoints. The guiding principles of (P)AR (see Wadsworth 1998) can be summarised in the following text.

Cyclical

The AR cycle involves: problem identification or situation analysis (including reflection), deciding on aims and objectives and planning the project; taking action (implementing interventions); observing and evaluating how effective the intervention is (including self-evaluation); and critically reflecting on the research (Reid *et al.* 2006). By learning from everyday practice through a series of reflective stages, researchers and co-researchers can develop a deep understanding of the ways social reality (and social change) result from contextual, reflexive interactions (Riel 2010). The specific stages are often less clearly reflected in actual action research reports because stages are often overlapping (Waterman *et al.* 2001). Nevertheless, in summary, AR is iterative in nature and at best follows several cycles of reflection on practice and action so that the research takes shape while it is being performed.

Emergent

One of the most interesting aspects of AR is its emergent property. Scientific research always begins with a clear research question, formalised into hypotheses and then tested. In contrast, AR mostly begins with a context of study and some fuzzy ideas about what problems might exist and might be interesting as the focus of work. As information gathering progresses and local knowledge is drawn on, the problem focus becomes clearer as the first stage of action is planned and research questions formulated. As the planning–action–reflection cycle progresses, research questions can be further crystallised, rejected or developed in order to better fit the emergent data and interpretations made of the situation. New directions can be pursued in the light of prior learning; new information collected and changes made to the research questions. This flexibility is a unique feature of AR.

Oriented to change

Action research centrally revolves around the concept of change – both as a paradigm of research dealing with the creation of change in real-world human systems, and as real-time processes and products to be evaluated for their capacity to service their stakeholders. As a problem-oriented approach, AR is grounded in the world of practice (Bradbury and Reason 1993). This means that AR can be described as an approach to improving social practice by changing it. The research element of change ensures that evolving issues can be recognised, understood and dealt with (as far as possible) and practices themselves can evolve. Epistemologically, AR fits within a paradigm of 'praxis' representing a strikingly pragmatic approach at the intersection of theory and practice (see Morgan 2007 for an overview of pragmatism with research).

Methodologically pluralistic

AR is generally qualitative in nature and primarily based on talk (interviews and focus groups, for example) but can involve quantitative methods such as surveys. Usually, methods are chosen to fit the task, rather than used because of a particular paradigmatic choice. Moreover, different and mixed methods can be used at different points within the cycle. Perhaps one of the most flexible aspects of AR is the capacity to develop new and adventurous ways of collecting data, moulded to the particularities of the context. AR has provided the impetus to reframe art forms as tools for data collection in order to broaden out the scope for new knowledge to form. For example, participatory theatre (Quinlan 2009), participatory photography (Prins 2010; Mountian *et al.* 2011) and artistic creation (Sixsmith and Kagan 2005) have been used to enable people to articulate their thoughts, experiences and feelings in interpretive ways. This is especially useful when articulation is difficult, such as for people unused to interviews or focus groups, or for issues which are highly sensitive (e.g. bullying – see Quinlan 2009) or difficult to imagine or visualise (such as the development of new care-related technologies for older people; see Pratesi *et al.* in press). Quinlan (2009: 117) argues that innovatory practices 'open up productive spaces for reflexivity and create knowledge that is grounded in immediate experience and direct experiment'. While methodological innovation has opened doors to such articulations, care should be taken that participants involved either as informants or co-researchers are protected from possible harms. Prins (2010) writes of the harms associated with participatory photography which were unanticipated because such a method had not been used in war/conflict zones before. Community suspicions of the purpose of taking photos, participant timidity in terms of asking for permissions and social ridicule of involvement in the practice were outcomes of the choice of method. This highlights the role of context and power in the experience of AR data collection as Prins (2010: 426) argues that participatory photography (and this may be extrapolated to other participatory methods) 'is a technology with contradictory potential for social control and surveillance, and for the recovery of marginalised groups' subjugated knowledge'. In this sense, insights attained were achieved at a rather high price.

Reflexivity and subjectivity

Reflexive critique lies at the heart of the research and learning components of AR. Simple reflection (i.e. thinking about why an intervention worked or didn't work, or why a relationship developed as it did) goes some way towards understanding the processes involved. However, a reflexive approach incorporates a more explicit critical edge as well as providing the platform from which researchers and other stakeholders can evaluate the impact they themselves have had on the research–action cycle (Riel 2010). This impact includes an evaluation of how the research findings and change process have been affected by personal characteristics (values, beliefs, experiences, and so on) and social structural positionality (such as gender, age, ethnicity or social class as well as roles such as researcher, co-researcher, organisational staff member, advocate for change, etc.) (see Gatenby and Humphries 2000; Ragland 2006). Clearly, this way of thinking about action research departs hugely from the more usual scientific tradition which encapsulates notions of objectivity. Instead, within the real-world grounding of action research and the iterative change and evaluation cycles, it is generally recognised that research is never objective, is always political in some sense and that the researcher is not a passive or objective participant. The role of the action researcher is to participate and facilitate discussion amongst the community or group involved, to work towards solutions, to think about how problems, change and solutions are all enmeshed within particular contexts and to tease out how such contexts, the people in them (including researchers) and events cohere together to create specific located and situational solutions.

Collaborative

People are seen as an important resource within AR and collaboration ensures that those responsible for action are actually involved in creating it. Collaborative partnerships are particularly evident in PAR and can develop within a number of different roles, often enhancing scholarly practitioner-community participant relationships (Bradbury 2010). Collaborative roles range from the minimal involvement of people as information 'recipients', or 'informants' by providing local information into the project. They can be more active as 'interpreters' by commenting on the meaning of data collected, 'planners' proving advice and taking part in design decisions or 'implementers' of planned actions. They can be 'facilitators' of the research process or, at its most participatory, they can be 'researchers' or 'co-researchers', being involved in all aspects of the AR cycle (Dick 1997). Co-researchers can be involved in all aspects of the research and action process including the framing of the issues to be addressed, collecting information, implementing action, reflecting on, analysing and interpreting data and writing reports. Intense collaboration has been used extensively in international development work, often involving disadvantaged people who are not typically involved in the research process. This provides them with a chance to look critically at their own problematic situations to allow some control over the framing of the problem, the information gathered, and on a deeper level, can involve an element of empowerment. Here, all collaborators can play an active role in developing the action and research, and this enriched degree of participation is seen as necessary to the building of long-term solutions, as the people involved know best what their problems are and how actions impact upon them. The value of this was shown in the work of Reid *et al.* (2006), whereby AR collaborators reported unanimously that they developed a sense of inclusion and belonging by meeting in a group, discussing their shared problems, and learning that they were not alone in their situations and desire for change.

However, working collaboratively can be extremely time-consuming and often progresses at its own pace to allow different stakeholders to make their contributions and enable ideas to build one upon another. This often happens through intense discussions and dialogue sessions in a process which values both experiential and research knowledge. In effect, action researchers work together with a group of stakeholders to identify a problem, consider outcomes and develop a procedure for reaching a mutually desired goal. They plan together to implement an intervention, record actions taken and accumulate evidence to determine the extent to which the goal has been achieved. Theoretically, all ideas from the range of collaborative stakeholders (including researchers as equal partners) are equally valid, open to discussion, acceptance and rejection. This is an important way of working since it avoids the so-called 'helicopter' style of scientific research whereby researchers assume control, impose their ideas, do the research themselves, get results and then leave the situation. Instead, by working collaboratively, PAR creates the conditions for ownership amongst affected communities of the social problems addressed, as well as enabling the establishment of 'self-critical communities' (Wadsworth 1998) based around enlightenment or 'conscientiousization' (Hanley 2005), where oppressive events and practices are recognised or exposed for what they are and this recognition is used to mobilise oppressed people to work together to fight against them.

Risky

However, because of the inherently collaborative nature of AR, practitioners need to balance competing sets of priorities and values. This necessitates a thorough understanding of underlying power structures within the context under scrutiny. This is particularly salient when AR is conducted within disadvantaged communities and the work takes an emancipatory approach. Here, there is a danger of conducting AR in a disempowering way if existing power structures are not considered and challenged. Time and effort need to be taken to provide ways through which seldom-heard groups can be involved as far as possible. If this is not recognised, there is a risk that important voices may be left out of the process (such as those unable to attend meetings or disempowered groups such as immigrants – see Ataov *et al.* 2010). Even when all those concerned do participate cooperatively, solving problems means that conflicts may arise since different people and different groups have different agendas. As Brown and Gaventa (2009) have shown in their work on a citizenship development research centre, securing 'buy in' from key stakeholder groups, establishing the mutual accountability of all involved for the change process and securing institutional embeddedness are key in making effective change and learning from it.

Quality and value

Action researchers emphasise that standard research criteria used to evaluate scientific forms of enquiry cannot appropriately be applied to action research. This means that questions of reliability, external validity, representativeness and generalisability are not relevant within the action research approach. Instead, emphasis is placed on establishing the trustworthiness of data and authenticity of findings. This can be accomplished through methodological triangulation (where multiple data sources provide information on the same issue), reflexivity (involving critical reflection on process and practice) and member checks to instil confidence in the data's authenticity (Meyer 2000; Waterman *et al.* 2001).

Action research has been criticised in the past for the lack of transferability or generalisability of the results because the AR cycle is particular to the situation it tries to improve. The localism of AR means that generalisation to a larger population does not make sense. Yet the wider value of AR is often sought, allowing it to reach beyond specific contexts and provide useful insights to a wider community. Here, a focus on the theoretical or practical generalisability of findings is possible whereby understandings generated as part of the AR process do have theoretical or practical resonance in other similar situations (Meyer 2000). Just as grounded theory develops out of people's experiences in a bottom-up process, in AR *theory, practice and transformation* go hand in hand. Theory informs practice and action, reflection on the impact of action is then used to refine theory in an iterative process. Understandings based on theory can then be applied in other contexts, again being subject to iterative refinements such that the essence of theory as applied in practice can be derived.

But perhaps the most powerful evaluation of the quality and value of AR lies in its capacity to meet its own goals, that is to transform a situation for the better while generating insights into the transformational process. Unfortunately as (Stocker 2009: 385) has shown in a review of 232 AR funding applications to the Sociological Initiatives Foundation: 'Grassroots community members, or organizations controlled by them, were rarely involved at the crucial decision stages of research, and instead limited to participation in collecting data. In addition, most research was proposed to produce papers, presentations or websites, rather than directly support action.' As such, it is argued that good quality and valuable action research, judged on its own merits, needs to be more participatory and integrally connected to action.

A word on ethics

Given the potential extended duration of the research process and the potential changing role expectations of participants throughout the AR cycle(s) (Blum *et al.* 2002), action researchers may be obliged to seek iterative longitudinal consent. This means several informed consent documents at different points of time may be employed to ensure the ongoing voluntary nature of participation. This is particularly important because action research requires substantial time investment and personal involvement and is transformative not just of situations but also of people, hopefully, but not always (e.g. Prins 2010) in empowering ways.

In addition, ethical concern with the well-being of all participants in AR is extremely important. In scientifically framed research, the impact of research practices on participant well-being is an issue and researchers are charged with ensuring that participants are not harmed by their involvement (BPS 2011). This is equally important within AR, but additionally the change process itself is likely to impact on well-being. After all, the focus of AR is to change the situation that people are grounded in, recognising that change can have both positive and negative outcomes. Finally, the expectations of increasingly positive change (i.e. AR's potential to solve problems and improve situations) that surround AR need to be kept under consideration as the AR cycles progress. Frustration with the pace of change, disillusionment with the extent of change or alienation from the change process itself (perhaps as power relations exclude some groups and not others) can be undesirable AR outcomes which require continuous discussion by participants. Additionally, the active involvement of the participants as co-researchers can lead to a sense of loss if the project does not result in action (Reid *et al.* 2006).

Finally, participants' vulnerability can be a barrier to research as it can prevent them from fully participating. For example, study participants have expressed concern over incurring penalties (such as retraction of their welfare benefits) if they speak or act against those in power. This was the case for Reid *et al.* (2006), who argued that '[f]or a group of stigmatized women to engage in collective action and to feel empowered to challenge the system contradicts the messages they have systematically received as welfare recipients – that they are unmotivated, reprehensible and contemptible'. Combating systemic abuse in this way within an AR project can take very many months of talk, preparation and support.

While it is not always possible to avoid potential negative outcomes, dealing with them in ways which minimise their impact is crucial. Here, the creation of trust is critical in order for participants to express their perspective in a safe and trusting environment. For example, Beukema and Valkenburg (2007) who applied an 'examplarian action research' cycle to investigate and support the implementation of demand-driven elderly care within selected organisations in the Netherlands created the opportunity for discussions in small self-selected groups which allowed participants to speak to people with whom they were already comfortable such that their perspectives were taken into account.

Having outlined the underpinning principles and practices of AR, distinguished it from more traditional scientific approaches and examined some of the quality, value and ethical issues arising as a result of AR, the following sections explore AR and its relation to evaluation approaches in the context of policy and programme initiatives.

Action research: finding its place

In the last ten years there has been a significant increase in the number of evaluations that utilise AR in attempting to better understand and improve practice. More recently, the emphasis on *participatory evaluation* (Lennie 2005; Smits and Champagne 2008; Plottu and Plottu 2009; Suárez-Herrara *et al.* 2009; Clough *et al.* 2010) has emerged strongly, marrying together the underlying principles of AR and programme evaluation. This may be a reaction to the request of governments both past and previous, to improve our policy evidence base. For example, the Department of Culture Media and Sport (2008: 16) has challenged the sector to 'develop a better mechanism for improving the overall evidence base by better co-ordinating the collection of impact evidence'. The Department for Health (2010: 6) is advocating a radical new approach demanding rigour and being 'professionally led, focussed on evidence and being effective'. The increased attention may be driven by academics trying to find a suitable environment for AR, a process once described as *'designing a plane while flying it'* (Herr and Anderson 2005, as cited in Smith *et al.* 2010: 3). Ironically, some of the earliest influential evaluation research was pioneered by Lewin in the 1930s as 'action research' studies (Rossi *et al.* 2004). With such deep-seated roots, it seems surprising that such approaches have been given little attention until recently. This chapter will attempt to critique recent approaches to evaluation and will focus on the developing role and emerging interpretation of AR when evaluating social programmes.

There are varied interpretations of evaluation. Weiss (1972: 1) once described it as 'an elastic word that stretches to cover many judgements of many kinds'. Pawson and Tilley (1997: 2) referred to evaluation as a term with 'so much baggage that one is in danger of dealing not so much with a methodology as with an incantation'. Similarly, as indicated above, AR remains open to interpretation depending on research settings, ideology and procedure (Whitehead *et al.* 2003). There are many that would defend this notion as both terms should remain elastic so as to be sensitive to a particular context or research environment, and also to remain perceptive to the dynamic setting within which many social research projects are placed and may indeed be caused by the evaluation itself. There is no single research strategy unique to both action and evaluation research. On this point all the literature agrees.

Conceptual clarifications

While AR has remained relatively unchanged in its interpretation and conceptualisation (see the principles outlined above), evaluation research has undergone significant evolution in its interpretation, leading to typologies and classifications that may best represent a given context at a given time. For example, early writings were heavily influenced by more objective, positivist thinking. Evaluation research was essentially the measurement of programme effectiveness in terms of reaching its desired goals (Bryman 2001). Evaluation was method-driven and pursued truth and causation. More recent thinking has led to the emergence of the importance of context and mechanism in explaining how a programme evolves and improves (Pawson and Tilley 1997). It is through this more modern philosophy that both action and evaluation have once again crossed paths.

Significant parallels can be made between the definitions of action and evaluation research. Replete in the literature are notions of stakeholder involvement, informing decisions and augmenting change. Perhaps the view of evaluation research of Weiss (as cited in Clarke and Dawson 1999: 2) demonstrates this analogous relationship with the greatest clarity, claiming that evaluation is:

> a type of policy research, designed to help people make wise decisions and choices about future programming. Evaluation does not aim to replace decision makers' experience and judgement, but rather offers systematic evidence that informs experiences and judgement. Evaluation strives for impartiality and fairness. At its best, it strives to represent the range of perspectives of those who have a stake in the programme.

By elaborating on elements of Weiss's view, the major themes and significant issues integral to the role of AR in programme evaluation can be highlighted.

Utility: informing decisions

In evaluation literature there is specific reference made to judging the worth of evaluation research based on its use and utility (Patton 1997), just as in AR. Of the similarities drawn between evaluation and AR, there are two that dominate. First, both methods produce information that should be directly useful to a group of people. Smits and Champagne (2008: 427) openly criticised less participatory forms of evaluation as their results were 'rarely used'. Second, the process of both evaluation and AR will empower people to be motivated to use that information and be implicit in its generation. This notion of evaluation shares the same attributes as AR as it is driven by all involved (Winter *et al.* 2001; McNiff and Whitehead 2006). However, providing meaningful evidence to inform decisions of stakeholders can be both a very complex process and a political minefield. Both AR and evaluation research assume that key stakeholders will value information simply because they were involved in its orchestration. This is not always the case. For example, some practitioners may fear judgements made of their projects to the point of ignoring any information gleaned, useful or not.

Utility is also very dependent on how we define or acknowledge success. In our own research we work with a sector driven by accountability and key performance indicators and rates of participation. The dichotomous relationship between quality and quantity is very apparent and the latter seems a far cry from the principles of evaluation and emancipatory values of AR. Helsby and Saunders (1993) advocate that if indicators are to be of any use then a participatory approach will be most effective. In their view this would improve the capacity of the research to capture unintended outcomes; improve the scope for success beyond the judgement of those directly (e.g. teachers) involved; promote the use of theory to try and explain findings – arbitrary indicators, usually based on quantity, satisfied or not, will do little to help explain the success or failures of our activities. Despite this, many practitioners are at the mercy of funding agencies that may already have a predetermined notion of success which could be very different from those of the stakeholder group. Rather than undermine participatory research in the sometimes interminable 'qualitative versus quantitative debate', participatory research allows for a multitude of approaches including the use of figures and quality indicators.

There is also something fundamentally flawed about literature that advocates the *doing with* approach without acknowledging the complexities of action researchers and evaluators becoming at one with the actors of social change and the research process. Despite the best intentions, consensus between all stakeholders is almost impossible to achieve (Pawson and Tilley 1997). This bond is essential and has to be made long before any AR or evaluation takes place. This brings into question the timing of the research. For example, where evaluation is a relatively new concept it often becomes an afterthought rather than integral to the design and development of an intervention. Consequently, the capacity to explain how the intervention worked becomes severely limited and its input into programme change is nullified.

An inherent problem in a collaborative philosophy is the readiness of the actors to accept a *level playing field*. In sectors where creating an evidence base for decisions is a relatively new concept – such as medical education (Vasser *et al.* 2010) and sport development (Long, as cited in Hylton and Bramham 2008) – it seems there is a long way to go in terms of establishing authentic stakeholder engagement. Pawson and Tilley refer to such research as having all the problems of a 'lumbering adolescent'. The point here is that despite all the good intentions of those who are interested, not all are ready to adopt the position of the social good against the realisation of personal agendas. There are also practitioners who are very interested in informed decisions and value their projects but simply have neither the intention, resource or expertise to involve themselves in the research process and instead are more comfortable with the *knowledge experts*' (i.e. researchers') view. In theory, enabling practitioners to investigate and evaluate their work has a fairly solid grounding. That stakeholders value the process increases the likelihood of their utilising the results to augment change. However, in reality AR and evaluation approaches can be challenged as too invasive, not scientific enough or simply not certain to deliver intended outcomes.

Representing a range of perspectives

Smith *et al.* (2010) acknowledge a gap between idealism and realism with AR projects where tensions between stakeholders are very apparent. These same issues are evident in evaluation research projects. The emancipatory and egalitarian principles that both action and evaluation research hold dear could challenge the effectiveness of the research outcome – to inform change and improve understanding. For example, both action and evaluation research normally work with groups or communities (stakeholders, actors, organisations) and within such groups hierarchical, managerial, and dominance relations differ. Stakeholders with such different agendas create problems when trying to maintain a fair and impartial approach to action and evaluation research. It cannot be assumed that all necessary stakeholders involved are around the table at the time of the problem identification and research design phases. If they are not, then equity is challenged. Also it cannot be assumed that those around the table will have an equally shared degree of responsibility and contribution. If not, then once again fairness is challenged and ultimately more problems are created than solved.

Those practising action or evaluation research approaches must negotiate and navigate among and between their collaborators, addressing power-sharing issues and establishing the identity of all involved. This brings into question who is or is not an appropriate member with the requisite stakeholder knowledge. Often a wide range of stakeholders are identified and attempts are made at inclusive involvement in all parts of the process. However, Brydon-Miller *et al.* (2003) challenge the notion that *all involved should determine everything*. The issue of ownership and empowerment over expertise is largely ignored in the action and evaluation research literature. As Weiss acknowledged, the aim is not to replace decision makers but to offer a systematic process in which each stakeholder brings their own expertise to the table and uses it effectively. This may take the form of guidance as to appropriate research methods, supervision (Plottu and Plottu 2009) or the provision of localised experiential knowledge of what works and in what circumstances. Different knowledge bases are then valued with stakeholders contributing from their own knowledge base.

The more stakeholders there are, the more resource-intensive the action research project or evaluation becomes. For example, a community sport and physical activity network involved a participatory evaluation research project that invited as many members of the community as possible to take part. This included representatives of the voluntary sector (in the form of local sports clubs) and the public sector (leisure services, local primary and secondary physical education teachers and the police). Project managers tasked with delivering on policy objectives and development officers responsible for delivering interventions and the potential participants who may benefit from the interventions were all involved in the research process. This level of participation was meant to allow those who did not normally have an equitable opportunity to contribute. However, such wide engagement led to delays in project start dates which cascaded into failure to meet deadlines.

Despite such complexity, greater stakeholder involvement remains central to action and evaluation research. In the case of the community sports network which represented local managers and delivery agents, regional and national representation were invited to contribute to the research planning and implementation phases. As in the best traditions of AR and evaluation, this would facilitate the utility of the research beyond the bounds of the local delivery agents and would help transfer knowledge and understanding to policy levels.

Chapter summary

- AR is underpinned by very different principles than those involved with scientific inquiry but has many similarities with evaluation research. These include a concern with the local context, involvement of a wide range of stakeholders in participatory processes, and cyclical and emergent processes. This means that AR can be applied in evaluation research but there is likely to be a greater influence and presence from the investigator where the research is driven by evaluation principles and a stronger collaborative emphasis from AR.

- Participatory forms of research, particularly AR and evaluation, will actively promote research in practice and modernise practitioners' approach to working with, improving and understanding the complexities of social issues.

- Action researchers embrace their own subjectivity, understand their positionality and what impacts that has on the people with whom they engage in AR.

- Community involvement is vital to attaining grounded, workable AR outcomes, but there are many challenges inherent in ensuring that involvement is effective and positive. Negotiation and ongoing dialogue are essential to keep AR stakeholders working together rather than pursuing individual agendas.

- AR opens the door to using mixed methods designs in research which evolves as it progresses. Moreover, the underpinning epistemological, ethical and practical basis of AR creates the conditions for emancipatory approaches, working with people who are marginalised within existing social systems, challenging the status quo and resisting oppression in order to make sustainable and positive change in people's everyday lives.

- In designing appropriate participatory approaches, all stakeholders, particularly the researcher, must consider the context, scope, readiness and resources to ensure as much useful evidence as possible informs action. The evidence base can be both qualitative and quantitative.

- Rather than undermine research through a paradigm war, participatory forms of research need to be assessed on their own merits, based more on developing workable solutions to social problems together with a solid understanding of why such solutions are effective. Improvements in practice and accompanying understandings can then inform theory and thus become transferable to new contexts.

References

Ataov, A., Brogger, B. and Hildrum, J. M. (2010) 'An action research approach to the inclusion of immigrants in work life and local community life'. *Action Research*, **8**(3), 237–65.

Bargal, D. (2008) 'Action research: a paradigm for achieving social change'. *Small Group Research*, **39**(17), 17–27.

Barnes, C. (2001) '"Emancipatory" disability research: project or process?' Accessed October 11, 2010. http://www.leeds.ac.uk/disability-studies/archiveuk/Barnes/glasgow%20lecture.pdf.

Beukema, L. and Valkenburg, B. (2007) 'Demand-driven elderly care in the Netherlands: a case of exemplarian action research'. *Action Research*, **5**, 161–80.

Blum, K., Perry, M., Rogers, J., Fadem, P., Minkler, M., and Moore, L. (2002) 'Ethical dilemmas in participatory action research: a case study from the disability community'. *Health Education and Behavior*, **29**(1), 14–29.

Bradbury, H. (2010) 'What is good action research?' *Action Research*, **8**(1), 930–1009.

Bradbury, H. and Reason, P. (1993) 'Action research: an opportunity for revitalizing research purpose and practices'. *Qualitative Social Work*, **2**(2), 155–75.

British Psychological Society (2011) *Code of Human Research Ethics and Conduct*. Leicester: British Psychological Society.

Brown, L. D. and Gaventa, J. (2009) 'Constructing transnational action research networks: reflections on the Citizenship Development Research Centre'. *Action Research*, **8**(1), 5–28.

Brydon-Miller, M., Greenwood, D. and Maguire, P. (2003) 'Why action research?' *Action Research*, **1**(1), 9–28.

Bryman, A. (2001) *Social Research Methods*. Oxford: Oxford University Press.

Clarke, A. and Dawson, R. (1999) *Evaluation Research: An Introduction to Principles, Methods, and Practice*. London: Sage.

Clough, G., Conole, G. and Scanlon, E. (2010) 'Using participatory evaluation to support collaboration in an interdisciplinary context', in *Proceedings of the Seventh International Conference on Networked Learning 2010*, 3–4 May, Aalborg, Denmark.

Department of Culture, Media and Sport (2008) *A Passion for Excellence: An Improvement Strategy for Culture and Sport*. London: Local Government Association.

Department of Health (2010) *Healthy Lives, Healthy People. White Paper: Our Strategy for Public Health in England*. London: Department of Health.

Dick, B. (1997) *Rigour and Relevance in Action Research*. Accessed February 2011. www. Scu.edu.au/schools/gcm/ar/arp/rigour.html.

Dick, B. (2009) 'Action research literature'. *Action Research*, **7**(4), 423–41.

Dick, B. and Swepson, P. (1997) 'Action Research: FAQ'. Accessed February 2011. www. Scu.edu.au/schools/gcm/ar/arp/arfaq.html.

Fals-Borda, O. (1987) 'The application of participatory action research in Latin America'. *International Sociology*, **2**, 329–47.

Freire, P. (1972) *Pedagogy of the Oppressed*. Harmondsworth: Penguin.

Freire, P. (1982) 'Creating alternative research methods: learning to do it by doing it', in B. Hall, A. Gillette and R. Tandon (eds) *Creating Knowledge: A Monopoly? Participatory Research in Development*. New Delhi: Society for Participatory Research in Asia.

Gatenby, B. and Humphries, M. (2000) 'Feminist participatory action research: methodological and ethical issues'. *Women's Studies International Forum*, **23**(1), 89–105.

Hanley, B. (2005) *Research as Empowerment? Report of a Series of Seminars Organised by the Toronto Group*. York: Joseph Rowntree Foundation.

Helsby, G. and Saunders, M. (1993) 'Taylorism, Tylerism, and performance indicators: defending the indefensible?' *Educational Studies*, **19**(1), 55–77.

Hylton, K. and Bramham, P. (2008) *Sports Development: Policy, Process and Practice*, 2nd edn. Abingdon: Taylor and Francis.

Kagan, C. and Burton, M. (2000) 'Prefigurative action research: an alternative basis for critical psychology?' *Annual Review of Critical Psychology*, **2**, 73–87.

Ladkin, D. (2005) '"The enigma of subjectivity": how might phenomenology help action researchers negotiate the relationship between "self", "other" and "truth"?' *Action Research*, **3**(1), 108–26.

Lave, J. and Wenger, E. (1991) *Situated Learning – Legitimate Peripheral Participation*. Cambridge: Cambridge University Press.

Lennie, J. (2005) 'An evaluation capacity-building process for sustainable community IT initiatives'. *Evaluation*, **11**(4), 390–414.

Lewin, K. (1946) 'Action research and minority problems'. *Journal of Social Issues*, **2**, 34–46.

McNiff, J. and Whitehead, J. (2006) *All You Need to Know about Action Research*. London: Sage.

Meyer, J. (2000) 'Evaluating action research'. *Age and Ageing*, **29**, 8–10.

Minkler, M. (2000) 'Using participatory action research to build healthy communities'. *Public Health Reports*, **115**, 191–7.

Morgan, D. (2007) 'Paradigms lost and pragmatism regained: methodological implications of combining qualitative and quantitative methods'. *Journal of Mixed Methods Research*, **1**, 48–76.

Mountian, I., Lawthorn, R., Kellock, A., Duggan, K., Sixsmith, J., Kagan, C., Hawkins, J., Haworth, J., Siddiquee, A., Worley, C., Brown, D., Griffiths, J. and Purcell, C. (2011) 'On utilising a visual methodology: shared reflections and tensions', in P. Reavey (ed.) *Visual Methods in Psychology: Using and Interpreting Images in Qualitative Research*. London: Routledge.

Patton, M. Q. (1997) *Utilization-Focussed Evaluation*, 3rd edn. Thousand Oaks, CA: Sage.

Pawson, R. and Tilley, N. (1997) *Realistic Evaluation*. London: Sage.

Plottu, B. and Plottu, E. (2009) 'Approaches to participation in evaluation'. *Evaluation*, **15**(3), 343.

Pratesi, A., Sixsmith, J. and Woolrych, R. (in press). 'Participatory design for future technologies: lessons from the Smart Distress Monitor Project'. *International Community Psychology: Community Approaches to Contemporary Social Problems*, **2**.

Prins, E. (2010) 'Participatory photography: a tool for empowerment or surveillance?' *Action Research*, **8**(4), 426–43.

Quinlan, E. (2009) 'New action research techniques: using participatory theatre with health care workers'. *Action Research*, **8**(2), 117–33.

Ragland, B. B. (2006) 'Positioning the practitioner-researcher: five ways of looking at practice'. *Action Research*, **4**(2), 165–82.

Reid, C., Allison, T. and Frisby, W. (2006) 'Finding the "action" in feminist participatory action research'. *Action Research*, **4**(3), 315–32.

Riel, M. (2010) 'Understanding action research'. Center For Collaborative Action Research. Pepperdine University. Accessed October 9, 2010. http://cadres.pepperdine.edu/ccar/define.html.

Rossi, P. H., Lipsey, M. W. and Freeman, H. E. (2004) *Evaluation: A Systematic Approach*. London: Sage.

Sixsmith, J. and Kagan, C. (2005) *Arts for Mental Health. Final Report.* Manchester: Manchester Metropolitan University.

Smith, L., Bratini, L., Chambers, D.-A., Jensen, R. V. and Romero, L. (2010) 'Between idealism and reality: meeting the challenges of participatory action research'. *Action Research*, **8**(4), 407–25.

Smits, P. A. and Champagne, F. (2008) 'An assessment of the theoretical underpinnings of practical participatory evaluation'. *American Journal of Evaluation*, **29**(4), 427.

Stoecker, R. (2009) 'Are we talking the walk of community-based research?' *Action Research*, **7**(4), 385–404.

Suárez-Herrera, J. C., Springett, J. and Kagan, C. (2009) 'Critical connections between participatory evaluation, organizational learning and intentional change in pluralistic organizations'. *Evaluation*, **15**(3), 321.

Wadsworth, Y. (1998) *What is Participatory Action Research? Action Research International, Paper 2.* Accessed September 7, 2006. http://www.scu.edu.au/schools/gcm/ar/ari/p-ywadsworth98.html.

Waterman, H., Tillen, D., Dickson, R. and de Koning, K. (2001) 'Action research: a systematic review and guidance for assessment'. *Health Technology Assessment*, **5**(23), iii–157.

Weiss, C. H. (1972) *Evaluation Research.* Upper Saddle River, NJ: Prentice-Hall.

Whitehead, D., Taket, A. and Smith, P. (2003) 'Action research in health promotion.' *Health Education Journal*, **62**(1), 5.

Winter, R., Munn-Giddings, C., Weaver, Y., Nicholls, V., Kennedy, N., Searson, F., *et al.* (2001) *A Handbook for Action Research in Health and Social Care.* London: Routledge.

Chapter 3

Positionalities

Dan Goodley and Sophie Smailes

Introduction

In this chapter we will explore the importance of positionality – from feminist and critical disability studies orientations – to qualitative research. Burns and Walker (2005: 67) consider positionality in terms of the 'implication of the researcher in the production of knowledge and a breaking down of the "masculinist" separation of the private [world of the researcher] through the public [activity of research]'. Positionality is located within this discussion as an ongoing engagement with contextual frameworks from which we (the writers and researchers) come, and their influence on the choices and approaches we make when embarking on research. In other words, we are interested in rendering visible the subjective and critically reflective frameworks to behind how we research, what we research and why we research. At a very fundamental level – we believe that no research is value free – and it is these values with which we are particular concerned. The chapter explores a number of key themes in relation to methodological, epistemological and ontological undergirdings of qualitative research using feminisms and critical disability studies as our points of location and reflection. We have chosen to write this as two parallel and interconnected accounts of our approaches and positions within this exploration as 'the differences in our experiences precisely underline the need to pay reflexive attention to the complex processes of doing research' (Jowett and O'Toole 2006: 456).

Viewpoint/sitpoint

We start by reflexively considering some of the origins of our research interests and why qualitative research is important to us not only as more than an idiographic approach but also as a space to understand the structural, cultural and political foundations of what is often known as the psychological.

A feminist viewpoint: Sophie Smailes

As a woman, academic, psychotherapist, feminist, white, able-bodied, middle-class, etc. etc. my 'fluid and constantly in flux identities' (Bordo 1990; Moulding 2006) have informed and been informed by how these positions reflect dominant discourses and positions. In qualitative research, the need to be open and aware of our position and impact on how we engage in the research process is a vital reflective action throughout all stages of the research. Both Willig (1999, 2008) and Lafrance and Stoppard (2006) write about the process of how we locate ourselves being drawn from particular prevailing discourses which 'contain a range of subject positions which in turn facilitate and/or constrain certain experiences and practices' (Willig 1999: 43). The structure of qualitative research, and in particular feminist research methodologies, is informed by this constant reflexivity and adds to the richness and transparency of the whole 'enterprise'.

With this in mind my reflections on my positioning and journey are a way of providing an insight into the how and why I engage with feminist qualitative research and its representational implications. My location is informed by a number of influences not least that I am female. I came to higher education with a background in British history where much of the material we covered was the preserve of men, power and patriarchy. So, the focus was on the kings (and the odd queen), the battles/crusades, the church versus state, the laws and legislature, urbanisation and industrialisation. The way in which this was taught, what we read and indeed the very essays we wrote were concerned with particular instrumental and power issues, which were the sphere of men. It was not just that these were considered the most relevant and important aspects to 'know' but also that these were universalised to all; and women, the poor and disenfranchised, disabled and homosexual, etc. were either invisible, peripheral or problematised.

What counts as legitimate knowledge, our ways of knowing and how we come to know what we know (Burns and Walker 2005), can reflect very rarefied perspectives. Notions of reality, knowledge and what was considered relevant, pertinent, worth knowing, and who recorded the knowledge, meant that the picture I had of British social history was partial at best. Stanley and Wise (1993) and Westmarland (2001) write about 'malestream methods' as being hierarchically located, legitimising only certain 'kinds' of data, information and sources. Willig (2008), O'Leary (2004) and Westmarland (2001) emphasise how what is presented/sourced as universal and worthy of note resides within patriarchal values and scholarship – hence the partiality.

My choice of degree was informed partly by my frustrations with this partiality and I endeavoured to choose one that would give voice to a far wider range of people/realities. I learnt that sources of data, what was considered as legitimate data, whose voices were heard and acknowledged were far more diverse than initially taught; and subject to the choices, interests and perspectives of the people who taught and wrote them (Jarviluoma *et al.* 2003). Feminist qualitative research is also concerned with opening up the arena of 'legitimate data and voices' and encourages the access of a wide variety of data sources/methodologies which allow for diverse voices, representations and constructions to be heard and acknowledged (Oakley 1981; Neilson 1990; Ramazanoglu with Holland 2003).

A further influential bed of knowledge/experience informing my approach to qualitative feminist research was my training in humanistic counselling/psychotherapy. This emphasises the relationship between the therapist and the client, centralising the voice, story and words of the client. Karniel-Miller *et al.* (2009) write about the importance, in qualitative feminist research, of the respondent's ownership of their story. The role of the researcher is to reflect/represent as closely as possible this story. Oakley (1981) writes about the need within qualitative feminist interviews to acknowledge and work with the power implicit within the relationship, and indeed engage with an active sense of reciprocity. In humanistic counselling reciprocity takes the form of being fully present, congruent and actively engaged in the client's process and its meanings (Geldard and Geldard 2003; Tolan 2003; Joseph 2010); explicitly valuing the person and giving space to their own realities.

Within such a person-centred reflexive training, little acknowledgement was given to social and political contexts except in the form of special 'add-on' sessions for gender, sexuality, disability and race. Lafrance and Stoppard (2006) and Kitzinger (2004) challenge this 'adding on' process within generalised normative discourses as implicitly positioning men as 'the norm' (Willig 2008). As with history, this approach rendered women (and indeed ethnicity, religion, class, sexuality, disability, etc.) as invisible and/or a problem (O'Leary 2004; Burns and Walker 2005; Watts 2006). Indeed, the intersectionalities between and within these various 'identities' were missed and often responses of tutors/students came from inadvertent pathologisation or elision.

Finally, as an academic I reside largely within the social sciences, qualitative research, feminist and critical theory and humanism. All of these strands, as well as my own lived experiences, feed into how I understand and engage with qualitative feminist research. Feminist qualitative research is transformative and ongoing; it situates 'knowledge' in ongoing debates and processes requiring 'awareness of the social context in which such accounts are expressed and of the social and cultural locations from which they are drawn' (Kerr *et al.* 1998: 114, cited in Jowett and O'Toole 2006: 453). As I continue to engage with these privileged and marginalised subjectivities, 'uncomfortable' and taken-for-granted areas become more visible. Critical research theory and feminism ask us to give voice to the experiences of ourselves and marginalised groups (Stephenson 2006; Salmon 2007) when engaging in qualitative research. More recently, feminist theorists like Watts (2006) emphasise the contested nature of our identities and the need to work with intersectionalities and diversities within; a commitment which can make the choices of methodologies and approaches in research even more challenging.

Critical research, including feminist methodologies, is not a static uncritical concept which is used to design qualitative research. These methodologies are various, ongoing, in a constant flux and always developing and responding to the contexts and constructions in/with which we reside. 'Feminism and feminist methodology are not monolithic but numerous, a contested terrain and source of continual debate among feminist scholars' (Burns and Walker 2005: 69). The second area of positionality we explore in this chapter resides in critical disability studies.

A critical disability studies sitpoint

When completing my undergraduate degree in psychology in 1993, I (Dan) felt let down by much of what I had been taught. Yes, there were highlights: the lectures on Marxism and psychoanalysis; sessions exploring feminism on the psychology of women course; some seminar discussions of discourse analysis and the opportunity to implement a qualitative dissertation project had given me access to some of the insights from critical and qualitative research. However, much of the psychology that I had come into contact with was positivistic, quantitative, individualistic and, frankly, dull. Moreover, my own personal commitments to what I came to know as the politics of disability seemed far, far away from the mainstream realities of much of what was considered to be "good psychology". When disabled people were addressed in psychology, this tended to be in terms of abnormality, as objects of cognitive and biopsychological research and intervention. Perhaps inevitably, this led me to leave psychology, to complete a PhD in a sociology department, to then work in departments of sociology and education. Throughout these times I became more and more immersed in critical disability studies and qualitative research. And then, in 2007, I returned to psychology and the department from which I had graduated. Two questions now occupy me: how can critical disability studies colonise psychology? To what extent can qualitative (psychological) research further the development of critical disability studies?

The notion of sitpoint (alluding to the disabled researcher and user of a wheelchair) is borrowed from the feminist disability studies scholar Garland Thomson (2005) who revises the feminist concept of standpoint in order to foreground disability. Recognising one's personal and political commitments – and reflexively accounting for their impact on the implementation of research – is an important element of qualitative research. While positivist researchers may identify such disclosure as evidence of the blatantly biased nature of qualitative research, we may turn the tables here back at positivists and remind ourselves, as Walker (1981: 153) did, that 'to choose to take on an objective, scientific or dispassionate stance is just as much a value position as to choose one's own subjectivity'. Foregrounding one's commitments to qualitative research – and qualitative research of specific issues of social justice – reminds us that research is often very much more than simply a data gathering exercise: it reflects assumptions, philosophical beliefs and ideological commitments (Rist 1977). Indeed, for Wright Mills (1970), the dominance of positivistic, quantitative research within social science disciplines such as psychology and sociology rendered a condition known as abstracted empiricism: a pronounced tendency to confuse what was being studied with the set of methods that were suggested for the study (Wright Mills 1970: 61). The dominance of science meant that social phenomena were only ever studied 'within the curiously self-imposed limitations of an arbitrary epistemology' (p. 65): namely positivism. For Jung (2002: 182) disability and feminist studies agree that objectivist and scientific approaches to knowledge production suppress and silence those who are marginalised or excluded. These silences in the academy are integral to the reproduction of unequal relations of power in the social world.

Inequality as a starting point for qualitative research

In this section we explore a shared assumption: that the social world is in conflict, that there are inequities and that qualitative research provides possibilities of tracing, mapping and challenging moments of discrimination, oppression and inequality.

Feminism and inequality

Inequalities in psychological research (Qin 2004; Lafrance and Stoppard 2006; Moulding 2006; Willig 2008) and indeed by association in our social world are deeply embedded in how knowledge and how men and women are constructed. McAlister and Neill (2007: 169) in their research with young Irish women's perceptions of self found that 'dominant patriarchal ideologies persist, but are more concealed'. These messages, or dominant discourses, impact on women's experience of self in increasingly complex ways. Feminist qualitative research's commitment to explore and recognise these inequalities allows the research to move from rather naïve, unexplored, taken-for-granted discourses to more rigorous socially inclusive research. Inequalities (a contested term in and of itself and one which can depend on what/who is 'defining/experiencing it') and the access to material/political/social opportunities and the power and 'freedom' they afford in terms of education, suffrage, employment, money, sexual 'freedom', etc. were at the heart of initial feminist movements. While some of these areas have opened up for some women, particularly in western contexts, notions of patriarchal privilege (and in this I take wider meanings in terms of white, middle-class, able-bodied, heterosexual, western, highly educated) still remain and serve dominant social and political structures (Westmarland 2001; Burns and Walker 2005; Watts 2006).

An area in which these 'structures' are particularly highlighted is psychological research on (and meanings of) women's depression. Lafrance and Stoppard (2006) and Ussher (1991, 2010) challenge the medicalisation of women's depression as first accounting for women's higher rates of diagnosed depression than men, as well as the discounting of women's lived experiences. They highlight the social and political context of women's lives, where women experience higher rates of poverty, continued unequal division of household labour and care in the home, higher levels of sexual assault and other abuse as compared to men, as being implicit in women's mental health and well-being. By locating women's experience of depression, where single mothers and young 'married' women with children are disproportionately represented (Lafrance and Stoppard 2006; Ussher 2010), within this context they dispute mainstream psychological research's claims that biological, psychological and behavioural differences between men and women account for this discrepancy (Lafrance and Stoppard 2006).

The background of both the researcher and researched is crucial in terms of working with inequalities and recourses to power and 'self-definitions'. So feminist qualitative research challenges the notion that we can do research without taking into account the cultural scripts which are imbued with power differentiations and meanings. Karniel-Miller *et al.* (2009) consider the centrality of the research relationship as renegotiating ownership of the research, and endeavouring to end the oppression of particular populations by attempting to 'democratize the relationship' and give voice to people who are or may be already marginalised. Hence, transparency, reciprocity and responsiveness and being able to be open to the challenges and transformative nature of the research process are part of that commitment. Salmon's (2007: 983) research with Aborigine women also discusses the need to democratise research relationships, particularly given the tendency of 'colonial and imperial practices [being reproduced in research] . . . when White scholars develop and undertake research in which Indigenous peoples and their customs, practices, and lived experiences are the sole *objects* of study'.

McAlister and Neill's (2007) research indicates that popular notions of equality are constructed increasingly in discourses of individualisation, where young women are blamed for either not living up to 'idealised womanhood' or derided for being duped. Lafrance and Stoppard (2006) emphasise the power and influence of these dominant messages which locate women's experience of depression in their biology and psychological make-up, despite the lack of conclusive and consistent evidence. Moulding (2006), Watts (2006) and Stephenson (2006) also point out that women's experiences and understanding of self have largely been constructed in opposition/comparison to men's – employing value-laden dualistic reason to make sense of differences.

Thus, gendered (and colonial, able-bodied) constructions of the 'ideal' as autonomous, rational and active serve to problematise women's (and other marginalised groups) experiences as being 'other', or indeed individual pathologies and/or weaknesses (Lafrance and Stoppard 2006; Moulding 2006), rather than subjective agencies.

If equality is defined in terms of choices, then clearly those available to women are within 'the confines of a constructed ideal of "feminine perfection"' (McAlister and Neill 2007: 172). Health-care practice around mental health, depression and eating disorders (two areas in particular where women far outnumber men) is often interested in containing and managing women and their experiences; invalidating and problematising women's subjective agencies which fall outside the idealised normative constructs. Feminist psychological methodologies are, as a result, interested in exploring the shifting category of 'woman' (Watts 2006) by not fixing them into particular essentialised positions but working with the respondents themselves in enabling as full a picture as possible of their experiences to emerge.

Disability and inequality

Disability and inequality are inextricably linked. The word 'disability' hints at something missing. Following Goodley (2011: 1–2), to be disabled evokes a marginalised place in society, culture, economics and politics. It is concentrated in some parts of the globe more than others, caused by armed conflict and violence, malnutrition, rising populations, child labour and poverty. Paradoxically, it is increasingly found to be everywhere, due to the exponential rise in the number of psychiatric, administrative and educational labels over the last few decades. Disability affects us all, transcending class, nation and wealth.

The notion of the TAB – Temporarily Able Bodied – recognises that many people will at some point become disabled (Marks 1999: 18). Most impairments are acquired (97 per cent) rather than congenital (born with) and world estimates suggest a figure of around 500–650 million disabled people, or one in ten of the population, with this expected to rise to around 800 million by the year 2015 (Peters *et al.* 2008). Currently, 150 million of these are children (Grech 2008) and it is estimated that 386 million of the world's working-age population are disabled. Eighty-eight per cent live in the world's poorest countries and 90 per cent of those in rural areas (Marks 1999). For example, India has a population of one billion and approximately 70 million are disabled (Ghai 2002). In the USA, 19.3 per cent or 49.7 million of the 'civilian non-institutionalised population of five years or older' are disabled (Quinlan *et al.* 2008). This makes disabled people the largest minority grouping in an already crowded theatre of multiculturalism (Davis 1995). Disabled people are more likely to be victims of rape and violence, less likely to receive legal protection, more likely to be excluded from mass education, under-represented in positions of power and more reliant on state benefits and/or charity (Meekosha 2008). As children they remain under-represented in mainstream schools, work, leisure and communities (McLaughlin *et al.* 2008). As adults, disabled people do not enjoy equitable access to human, economic and social capital resources. If we accept Marx's view that charity is the perfume of the sewers of capitalism, then disabled people are subjected to the bittersweet interventions of charity. Of the nigh on 200 countries in the world only a third have antidiscriminatory disability legislation, and many of these laws are questionable in terms of their legislative potency (UN Department of Public Information 2008).

Structurally, culturally and relationally disabled people continue to face oppression and marginalisation. Critical disability studies respond to the inequities faced by disabled people in contemporary society. Critical disability studies constitute a transdisciplinary space which breaks boundaries between disciplines and creates inroads into disciplines that have historically marginalised disabled people such as medical sociology (Thomas 2007), philosophy (Kristiansen *et al.* 2008) and psychology (Goodley and Lawthom 2005).

Sketching out feminisms and critical disability studies

In this section we introduce these two transdisciplinary spaces as reactions and resistances to dominant theories of gender and disability.

Gender politics

As an opening position, Ramazanoglu's (1992: 208) understanding of 'what one takes by feminist methodology depends in part on which authors one takes as examples' is a useful one. Qualitative research methodologies and critical approaches in particular are always concerned with locating the interpretations and reflexivity of the researcher as being implicated within the purpose, structure and design of research endeavours. Thus, the range and variety within feminist methodologies are reflective of shifting and multiple epistemologies (Stephenson 2006; Watts 2006). Banister *et al.* (1997) write that feminist methodologies are also identified by their purpose, how they engage with phenomenon and research itself, what the hoped for outcomes may be and how these outcomes might be used. Burns and Walker (2005: 66) also consider these commonalities in terms of 'a shared commitment to drawing attention to the deep and irreducible connections between knowledge and power (privilege), and to making problematic gender in society and social institutions in order to develop theories that advance practices of gender justice'.

As already noted, feminist methodologies are informed by a desire to challenge and render visible deeply embedded, taken-for-granted discourses of inequality, hegemonic 'knowledges' and power. Positivism's assumed position of reason, universality and objective 'truth' is one that feminist methodologies challenge (Stephenson 2006; Watts 2006; Willig 2008), particularly as this knowledge has been constructed on the (white, middle-class, able-bodied, heterosexual, western) male as being what Willig (2008) calls the 'protypical human subject'. As Oakley (1974), Stanley and Wise (1993), Ramazanoglu (1992) and Westmarland (2001) all point out, this positioning of knowledge impacts on how and what research has been done and is being done in ways which negate the need to consider the social/political/economic contexts in which research takes place.

Wilkinson (1998) and Jowett and O'Toole (2006) both write about feminisms in terms of 'disrupting' the power imbalances, challenging them and then seeing where the research goes and what emerges. Salmon (2007: 983) emphasises that 'feminist, antiracist, and anti-colonial [this could equally apply to critical disability, queer theory, etc.] have underscored the need to transform the oppressive relations inherent in standard [psychological] research methods' by disturbing this limited normative approach to research and recognising the relationship between the researcher and researched. Fay (1987: 23, 27) emphasises how feminist methodology 'explains social order or explains social reality, criticises it and empowers people to overthrow it, or in milder forms, helps to understand social reality'. In terms of designing and engaging with qualitative research then, it is not just about what emerges and how realities are constructed between and within the research relationships, but how the process and findings are put into active use (Watts 2006). Thus, a core element to feminist methodologies is validating the knowledge of marginalised groups with the view to challenging the status quo and existent power structures.

Burns and Walker (2005) emphasise the challenge of feminist methodologies to what is seen as the silencing/sidelining of women's voices, assigning women passive roles (no agency), with little 'reasoning'. The research with women of McAlister and Neill (2007), Moulding (2006) and Lafrance and Stoppard (2006) highlights how existent patriarchal underpinnings of mental health, idealised womanhood and depression act in ways which serve to limit women's choices within the 'confines of a constructed feminine perfection' (McAlister and Neill 2007: 172). Jowett and O'Toole's (2006), McAlister and Neill's (2007) and Lafrance and Stoppard's (2006) research are all concerned, in various ways, in engaging with women's voices; while the work of Moulding (2006) filters women's experiences through the lens of practitioners who work 'on' anorexic young women. The research of Lafrance and Stoppard (2006) and McAlister and Neill (2007) worked with their respondents in ways which allowed emergent realities and contradictions to be highlighted and acknowledged. Thus, their work 'revealed' that dominant messages about social, relational and maternal identification and 'the good woman' 'are concealed in visions, messages and text concerning the empowerment of women, the celebration of womanhood, choice, individuality, freedom and a breaking from age-old gender inequalities and assumptions' (McAlister and Neill 2007: 169). Methodologically feminist research can enable this unveiling process, where the contradiction and double binds of increasingly dominant messages of individualisation are seen to work alongside existing structures of inequality in complex ways – ways which reflect some of the wider 'cultural contradictions' around femininity, class, race, sexuality and disability (Moulding 2006; Salmon 2007).

The politics of disability

Critical disability studies emerged as a response to the growing politicisation of disabled people across the globe. With politicisation came conscientisation: a realisation that societies tended to view disability – and treat disabled people – in terms of an individual pathology, a tragedy, a problem of a deficient body or mind. This approach is heavily reliant upon medicalised views of the disabled-person-as-broken. Linton (1998) and Sherry (2006) suggest that this individualizing discourse creates a number of 'fault lines': disability is cast as an essentialist condition (with organic aetiologies); disabled people are treated as objects rather than authors of their own lives; 'person fixing' rather than 'context changing' interventions are preferred; the power of health and social care professionals becomes ever increasing as they seek to rehabilitate, educate or normalise disabled people. Disabled people are infantilised, constructed as helpless and viewed as asexual and incompetent. Out of this growing awareness that dominant ideas have individualised the problems of disability emerged alternative views of disability that were more social, cultural and structural in orientation (Goodley 2011).

From the 1970s onwards, critical disability studies emerged as a transdisciplinary space for the development of theory, research and practice that responded to the perspectives and ambitions of the disabled and cast disability not as a problem intrinsic to individuals with sensory, physical or cognitive impairments, but as a sociocultural and political problem through and through.

These ideas did not remain in academia but fed into and were informed by the politicisation of disabled people. This new discourse of critical disability studies gave rise to alternative definitions which recognised the cultural and social responses to people with impairments:

> **IMPAIRMENT**: is the functional limitation within the individual caused by physical, mental or sensory impairment.
>
> **DISABILITY**: is the loss or limitation of opportunities to take part in the normal life of the community on an equal level with others due to physical and social barriers.
>
> (Disabled People's International 1982)

These definitions acknowledge impairment but politicise disability. For Sherry (2007: 10), impairment can be understood as a form of biological, cognitive, sensory or psychological difference that is defined often within a medical context. Disability, however, is the negative social reaction to those differences associated with impairment. Thomas (2007: 73) extends this analysis further in her definition of *disablism* as 'a form of social oppression involving the social imposition of restrictions of activity on people with impairments and the socially engendered undermining of their psycho-emotional well being'. Disablism therefore sits alongside other forms of oppression including hetero/sexism and racism. Critical disability studies theory and research aim to expose the conditions of disablism as they work at the level of psyche, culture and society (Goodley 2011: xii–xiii).

A key issue for qualitative research is focus: does disability studies research focus on understanding disabling society or the meaning of impairment (Goodley and Lawthom 2005)? While both are important questions to ask, critical disability studies is mindful of the fact that much disability-related research has tended to be impairment-obsessed: individualising the problems of disability in terms of pathological, individualised and deficient understandings of the disabled body and mind. Indeed, qualitative research in the field of medical sociology and health psychology, for example, has been criticised for attending too often to the embodied experience of living with particular impairments rather than casting the net wider to qualitatively analyse the conditions of disablism (see, for example, Thomas 2007). That said, critical disability studies encompass a multitude of research questions and qualitative studies that, in their broadest sense, aim to understand the meaning of impairment and disablism.

The 'ologies': epistemology, ontology and methodology

We now consider the ways in which these key concepts of qualitative research can be understood from our two positions. In particular we will consider the ways in which feminisms and critical disability studies offer new epistemologies, ontologies and methodologies to dominant ones associated with essentialism, medicalisation, individualism, psychologisation and functionalism.

Feminist theories

Reflexivity, situational knowledge and an ongoing dynamic critique of how knowledge is constructed, and who does the 'constructing', weave throughout much of what is positioned as feminist epistemologies. May (2003) explores critical research theory's interest as to how our common-sense meanings have been constructed, what process takes place and how these meanings are operated upon by political, social and economic powers within society. 'All knowledge is produced in someone's interest so all knowledge is generated from positions of power/ powerlessness' (Skeggs 1997: 50). Thus, it challenges positivism's position that 'facts' exist separate from the ideologies, beliefs and invested self-interests of dominant groups (Gray 2004).

O'Leary (2004) also emphasises this critical epistemological position, noting that we are all part of this socialisation, that we are all products of this process and these discourses influence and inform how we position ourselves within research, how we position our respondents and what we consider 'relevant and meaningful'. 'All knowledge, including women's knowledge, is . . . partial and situated' (Burns and Walker 2005: 68). According to Travers (2001) and Ramazanoglu with Holland (2003) the role of the feminist researcher is to engage with these contested issues, recognising their own part within this. Jowett and O'Toole's (2006) research explores this when they acknowledge, in the process of their own research, how their [privileged] assumptions materialised in ways which were implicated within their choices of methodology as well as how they engaged. The flexibility and responsiveness of their research designs allowed these assumptions to emerge and, as a result, the researchers were able to re-adjust their design so that the subjective agencies of their respondents were recognized, and responded to, in ways they had not anticipated.

Qualitative feminist research requires a rigorous critical positioning of self 'within' the research rather than 'with out' it. So the place of the researcher is central to how the research proceeds on all levels. Travers (2001: 138) goes on to say that it is not just about producing 'emancipatory knowledge' for others but also 'to demonstrate that [she] has come to view [her] own life differently through conducting empirical research'. Thus for feminist methodologies we are co-creators, co-'responders', co-meaning makers with the people with whom we research. Epistemologically it also works with some of the contested notions that the individual is a 'relatively autonomous, self-contained and distinctive entity, who is affected by external variables like "socialisation" and "social context" but is in some sense separate from these "influences"' (Kitzinger 1992: 229). The challenge for feminist and indeed all critical researchers working within postmodernist discourses is to find ways of working with 'difference and complexity while not losing sight of the bigger issues around women's (and some men's) oppression' (Burns and Walker 2005: 68). McAlister and Neill's (2007) research with young women is particularly revealing of this ongoing epistemological challenge to both individualisation and essentialism. By highlighting women's accounting of their relationships to and with their bodies, they draw attention to how the young women pathologise and 'other' experiences of body dissatisfaction and objectification. The larger contradictory cultural and structural processes and messages are thereby lost in discourses of individual responsibility and choice.

Watts (2006) and Stephenson (2006) also consider how feminist methodologies provide opportunities for exposing particular subtle dominant messages which are still informed by phallocentric ideals of autonomy and responsibility – situating the individual in charge of their lives and eliding processes of individualisation and 'the personal' into depoliticised concepts of 'freedom'.

Theories of disability

One way of pitching an analysis of theory – or the epistemological, ontological and methodological approaches of theory – is to draw on the work of Burrell and Morgan (1979). Clough and Nutbrown (2002: 30) provide a helpful definition of these terms: an *ontology* is a theory of what exists and how it exists; an *epistemology* is a related theory of how we can come to know these things; *methodology* is the approach to how we investigate these things. Burrell and Morgan (1979) consider these components of theory through the mapping out of distinct theoretical positions across two overlapping axes (see Figure 3.1 and Goodley, 2011 for a more elaborate expansion of this work).

The horizontal axis of subjectivity and objectivity is underpinned by distinct assumptions. Epistemologically, an objectivist approach would be closely related to a positivist approach (an objective deductive engagement with observable real things), while a subjectivist approach is associated with an anti-positivist perspective (a subjective inductive engagement with the processes of meaning making). In terms of ontology, subjectivists would be characterised as nominalists; focused on the often elusive properties of individuals. Objectivists, in contrast, are realists; focused on the real things that exist independently of the observer in the world. Methodologically, then, it would follow that an objectivist position would be aligned with nomothetic approaches to research (including scientific, quantitative, experimental approaches to research that measure variables), while subjectivists would adopt idiographic methodologies (such as non-scientific, qualitative research that engages with meaning making). In addition, following Burrell and Morgan (1979), each position would view human nature in contrary ways. Objectivists would tend to understand human nature in terms of determinism (human nature is the product of biological or social structures), while subjectivists would be sympathetic to the stance of voluntarism (human nature is the product of individual and relational agency).

The vertical axis of radical change and regulation reflects what Burrell and Morgan (1979) define as the concerns of theory. Regulation theorists adopt a consensual view of the social world and are interested in notions of status quo, social order, consensus, social integration, solidarity and need satisfaction. Conflict theorists adopt a different view of society and culture and are interested in notions of radical change, structural conflict, modes of domination, contradiction and deprivation.

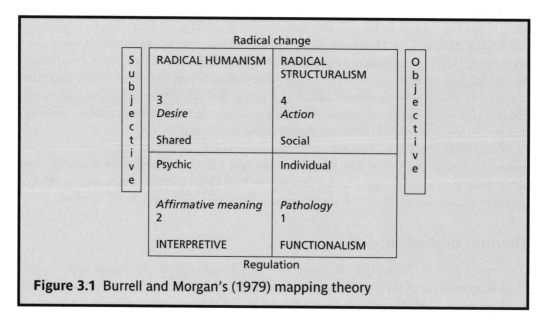

Figure 3.1 Burrell and Morgan's (1979) mapping theory

Placed against one another, these two axes allow us to locate particular approaches to the study of social and psychological factors. Critical disability studies has undergone some major theoretical shifts from a view of disability as the product of an individual's mental functioning and behaviour (functionalism) to an engagement with the structures and institutions of society that disable (radical structuralism). Along the way, researchers have illuminated the primacy of experiences of disabled people to an understanding of the social world (interpretivism), while others have contested ideologies of disablism (radical humanism). To exemplify this further, following Goodley (2011: 51–2), a *functionalist* view of the world sees society as regulated and ordered, promotes objective measures of (dys)functional mental states and behaviours and, inevitably, views disabled people as adherents of a 'sick role' (Barnes 1998). From this worldview, disabled people have inherited pathological conditions that can be objectively diagnosed, treated and in some cases ameliorated. A functionalist position assumes that disability has a biological, social and experiential component (Wendell 1996: 23).

An *interpretivist* stance understands the social world as an emergent social process, created by individuals and their shared subjective understandings (Goodley 2011: 52). Disabling or enabling identities and attitudes are made by and between voluntaristic individuals in a coherent and regulated world. An interpretivist position is adopted by Ferguson *et al.* (1992) who draw on qualitative research with disabled and non-disabled people to explicate the ways in which, for example, the attitudes of non-disabled people threaten to stifle the participation of disabled children in school settings.

Radical humanism situates knowledge production in the elusive shared subjective creation of dominant disability discourses, hegemonies and social meaning-making processes of wider society (Goodley 2011: 52). Langness and Levine (1986) demonstrate that the entire concept of mental retardation is bound up with capitalist and modern ideologies that mark some people as productive, contributory citizens and others as passive dependents.

Radical structuralism sees the social world as constantly in conflict, where economic and political structures can be objectively observed and in which certain social groupings are always at risk of alienation, oppression and false consciousness (Goodley 2011: 52). For example, Finkelstein (1981) argues that while early capitalism (phase 1) offered some inclusion in the community through disabled people's involvement in small-scale cottage industries, the rapid growth of manufacturing and machinery supplanted their contribution to a growing labour force. Phase 2 saw manufacturing industries such as coal and steel expanding. Mass migration from rural to urban areas increased exponentially. Industrialisation deskilled and impoverished disabled people who had previously worked in agrarian communities. Many disabled people, deemed incapable of offering labour quickly joined the unemployed in the cities. Industrialisation demanded fit workers. Factories exposed uncompetitive workers. Institutionalisation provided a means of controlling non-viable workers and, in contrast, developed new forms of labour for those working in them. Phase 3, late capitalism, offers more opportunities for consumer groups and disabled people's organisations to challenge their exclusion from mainstream life.

Politics of embattlement

The peripheral location of feminisms and critical disability studies in relation to more mainstream (psychological) uses of qualitative research situates them as, potentially, transformative spaces. We will consider this peripheral location as a limitation (exclusion) and as a place of possibility (offering deconstruction).

Feminist encounters

'Psychology does politics when it tests the current normative constraints of the personal realm' (Stephenson 2006: 82). Qualitative research facilitates the exploration and emergence of these normative processes, not just giving space to the voices of marginalised groups but noting the impact of these processes on our understandings and experiences. The researcher's role within these approaches is to explore and investigate, to extend the reaches of knowledge construction, to be able to challenge and work with their own perspectives and impacts, the choices they make and the language they chose. Jarviluoma *et al.* (2003) question the limitations of mainstream research in terms of its non-acknowledgement of differential power and cultural constructions, while McAlister and Neill (2007) and Lafrance and Stoppard (2006) highlight how constructions of femininity and masculinity are contained within particular discourses which serve to constrain women (and men) in particular ways.

O'Leary (2004: 45) considers that the engagement with these ongoing structures enables far more rigorous research as 'being aware of your own social status and the social status of the researched puts you in a position to manage any potential power related issue that might influence your research'. This ethical commitment to non-exploitative research (Neilson 1990; Travers 2001; Letherby 2003; Salmon 2007) is about not simply *using* our respondents as a resource for our knowledge construction, *using* their experiences and perspectives as a way of, to put it bluntly, increasing our *own* academic portfolios, developing our *own* theories, improving our *own* status and so on – it goes to the fundamental ethical principles of shared emancipatory knowledge and action. De Laine (2000: 110) explains it well when she claims that for qualitative feminist researchers 'a key to ethically and morally responsible fieldwork resides with participating more fully in social relations' and endeavouring not to replicate the unequal power relations existing in social and political structures. Thus critical qualitative research can be designed to open up and disrupt these implicit, and explicit, power relations (Jowett and O'Toole 2006; Lafrance and Stoppard 2006). Respondents are located as the 'experts' (Oakley 1981; Stanley and Wise 1993) of their own lives and 'allowed' to name their priorities and represent their subjective agencies, a process which can help redress some of the power imbalances. Perhaps at the core of qualitative critical researchers' practice is this working with subjective agencies. The 'freedom' of individual voices and groups to experience, practise and engage with power is informed by 'the freedom to position oneself in discourse [being] contingent upon access to power' (Parker 1992: 795).

Within this more recent debate is the acknowledgement of the complexities and intersections of particular positions, which requires feminist researchers to work across and within these multiple constructions without losing sight of the political and power dimensions of oppressive structures (Westmarland 2001; Watts 2006). 'The contested and shifting identity of this category (i.e. women as a category, being highly fragmented and amidst the cultural, racial, social and political plurality) gives insight into the tensions inherent in the choice of "appropriate methodology" (Watts 2006: 386). Personal is indeed political, and as Stephenson (2006) and Watts (2006) discuss, the danger with deconstruction is that feminist researchers become complicit in the 'depoliticisation of the personal . . . feminist attempts to realize the political dimensions of the personal realm can produce unwanted effects – subjective experiences being continuously retied to neoliberal individualization' (Stephenson 2006: 79). The balance between deconstruction and contextualisation is a challenging one, and one which McAlister and Neill's (2007: 175) research rendered very clear when they found that the messages which young women were receiving and engaging with were ones of 'freedom, choice, power and individualism – yet within clear constraints – and the dominance of these messages means that larger structures of inequality and reproduction of gender messages are less obvious'.

The deconstruction of disability

While critical disability studies has developed theoretical weight to the growing politicisation of disabled people, the peripheral place of disabled people in mainstream life ensures that when they do enter the research context and academy then this can be met with resistance. As Shildrick and Price (1999) suggest, the disabled or devalued body is capable of generating deep ontological anxieties on the part of the non-disabled majority. Coming out as a disabled researcher presents possible dilemmas: 'to identify as blind is to invite and perhaps amplify the objectifying look of sighted researchers' (Mintz 2002: 163). Qualitative research is not immune to disabling discourses that circulate in wider society. This is particularly the case in psychology – which has contributed to dominant functionalist understandings of disability and impairment. As Henriques *et al.* (1984: 1) contend, psychology does not simply describe individuals, it regulates, classifies, administers and constitutes the subjectivities as well as the objects of psychological science. The objects of disability, then, are often understood in terms of pathology, deficit and lack. The associated subjectivities – what it must mean to be disabled – are understood in similarly deficient ways. Critical disability studies therefore intervenes at a point of conflict: challenging dominant epistemologies, ontologies and methodologies typically associated with the psychopathology of disability.

A classic example of such an intervention is provided by Bogdan and Taylor (1976, 1982). Their earlier paper, published in the *American Psychologist*, and the book written thereafter, reveal the embattled nature of two debates; the conceptualisation of disability and the merits of qualitative research. In their work they present the story of a man named Ed Murphy who had been given the label of mental retardation. Drawing on a number of in-depth interviews with Ed, the story, which is told in the first person, retraces his experiences of diagnosis and institutionalisation and its impact on his sense of self and the perspectives of family members. This powerful narrative served to demonstrate the subjective richness of a qualitative methodology and a very different view of disability afforded through an interpretivist epistemology to a psychological community that was still very much preoccupied with the arbitrary epistemology of positivism, the methodology of experimentation and quantitative analysis and a stance of functionalism in relation to disability. Retrospectively, we can read Ed's story as enacting a form of what Henriques *et al.* (1984: 2) describe as deconstruction: challenging and teasing apart 'taken-for-granted, common-sense' understandings of, specifically, mental retardation:

> The word 'retarded' is a word. What it does is put people into a class. I like mental handicap better than mental retarded. The other word sounds nicer . . . my day's gonna come through . . . I'm gonna tell them the truth. They know the truth. All this petty nonsense.
>
> (Ed Murphy, Bogdan and Taylor 1982: 77)

Following Henriques *et al.* (1982: 2), Bogdan and Taylor intervene in a process of prising apart the meanings and assumptions that are fused together in the ways that people use to understand themselves, to reveal these meanings and assumptions not as timeless and inconvertible facts but historically specific products.

Subjectivities

We now consider how subjectivity can be considered as the resource for qualitative research – with a specific focus on voice, ownership, participation and emancipation in research.

Doing feminist qualitative research

It is hopefully fairly clear by now that critical qualitative research works with and acknowledges the important role that positional subjectivities have in the 'doing' of research. The transdisciplinariness of subjectivities, ours and our respondents, is seen as a great source of richness and rigour. Indeed Stanley and Wise (1993) see this as a crucial aspect to the research process, allowing the knowledge that is produced from the researcher's position to be less distorted, more transparent and more thorough than when diverse subjectivities are not acknowledged or worked with. It is important, however, not to fall into a practice of fixing these subjectivities and/or categories into essentialised constructs. Notions of subjectivity are, therefore in a constant flux, being both unstable and often opaque (Stephenson 2006) and can be paradoxical, conflicted and in constant disharmony. Burns and Walker (2005), Watts (2006) and O'Leary (2004) consider this ongoing process as being one of reconstructing/deconstructing dualism, essentialism and individualism. For O'Leary (2004) in particular, the role of subjectivity in feminist qualitative research is fragmentary, revealing and enlightening for both the researcher and researched, while Salmon (2007) highlights the importance of reciprocity and mutuality when engaging with multiple subjectivities in research.

A key to feminist research is this ongoing acknowledgement and openness to the impact and influence of our own value-laden subjectivities, challenging the notion that we are separate from what we produce, how we research, how we interact, how we interpret and understand our research field:

> We can speak ourselves into different ways of being, but only within the parameters of the discursive resources, or sets of meaning available within a cultural context. . . . Individuals draw on discourses to account for themselves and their experiences while, at the same time discourses contain a range of subject positions which in turn facilitate and/or constrain certain experiences and practices.
>
> (Lafrance and Stoppard 2006: 310)

Within this debate is the challenge to dualistic notions of subjectivity and objectivity and the values that are attached to each – so instead of deriding, disavowing, or denying subjectivities it would be far more 'logical' (Ramazanaglu with Holland 2003) to work with them, acknowledge them, be open to them and recognise their impacts in order to produce/engage with rigorous ongoing research. More specifically O'Leary (2004: 44) sees the richness of working with our own and our respondents' subjectivities:

People will likely respond to you as a 'gendered' ['disabled', 'racial', 'heterosexual', etc.] individual and, without even realizing it, you will most likely respond as a 'gendered' self . . . the power of our sexuality is often underplayed and unseen. Yet, the rapport and trust you will build with respondents, the slant on stories you will hear, and the memories you will extract can be very dependent on gender.

Doing disability research

Subjectivity is viewed as a resource in qualitative research (Banister *et al.* 1997). Researchers and participants bring to the research encounter their subjectivities: their preoccupations, ambitions, perspectives, stories, reflections and implicit as well as explicit theories. Researchers and participants are the key research tools of qualitative research (Taylor and Bogdan 1984: 77). Critical disability studies approaches to qualitative research have raised some interesting questions about the power of the researcher and participant and the modes of research productions that operate. From this we can ask: whose subjectivities shape qualitative research? In reviewing critical disability studies research papers Goodley and Lawthom (2005) identify a number of key questions:

- *Inclusion* – to what extent does research include disabled people?
- *Accountability* – who are disability studies researchers accountable to?
- *Praxis* – does disability research make a positive difference in the lives of disabled people?
- *Ontology* – whose knowledge and experiences count?
- *Partisanship* – whose side is the disability researcher on?
- *Analytical levels* – does research investigate politics, culture, society, relationships or the individual?

Appropriating and adapting Goodley (2011: 24), Figure 3.2 is presented to capture different approaches to research. The left-hand side of Figure 3.2 captures an approach to research which tends to dominate most approaches to qualitative research from undergraduate to funded research projects. Here the subjectivity of the researcher is central: she develops the research ideas, the research questions, makes decisions about the methodology, method and analysis and takes the lead in the writing up of the findings. Langness and Levine (1986) exemplify this approach: an edited collection of texts which draw on qualitative data (including ethnography, interviews, documentary analysis) to develop the argument that intellectual disability is a creation of social and cultural practices.

The middle approach, represented in Figure 3.2, places more onus on the subjectivities of researcher and participants. Here qualitative research involves researcher and participants working together in collaboration through the various stages of identifying research questions, carrying out the qualitative work and sharing the analyses. Doherty *et al.*'s (1995) research captures this mode of production well: where researchers with and without the label of intellectual disabilities explore the use of qualitative methodologies. They conclude that researchers must seriously reconsider how they approach research; to move away from a reliance on researcher-led research (which benefits the researcher only) to an inclusive approach to research (which also promotes the expertise of disabled researchers with intellectual disabilities).

Knowledge	Shared knowledge	Action research
e.g. An academic analyses the constitution of normalcy (Langness and Levine 1986)	e.g. Researchers work with a self-advocacy group to develop inclusive research practices (Docherty *et al.* 2005)	e.g. Disabled people's organisations work with researchers to measure and eradicate disablism (Arthur and Zarb 1995)
Non-participatory	**Participatory**	**Emancipatory**
Researcher-led	Researcher invites participants into research	Co-researchers

Figure 3.2 Research as participatory and emancipatory

Disability studies research can be conceived as a continuum

The third approach taken by Arthur and Zarb (1995) reflects on the 'Measuring Disablement in Society' project which set out to address this problem by providing a systematic empirical analysis of the barriers to disabled people's participation in mainstream community life in 1990s Britain. This research included interviews with key people in relevant local authority departments and local disability organisations (Barnes 1995). The work brought together disabled researchers and disabled people's political organisations to assess qualitatively (and quantitatively) the extent to which people with impairment are disabled by mainstream life and to identify policies, practices and interventions which would reduce this disablement. This is an example of emancipatory disability studies research: where research not only makes sense of the world but proposes changes that eradicate conditions of marginalisation. Clearly, such an approach has much in common with critical theory and Marxist orientations (Giroux 2009) and, indeed, many early examples of critical disability studies research shared this approach (see Barnes and Mercer 1997).

Chapter summary

In this last section we will reflect on each other's approach to consider possible tensions and commonalities between feminisms and critical disability studies.

Following Goodley (2011), disability studies might be seen as *paradigm busting*: subverting the normative tendencies of academic disciplines, testing respected research encounters and challenging theoretical formations. With these conceptions in mind, how would critical disability studies read the feminist orientations outlined in this chapter and vice versa?

First, it is important to recognise tensions. As Reeve (2008: 188) notes, when disabled women express their desire for activities such as motherhood, being a housewife, cleaning the house – which are often denied to them – then this might jar with some feminist work that has historically aimed to support women's exit from domestic feminised settings. Feminism and disability will, at times, disconnect.

Second, we acknowledge that the hugely different styles in writing, the language we use, the concepts we draw on to make sense of our approaches are reflective of our positionalities and the resources we have available to us:

> The researcher's personality, world view, ethnic and social background, perceptions derived from the researcher's professional discipline, the qualitative paradigm, the theoretical base of the research, the type of the research and its goals, the research methodology, and the researcher's own perception of the place and role of the subject/participant/collaborator/coresearcher.
>
> (Karniel-Miller *et al.* 2009: 280)

These are all interwoven within our engagements with this project, with one another and as part of an ongoing process of the writing up and exchange of ideas.

Third, these differences in our approaches provide a rich source for ongoing reflection and reflexivity. The transformative nature of engaging with feminist/critical disability qualitative research (Stephenson 2006) is indicative of the responsive and ongoing debates around critical theory and qualitative research. It is perhaps only through acknowledging diverse positions that we begin to fully recognise the wide reach of qualitative research in and outside of psychology.

References

Arthur, S. and Zarb, G. (1995) *Measuring Disablement in Society: Working Paper 3. Disabled People and the Citizen's Charter*. Accessed May 1 2009. http://www.leeds.ac.uk/disability-studies/archiveuk/Zarb/meas%20work%20paper%203.pdf.

Banister, P., Burman, E., Parker, I., Taylor, M. and Tindall, C. (1997) *Qualitative Methods in Psychology: A Research Guide*. Maidenhead: Open University Press.

Barnes, C. (1995) 'Measuring disablement in society: hopes and reservations'. Accessed May 1, 2009. http://www.leeds.ac.uk/disabilitystudies/archiveuk/Barnes/measuring%20dis.pdf.

Barnes, C. (1998) 'The social model of disability: a sociological phenomenon ignored by sociologists', in T. Shakespeare (ed.) *The Disability Reader: Social Science Perspectives*. London: Continuum.

Barnes, C. and Mercer, G. (eds) (1997) *Doing Disability Research*. Leeds: Disability Press.

Bogdan, R. and Taylor, S. (1976) 'The judged not the judges: an insider's view of mental retardation'. *American Psychologist*, **31**, 47–52.

Bogdan, R. and Taylor, S. (1982) *Inside Out: The Social Meaning of Mental Retardation*. Toronto: University of Toronto Press.

Bordo, S. (1990) 'Reading the slender body', in M. Jacobus, E. F. Keller and S. Shuttleworth (eds) *Body/Politics: Women and the Discourses of Science*. New York: Routledge.

Burns, D. and Walker, M. (2005) 'Feminist methodologies', in B. Somekh and C. Lewin (eds) *Research Methods in the Social Sciences.* London: Sage.

Burrell, G. and Morgan, G. (1979) *Sociological Paradigms and Organisational Analysis: Elements of the Sociology of Corporate Life.* London: Heinemann.

Clough, P. and Nutbrown, C. (2002) *A Student's Guide to Methodology.* London: Sage.

Davis, L. J. (1995) *Enforcing Normalcy: Disability, Deafness, and the Body.* New York: Verso.

de Laine, M. (2000) *Fieldwork, Participation and Practice: Ethics and Dilemmas in Qualitative Research.* London: Sage.

Disabled People's International (1982) *Proceedings of the First World Congress.* Singapore: Disabled People's International.

Docherty, D., Hughes, R., Phillips, P., Corbett, D., Regan, B., Barber, A., Adams, P., Boxall, K., Kaplan, I. and Izzidien, S. (2005) 'This is what we think', in D. Goodley and G. Van Hove (eds) *Another Disability Reader? Including People with Learning Difficulties.* Antwerp: Garant.

Fay, B. (1987) *Critical Social Science: Liberation and its Limits.* Ithaca, NY: Cornell University Press.

Ferguson, P. M., Ferguson, D. L. and Taylor, S. J. (ed.) (1992) *Interpreting Disability: A Qualitative Reader.* New York: Teachers College Press.

Finkelstein, V. (1981) 'Disability and the helper/helped relationship: An historical view', in A. Brechin, P. Liddiard and J. Swain (eds) *Handicap in a Social World.* London: Hodder and Stoughton.

Garland Thomson, R. (2005) 'Feminist disability studies'. *Signs: Journal of Women in Culture and Society*, **30**(2), 1557–87.

Geldard, K. and Geldard, D. (2003) *Counselling Skills in Everyday Life.* Basingstoke: Palgrave Macmillan.

Ghai, A. (2002) 'Disabled women: an excluded agenda for Indian feminism'. *Hypatia: A Journal of Feminist Philosophy*, **17**(3), 49–66.

Giroux, H. (2009) 'Critical theory and educational practice', in A. Darder, M. P. Baltodano and R. D. Torres (eds) *The Critical Pedagogy Reader*, 2nd edn. New York: Routledge.

Goodley, D. (2011) *Disability Studies: An Interdisciplinary Introduction.* London: Sage.

Goodley, D. and Lawthom, R. (2005) 'Disability studies and psychology: new allies', in D. Goodley and R. Lawthom (eds) *Psychology and Disability: Critical Introductions and Reflections.* London: Palgrave.

Gray, D. (2004) *Doing Research in the Real World.* London: Sage.

Grech, S. (2008) 'Living with disability in rural Guatemala: exploring connections and impacts on poverty'. *International Journal of Disability, Community and Rehabilitation*, **7**(2), online.

Henriques, J., Hollway, W., Urwin, C., Venn, C. and Walkerdine, V. (1989) *Changing the Subject: Psychology, Social Regulation and Subjectivity.* London: Methuen.

Jarviluoma, H., Moisala, P. and Vilkko, A. (2003) *Gender and Qualitative Methods.* London: Sage.

Joseph, S. (2010) *Theories of Counselling and Psychotherapy.* Basingstoke: Palgrave Macmillan.

Jowett, M. and O'Toole, G. (2006) 'Focusing researchers' minds: contrasting experiences of using focus groups in feminist qualitative research'. *Qualitative Research*, **6**(4), 453–72.

Jung, K. E. (2002) 'Chronic illness and educational equity: the politics of visibility'. *NWSA Journal*, **14**(3), 178–200.

Karniel-Miller, O., Strier, R. and Pessach, L. (2009) 'Power relations in qualitative research'. *Qualitative Health Research*, **19**(2), 279–89.

Kerr, A., Cunningham-Burley, S. and Amos, A. (1998) 'Drawing the line: an analysis of people's discussions about the new genetics'. *Public Understanding of Science*, **7**(2), 113–33. Cited in M. Jowett and G. O'Toole (2006) 'Focusing researchers' minds: contrasting experiences of using focus groups in feminist qualitative research'. *Qualitative Research*, **6**(4), 453–72.

Kitzinger, C. (1992) 'The individuated self concept: a critical analysis of social contructionist writing on individualism', in G. M. Breakwell (ed.) *Social Psychology of Identity and the Self Concept*. Guildford: Surrey University Press.

Kitzinger, C. (2004) 'Feminist approaches', in C. Seale, G. Gobo, J. F. Gubrium and D. Silverman (eds) *Qualitative Research Practice*. London: Sage.

Kristiansen, K., Vehmas, S. and Shakespeare, T. (eds) (2008) *Arguing about Disability: Philosophical Perspectives*. London and New York: Routledge.

Lafrance, M. N. and Stoppard, J. M. (2006) 'Constructing a non-depressed self: women's accounts of recovery from depression'. *Feminism and Psychology*, **16**(3), 307–25.

Langness, L. L. and Levine, H. G. (eds) (1986) *Culture and Retardation*. Amsterdam: Kluwer.

Letherby, G. (2003) *Feminist Research in Theory and Practice*. Maidenhead: Open University Press.

Linton, S. (1998) 'Disability studies/not disability studies'. *Disability and Society*, **13**(4), 525–39.

Marks, D. (1999) *Disability: Controversial Debates and Psychosocial Perspectives*. London: Routledge.

May, T. (2003) *Social Research: Issues, Methods and Process*. Maidenhead: Open University Press.

McAlister, S. and Neill, G. (2007) 'Young women's positive and negative perceptions of self in Northern Ireland'. *Child Care in Practice*, **13**(3), 167–84.

McLaughlin, J., Goodley, D., Clavering, E. and Fisher, P. (2008) *Families Raising Disabled Children: Enabling Care and Social Justice*. London: Palgrave.

Meekosha, H. (2008) 'Contextualizing disability: developing southern theory'. Keynote presentation, Disability Studies Association 4th conference, Lancaster, 2–4 September.

Mintz, S. B. (2002) 'Invisible disability: Georgina Kleege's sight unseen'. *Feminist Disability Studies*. *NWSA Journal*, **14**(3), 155–77.

Moulding, N. (2006) 'Disciplining the feminine: the reproduction of gender contradictions in the mental health care of women with eating disorders'. *Social Science and Medicine*, **62**, 793–804.

Neilson, J. M. (ed.) (1990) *Feminist Research Methods: Exemplary Readings in the Social Sciences*. London: Westview Press.

Oakley, A. (1974) *The Sociology of Housework.* London: Martin Robertson.

Oakley, A. (1981) 'Interviewing women: a contradiction in terms', in H. Roberts (ed.) *Doing Feminist Research.* London: Routledge and Kegan Paul.

O'Leary, Z. (2004) *Essential Guide to Doing Research.* London: Sage.

Parker, I. (1992) *Discourse Dynamics: Critical Analysis for Social and Individual Psychology.* London: Routledge.

Peters, S., Wolbers, K. and Dimling, L. (2008) 'Reframing global education from a disability rights movement perspective', in S. Gabel and S. Danforth (eds) *Disability and the International Politics of Education.* New York: Peter Lang.

Qin, D. (2004) 'Toward a critical feminist perspective of culture and self', *Feminism and Psychology,* **14**(2), 297–312.

Quinlan, K., Bowleg, L. and Faye Ritz S. (2008) 'Virtually invisible women: Women with disabilities in mainstream psychological theory and research'. *Review of Disability Studies,* **4**, 4–17.

Ramazanoglu, C. (1992) 'On feminist methodology: male reason versus female empowerment'. *Sociology,* **26**(2), 207–12.

Ramazanoglu, C. with Holland, J. (2003) *Feminist Methodology.* London: Sage.

Reeve, D. (2008) 'Negotiating disability in everyday life: the experience of psycho-emotional disablism'. Unpublished PhD thesis, Lancaster.

Rist, R. C. (1977) 'On the relations among educational research paradigms: from disdain to détente'. *Anthropology and Education,* **8**(2), 42–9.

Salmon, A. (2007) 'Walking the talk: how participatory interview methods can democratize research'. *Qualitative Health Research,* **17**(7), 982–93.

Sherry, M. (2006) *If I Only Had a Brain: Deconstructing Brain Injury.* London: Routledge.

Sherry, M. (2007) '(Post) colonising disability'. *Wagadu, Journal of Transnational Women's and Gender Studies,* **4**, 10–22.

Shildrick, M. and Price, J. (1999) 'Openings on the body: a critical introduction', in J. Price and M. Shildrick (eds) *Feminist Theory and the Body.* Edinburgh: Edinburgh University Press.

Skeggs, B. (ed.) (1997) *Feminist Cultural Theory.* Manchester: Manchester University Press.

Stanley, L. and Wise, L. (1993) *Breaking Out Again: Feminist Ontology and Epistemology.* London: Routledge.

Stephenson, N. (2006) 'Breaking alignments between "the personal" and "the individual": what can psychology do for feminist politics?' *Feminism and Psychology,* **16**(1), 79–85.

Taylor, S. J. and Bogdan, R. (1984) *Introduction to Qualitative Research Methods: The Search for Meanings,* 2nd edn. New York: Wiley.

Thomas, C. (2007) *Sociologies of Disability, 'Impairment', and Chronic Illness: Ideas in Disability Studies and Medical Sociology.* London: Palgrave.

Tolan, J. (2003) *Skills in Person-Centred Counselling and Psychotherapy.* London: Sage.

Travers, M. (2001) *Qualitative Research Through Case Studies*. London: Sage.

United Nations Department of Public Information (2008) *Backgrounder: Disability Treaty Closes a Gap in Protecting Human Rights*. Accessed March 3, 2009. http://www.un.org/disabilities/default.asp?id=476.

Ussher, J. (1991) *Women's Madness: Misogyny or Mental Illness?* Harlow: Prentice Hall.

Ussher, J. (2010) 'Are we medicalizing women's misery? A critical review of women's higher rates of reported depression'. *Feminism and Psychology*, **20**(9), 9–35.

Walker, R. (1981) 'On the uses of fiction in educational research', in D. Smetherham (ed.) *Practising Evaluation*. Driffield: Nafferton.

Watts, J. (2006) '"The outsider within": dilemma of qualitative feminist research within a culture of resistance'. *Qualitative Research*, **6**(3), 385–402.

Wendell, S. (1996) *The Rejected Body: Feminist Philosophical Reflections on Disability*. New York: Routledge.

Westmarland, N. (2001) 'The quantitative/qualitative debate and feminist research: a subjective view of objectivity'. *Forum: Qualitative Social Research*, **2**(1), Art 13. http://nbn-resolving.de/urn:nbn:de:0114-fqs0101135.

Wilkinson, S. (1998) 'Focus groups in feminist research: power, interaction, and the co-construction of meaning'. *Women's Studies International Forum*, **21**(1), 111–26.

Willig, C. (1999) 'Beyond appearances: a critical realist approach to social constructionist work', in D. J. Nightingale and J. Cromby (eds) *Social Constructionist Psychology: A Critical Analysis of Theory and Practice*. Buckingham: Open University Press.

Willig, C. (2008) *Introducing Qualitative Research in Psychology*. Maidenhead: Open University Press.

Wright Mills, C. (1970) *The Sociological Imagination*. Oxford: Oxford University Press.

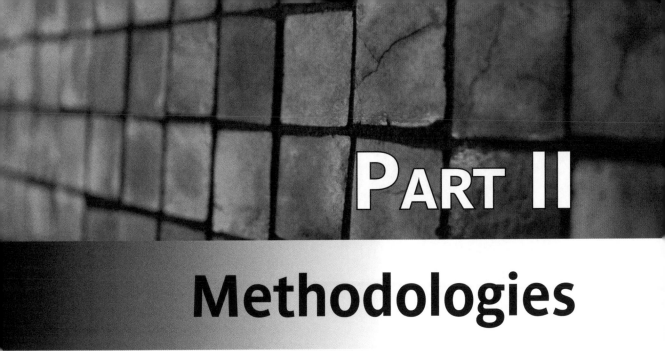

PART II

Methodologies

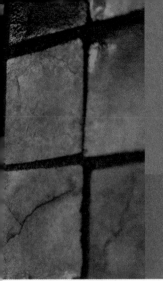

Chapter 4

Observation

Peter Banister

Introduction

In this chapter, we turn to what is probably the most basic method in the whole of psychology, one which is involved throughout the discipline. Observation is a process we are all engaged in, and in the eyes of the public, psychologists are notorious for spending their time watching (not to mention analysing) other people. Even when we are not working as psychologists, we are always forming hypotheses, making inferences and trying to impose meaning on our social world, based on our observations.

All psychological research involves at least some element of observation. This may be something as simple as reading a dial on a machine, or as complex as observing group interactions. Many of the major developments within psychology have come from the initial observation of a serendipitous event, where something is found whilst looking for something else. Examples here include Pavlov, Skinner and superstitious behaviour, Piaget's observations of the systematic failure of children on intelligence tests (which led to his theories on cognitive development) and Freud's insights, which developed from observations of systematic links between earlier experiences and current problems in his patients. Sometimes, observations of a single event have sparked off a whole series of related studies, and have opened up new areas of psychological research. An example here is the Latané and Darley (1970) research on 'bystander apathy', which was initially inspired by the tragic death of Kitty Genovese in New York.

In any psychological study, quantitative or qualitative, the researcher should always be alert to unexpected as well as expected reactions of participants to the situation; often such reactions may provide vital pointers to future research. Qualitative methods have the advantage of focusing in on real-life problems, of reflecting the world as it actually is, and are more likely to come up with unexpected results. This chapter will include a small-scale observational study based on an everyday occurrence which nonetheless produces interesting findings. Ethnography will be dealt with separately in Chapter 5.

Background

The term 'observation' derives from Latin, meaning to watch, to attend to. Dictionary definitions stress the accurate watching and noting of phenomena as they occur in nature (note 'in nature', as opposed to an experiment, which concentrates on the deliberate manipulation of conditions, often in artificial circumstances). The essence of observation in the context of this book is that it is concerned with naturally occurring behaviour, which can take place in any setting. Variables can nonetheless be examined, for instance, by looking at different settings or by selecting people to observe who have different demographic characteristics. A more specific definition to use in this context (although not without problems of its own) is that of Marshall and Rossman (1989: 79), who define observation as 'a systematic description of events, behaviors and artifacts in the social setting under study'. In common with other qualitative methods there is a commitment to try to understand the world better, usually from the standpoint of individual participants. Thus we are concerned with such aims as getting to understand 'real' people in their everyday situations, to learn about the world from different perspectives, to experience what others experience, to unravel what is taken for granted, to find out about implicit social rules, etc. It must be noted, however, that our 'findings' can be divorced from the experiential knowledge of those being observed. Indeed, at times one may be looking at aspects of behaviour (e.g. non-verbal) of which the person being observed is not consciously aware. In this context, it must also be stressed that observation, unlike many other qualitative methods, does tend to be from an outsider rather than an insider perspective. In addition, the method can be used as a very useful precursor to later studies, opening up possibilities and making suggestions for future research.

It must be pointed out that observational methods are not necessarily within the Reason and Rowan (1981) conceptualisation of 'new paradigm' research, their ethos of collaboration and participation being not always applicable to this approach. The method can be very much 'objectivist' in its standpoint, with the researcher sometimes using the material gained very much for their own ends. There are obvious ethical problems here, which can be compounded by the tendency of psychologists not to feed back and share findings with those who have been observed. Some have called the method a potential 'act of betrayal', where what is private is made public, and those observed may have to take the consequences of what has been written about them. There are ethical guidelines that must be adhered to, and this area is so important that it is considered in detail in Chapter 13.

As has been suggested above, the typical observation is a field one, where one attempts to record in a relatively systematic fashion some aspect of the behaviour of people in their ordinary environment, in as unobtrusive a fashion as is possible. It is thus basically a 'watching' operation, but does embrace a whole variety of different approaches and techniques. There are very different methods in approaching observation, and it is beyond the scope of this chapter to consider all the possible permutations. Nonetheless, it is important for the reader to be aware of the range here. Among different approaches are the following:

1 *Structuring of the observation*, which can range from highly structured, detailed observation to very diffuse unstructured description.
2 *Focus in observation*, ranging from a very narrow concentration on specific aspects (such as a single non-verbal cue) to a broad focus.

3 *Knowledge of those being observed about the process*, which can vary from being known to all (for instance, in the observation of a teacher's classroom technique) to being known by none (where one is, for instance, secretly observing people interacting in a public social setting).

4 *Explanations given to those being observed for the observation.* These can vary from full explanations to no explanations, and may even include highly ethically dubious false explanations, where participants are told that the observer is watching something different from that which is really of interest.

5 *The time scale of what is being observed*, varying from one-off observations to extended observations over time.

6 *The methods used*, which can vary from simple note taking to the use of devices such as audio and video taperecorders, from checklists to stopwatches.

7 *Feedback given to those observed*, which can range from a full sharing of observations and interpretations to no further contact at all with the participants.

These approaches can obviously be permutated in a variety of ways, and it must be noted that there are even set techniques which can be used. These tend to be on the more quantitative side of the discipline, but mention of them may be useful here. There are a number of examples.

Bales (1950) developed techniques for analysing group interactions, where specific instances of verbal behaviour are recorded in terms of whether the contribution is positive or negative, whether it is asking for or giving suggestions, etc., with the aim of attempting to look at group participants in terms of labelling them as 'task' or 'socio-emotional' specialists.

Minuchin (1974) divided family dynamics in terms of up/down, near/far and in/out relationships, as a first step towards family therapy. Here, the interaction and interdependence of participants are concentrated on, looking at characteristic patterns and strategies adopted by participants to cope with others in the family.

Webb *et al.* (1981) advocated the development of 'unobtrusive measures', where one attempts to establish findings on the basis of observing evidence left behind by people. Their research includes the examination of carpet wear and 'nose-prints' on glass protecting screens as indicators of the relative popularity of art at exhibitions. They also cite discarded rubbish studies, where the contents of people's rubbish bins are looked at in terms of such variables as their consumption of alcohol.

Examples abound in the literature of interesting and important studies which have been based on observational methodology. Three are given here.

First, Albert and Kessler (1978) examined greeting rituals on telephones, including the methods used to end personal telephone conversations. They found that in general there was a four-part ritual, including a summary of the call, a justification for terminating the call, some positive comment and some indication that the relationship would continue.

Second, Argyle (e.g. 1987) has published myriad studies on non-verbal behaviour, including such important areas as postural moulding and eye gaze in the regulation of social encounters. He suggests that postural moulding (i.e. the copying of body posture) often indicated that the dyad concerned were getting on well with each other, while eye gaze (and the breaking of eye contact) were important in synchronising conversations, signalling to the other when you wished him or her to take over, for example.

LIVERPOOL JOHN MOORES UNIVERSITY
LEARNING SERVICES

Third, Cary (1978) looked at the procedures of pedestrians in the public use of pavements, finding (in this study using students on a university campus) little support for Goffman's (1963) notion of 'civil inattention', where two pedestrians are meant to look at each other until they are about 2.5 metres apart, and then to look away when actually passing. Such social rules might well change with different populations.

How to carry out a qualitative observation

The method has a lot of potential, and could be used in many settings. As has been highlighted above, there are many different ways of carrying out observational qualitative research. This section will start by talking about general considerations, before going on to take the reader through a particular example. The assumption underlying this chapter is that the reader is interested in carrying out conventional, non-intrusive, non-participating qualitative observation.

Obviously, specifics will vary, but in general there are three crucial questions that need to be considered initially. First, 'why' is the research being carried out; what is the research question that is being considered? This can be formally stated in terms of a hypothesis (e.g. that more active play will be observed in male children than in female children), or may more usually be formulated in terms of a statement of intent (e.g. 'the activity play of children will be observed'). Often, this may initially arise from personal interest or concern, informal observation, the interests of others, other research, experience, etc., which leads to a literature search. Ideally, it should be rooted in the relevant literature; otherwise, the absence of relevant literature (and possible reasons for such an absence) should be discussed.

Second, 'who' is the research to be carried out on, or (better) who is the research about? This includes not only the actual sample of people to be used (e.g. what age children to use, how many to observe), but also where the study will take place (e.g. in a nursery, in their homes), over what period of time, etc. Decisions will be needed as to ethical and other concerns, such as how much ought to be revealed to those being observed or how to disengage oneself from the field.

Third, 'what' is to be recorded? How, for instance, is 'active play' to be defined? Are time samples to be taken (e.g. just the first ten minutes will be observed), is only play alone to be recorded, what environmental and other constraints will be needed to be taken into account? What recording methods are going to be utilised? Will a single child be concentrated on or will single instances be taken from different children?

Other general points to keep in mind include the following. Pilot studies are strongly advisable, to discover and smooth out problems and to refine techniques. Here, you might start by informally observing the area of interest, and then go on to carry out a preliminary observation using the methods which you are intending to employ subsequently, checking to see if the chosen method is feasible, that it is producing useful material, etc. It may not be possible to videotape in a particular nursery, for instance, because the cameras cannot cover all the potential play area and behaviour may arise that is difficult to record, or it may be found that too much is lost by only using pencil and paper recording methods.

Observational research is often best done with at least one other observer, and the comparison of independent observations may help to indicate if there are any reliability problems in terms of recording. It is also useful to discuss findings with another person, which may help to avoid idiosyncratic recordings and interpretations.

Notes need to be taken at the time, and subsequently written up systematically and quickly. They are usually useful in addition to any more formal recording (such as a videotape, which might miss out crucial material). Such notes should include reflections, personal feelings, hunches, guesses and speculations as well as the observations themselves and anything else observed (and these different aspects should be clearly differentiated). Descriptions should be reasonably full, allowing the writer to remember the observation from the account later, and the reader should be able to visualise it reasonably accurately. It is often useful to take two copies of such notes, to allow one to be cut up, to simplify any subsequent analysis. Writing up is likely to take several drafts.

Ethical considerations are always crucial in research, and must be carefully considered. Observations in natural settings are often made without participants being aware of the process, and they are usually unable to say that they do not wish to take part in the research. Individuals should not be identifiable from the research report and should not be harmed by the publishing of the data. Research generally should not be carried out if the researcher has reason to believe that participants would refuse if given the opportunity to do so.

When it comes to writing up observational research reports, there are no standard ways in which this should be done. Chapter 13, on research report writing, makes general comments that are useful here. The example that follows is based on an attempt to provide a systematic narrative account of a particular observation carried out in a chosen social setting to answer a specific research question. An important point to bear in mind is the criterion of replicability: ideally, sufficient detail should be provided to allow the reader to follow precisely what has been done, which should be in sufficient detail to allow the study to be repeated from what is provided. Often, we take many things for granted, and we are not aware that we are doing so. One way to aid thinking here is to make notes under the following headings:

1 *Describe the context*, including the physical setting. Do remember that aspects such as the date, the time, the weather or the lighting may be of crucial importance, and noticing these things will certainly aid replicability.

2 *Describe the participants*. Who they are needs to be noted, including such potentially important variables as age, gender, ethnicity, clothing and physical description. Note that the boundary between description and interpretation is often a fuzzy one: how do we 'know' the ages of others just by looking at them, and how accurate can we be?

3 *Describe who the observer is*, as this is likely to affect what is seen, what is recorded and subsequent interpretations. If the observer has any prior links with those observed (and thus insider knowledge), this should also be made clear.

4 *Describe the actions* of the participants, including both verbal and non-verbal behaviours (where this is possible). Some coding may be needed for some of the variables (e.g. body posture) to aid recording. The sequence of actions over time is likely to be important and needs to be carefully noted.

5 *Interpret the situation*, attempting to give an indication of its meaning to the participants and to the observer, what their experiences are likely to be, what their background might be, etc. In this, the evidential basis for the interpretations must be made as clear as possible; these could be from direct observations, from the observer's own experience or from the observer's projection of their own expectations or habits. Often, this is very difficult to do, as we may

not be consciously aware of how social reality is constructed until our social expectations are violated in some way or other. Metaphors are sometimes useful here, to aid the explanation that is being put forward; for example, 'waves of people' may convey a lot more than a simple record of the number of people and how they were moving.

6 *Consider alternative interpretations of the situation*, again giving reasons for the conclusions arrived at. If one looked at the situation from another perspective, might this affect the conclusions reached? Would a child view the situation in the same way, or somebody from the Amazon jungle, or a Freudian, or a behaviourist? It does not matter how far-fetched these examples may seem. It is most important to recognise that many alternative interpretations may be possible in any given observation.

7 *Explore your feelings in being an observer* (reflexive analysis is always important in qualitative research), including your experience of the observation. Again, ethical considerations are useful here, especially in highlighting the ways in which we may affect what we study, with consequences that are often beyond our control.

A particular example will now be given, and worked through. Let us say that we are interested in observing people's queuing behaviour.

Why

We are interested in following up work done by Mann (1977) on queuing behaviour. He found in field experiment-based studies in Jerusalem that queues only formed when there were six or more people waiting for the same bus. We are particularly concerned to see not only whether this finding holds good for the UK, but also what other variables may affect queuing in a 'real-life' setting. Mann's use of a field experiment can be criticised, for instance, for producing the results that he claimed to have found: what he might have discovered is solely what people in Jerusalem do when presented with a queue of strangers, and may bear no resemblance to their normal queuing behaviour, which could possibly be a lot more anarchic. A real-life observational study may help to uncover all sorts of other behaviours and variables which need to be taken into consideration when we look at queuing in the real world. Work of this nature might provide interesting cross-national findings, indicating differences in social rules that might be of interest to people travelling to other countries. In addition, work of this nature might help in the design of street furniture, and might perhaps have implications for the design of social skills courses for, *inter alia*, people re-entering the community after having been institutionalised for some length of time.

Who

In order to compare our findings with those of Mann (1977), we decided to concentrate on queuing at bus stops. After some pilot work, we decided to concentrate on a particular bus stop in Manchester, where there is limited shelter (as the restricted space affects how people stand to wait), and where there is plenty of pavement space (so people are free to queue or not). Our earlier work found that rain affects queuing (people often shelter nearby, and then rush for the bus when it arrives), so we decided to carry out the study at a dry time, in the early afternoon, when the buses are reasonably well used. This example merely reports the results for the observation of one particular queue over the five minutes immediately before a bus is scheduled to come (the stop is the start of the route, so we know that it is likely to be on time). All the people who turn up to catch the particular targeted bus will be recorded. We decided that ethical concerns are minimal, as we are merely watching naturally occurring behaviour from a window overlooking the bus stop, where our presence will not affect what is being watched. We felt that it was not necessary to tell our participants about our study; indeed, in this case, it may well be virtually impossible to find them again.

What

We decided to attempt to take detailed paper and pencil-based notes, as it was felt that a video-camera might be observed. Moreover, because of the distance involved, it would have to be selective or produce images that would be too small to provide useful material. Pilot studies indicated that it is impossible to hear conversations, so we concentrated on the non-verbal behaviour of all the participants. This was a relatively unstructured observation, where we attempted to record all that occurred during the five-minute period. Observation was undertaken alone, as no other observer was currently available. What follows is the detailed written account produced imme-diately after the observation period, following the format outlined above.

The observation

Description of the context

The observation was carried out from 14.35 to 14.40 on Friday 8 October 2010 in Oldham Street, Manchester; the weather was dry, calm and overcast. Oldham Street is a one-way street, the traffic coming in 'waves', being governed by traffic lights throughout the street. The 184 bus stop for Uppermill was observed from the first floor window of a building directly opposite the bus stop (but about seven metres away) by the observer.

Description of the participants

In all, 19 people were observed during the observation; to avoid needless replication, their details are provided in the next section.

Description of the observer

The observer was a man in his sixties from the Manchester Metropolitan University psychology staff who regularly uses the buses.

Description of the actions of the participants

At the start of the observation period, nobody was standing at the bus stop. After one minute, two young men wearing tracksuits came up, and stood right by the stop, on the south side of it; they stood looking around and talking, particularly up Oldham Street, where the bus comes from.

They were followed after another minute by two well-dressed women in their fifties carrying shopping bags, which they put down on the pavement two metres from the first person, to the north side; they turned to face each other, and one started to speak, while the other nodded her head. The men glanced at them, but ignored them. At three minutes, two more smartly attired women in their early twenties arrived, each carrying a black briefcase. They stood one metre away from the last two, well back from the pavement, and started talking to each other, both facing up Oldham Street. They were followed in rapid succession by a single man in his fifties wearing a black overcoat and carrying a briefcase, five women in their teens in casual clothes, and two more men in their twenties wearing city suits. Each stood in a vague line from each other, at variable distances from each other, those furthest from the bus stop standing closer to the next person. The bus, which was driven by a male bus driver, came down the street, bags were picked up and the queue filled up the gaps, becoming more orderly. The bus stopped marginally short of the head of the queue, and the bus doors folded inwards. The two older women got on it first, followed by the two younger women. The young men who were first to arrive then boarded, followed by the remainder of the queue. Order was not entirely maintained as five further younger women in casual clothes rushed up from elsewhere and pushed in before the two men who were at the end of the queue.

Interpretation of the situation

This was an everyday situation for the participants, who were a varying batch of people. It might be assumed, bearing in mind variables such as the time, the age and gender of those observed, their clothing and the location of the observation, that some were shoppers, some city office workers, some shop assistants, some unemployed. All seemed familiar with catching buses, and appeared to be holding some implicit rules about queuing, which broke down slightly in this context. It must be noted though that none of the participants seemed to be particularly upset at what might have been construed as queue jumping in this study. In terms of the original interests, this research indicates that queuing behaviour in the UK seems to occur (in marked contrast to Mann's research), but it also suggests that there is a need to investigate other variables, especially as the queue order was not the same as the bus boarding order. It could be that there are social rules as to who is given preference in such settings (what is the impact of age and gender, for instance?), or differing expectations by the participants as to the social expectations and rule following of others (should those carrying heavy bags or using season tickets be given precedence, for instance?). Further investigation is obviously needed as to whether these results are replicated in other similar observations.

Alternative interpretation of the situation

It could be suggested that the bus driver deliberately stopped the bus before the stop, as he wanted to give preference to the two older women who were laden down with shopping bags, or he thought that the young men at the head of the queue were just hanging around, or wanted to catch a different bus. It may be that he resents picking up young males in tracksuits, as they have caused problems on his bus in the past. It could be that some of the potential passengers were smoking when the bus came up, and lost their place in the queue while they extinguished their cigarettes. The younger females who rushed up at the last moment could have been psychology students who were carrying out a field experiment on the effects of queue jumping. There may also be relationships between other variables, such as gender, age and preferred interpersonal distance, which could account for the results found. Moreover, there could be possible different types of personality or cultural codes (Manchester is a multicultural city) that are related to queuing behaviour.

Feelings as an observer

The presence of the observer seemed to have had no effect on the behaviour of the participants, and the observation felt ethically comfortable, as it was watching people in their everyday situations. This method produces a rich wealth of data, and sometimes unexpected results. What is clear is that the observation above is only a selection of non-verbal behaviours, it being impossible physically to record all the observable actions of some 19 people over even a five-minute period. No record was kept of smoking behaviour, which (as has been suggested in the 'alternative interpretations' section) could have been crucial. Over even a brief period of time the relative positions and body postures of participants will change with respect to each other: participants will need to monitor whether the bus is coming on a fairly continuous basis, as well as converse with and/or watch others. As the number of people increases, the detailed amount recorded decreases; a video recording might be of assistance here, but is likely to pose further problems. Interestingly, the sample of people seen in this study was somewhat atypical in terms of demographic characteristics of Manchester bus users, with more males and less older people than would normally be expected; this could be related to the particular time of day and/or route chosen for observation. As well as the questions raised above, it might be interesting to speculate as to whether these findings would be replicated elsewhere in the country (or in Manchester). The fact that there was obviously sufficient room on the bus for everyone queuing may have meant less concern at queue jumping. What is also worthy of note is that the observation provides detailed estimates of gender, age and clothing, but says nothing about ethnicity. This could be a reflection of biases of the observer, which could be conscious or unconscious.

There is often a taken-for-granted element that is difficult to avoid. Often, we are so rooted in our own culture, time and background that we do not realise how myopic we are. What led, for instance, to the interpretation of 'unemployed' made above? Whether somebody from another culture would notice, record and emphasise the same features is an interesting point; even another viewer from the same culture may well have recorded the scene differently. Age estimates are particularly problematic, but in certain circumstances gender assumptions may also be incorrect. At best, this is an interesting observation, but one that needs to be looked at in the context of considerable further research.

Assessment

Advantages of observation as a method

Although this very short observation only provides the briefest description of five minutes of queuing behaviour, it has produced much material that can be related to previously published literature in the area. It has provided some unexpected results, it is open-ended and it has suggested many avenues for further research. A picture is provided of a 'real-life' naturalistic setting (with no problems of ecological validity), and many interesting questions are raised. The research results are generally accessible. Though there may be problems with the recording of the observation and its interpretation, the researcher intrudes very little into the situation, and his presence is not obviously reactive. It is hoped that sufficient details are provided to allow readers to make their own judgements about the findings, and how they can be interpreted. The method can tell us not only what is going on, but also who is involved, when and where things happen. It can illuminate processes and it can examine causality, suggesting why things happen as they do in particular settings. It can give access to phenomena that are often obscured (e.g. non-verbal cues) or not amenable to experimentation (it would be difficult to replicate the findings of the observation above in a laboratory-based study). Situations can be examined that cannot be replicated in a laboratory, such as weddings, political meetings, prisons, behaviour in bars, and football crowds. The chronology of events can be taken into account, and continuities over time can be looked at. The use of technological equipment such as video recorders (though not without their problems, an issue we will take up below) allows permanent records to be made, which can be independently analysed and re-analysed in detail, ensuring some reliability of interpretation. Observation can, of course, be part of a more mixed method approach, where a variety of different techniques is used, focusing in on a common research question.

Disadvantages of observation as a method

There may be external validity problems. At times the results can end up being very subjective, depending more on who the researcher is (and their biases) than the situation being observed. Researchers may well notice different aspects of the situation. In the example above, a strong anti-smoker may have noticed smoking behaviour to a greater extent, while somebody who was more fashion conscious might form different opinions about the likely background of the participants based on a keener observation of the clothes worn. A researcher can produce results that are over-impressionistic, careless or just idiosyncratic. The fact that somebody is known to be interested in a particular phenomenon may well affect people's behaviour, and this is likely to be different when the observer is present. There have been cases in educational research where a school has carried on utilising a method that was being researched when in the ordinary course of events (when it was not being observed) it would have been abandoned.

As well as selectivity in terms of the observation, inferences within interpretations are obviously subject to research bias. Although the example in this chapter avoided reactivity of the observer on the situation, there is always the possibility that the observer may have been influenced in some way by the situation. Given that the social world is socially created (as Berger and Luckmann 1967 suggest), it is often very difficult to be able to stand back from a process that one is already part of. Moreover, perceived reality may be structured through the very framework being utilised.

The 'why' may be poorly formulated, leading to a concentration on the wrong (or unimportant) aspects of a situation. As has been mentioned, one should be aware of the likely interdependence of observations and interpretations.

The 'who' may be a poor sample, the time chosen may be inappropriate. As suggested above, early afternoon may sample from a different population of bus users. This is likely to be a particular problem if the observation is carried out in a setting with which the researcher is unfamiliar. Special care needs to be taken in cross-cultural settings, where the implicit social rules are likely to be unfamiliar to the observer. The observation may be for too short a time, thus missing out crucial material. It may be for too long a time, ending up simply skimming the material, or being overwhelmed by too much information.

The 'what' may also be problematic, as there may well be internal validity problems. The observer may be blind to what is being looked at, may not understand it, may think that they have seen something or may influence the ongoing process both consciously and unconsciously. Although video cameras and recorders have been heralded as the way of ensuring that accurate records are available, it must be realised that they also have disadvantages. They are inevitably selective, giving at best only a partial view. They only represent one particular viewpoint and the angles taken may influence interpretations (for instance, a standing figure may be evaluated differently if a camera goes from head to toe, rather than from toe to head), and they are likely to be reacted to. Even using paper and pencil recording has problems: as the above example indicates, it is inevitably selective, and the very act of note taking will lead to material being missed. Our sense organs and attentional mechanisms are inadequate for the task.

Observation as a method can be very time-consuming and labour-intensive, especially as it creates an enormous amount of data which then becomes very hard to winnow. It is therefore important to decide how much is likely to be needed, and to consider carefully what precisely it is that will be analysed.

In common with many other methods and theories in psychology, the approach is imbued with assumptions that people do make sense of their social world, do carry around with them (albeit probably at an unconscious level) a set of implicit social rules, do behave purposively, etc. But people may be inconsistent or behave in an unthinking manner in social situations, sometimes even following inappropriate scripts. Langer (1978) suggests that for a lot of the time in social interactions we do not behave in a thoughtful fashion, but rather act 'mindlessly'. Control by the observer over the phenomena being observed is usually minimal, and it may not be possible to predict when certain events are going to occur.

All research should involve the careful consideration of ethical problems. This has been touched upon above, and will be discussed further in Chapter 13. It is often assumed that there are fewer ethical problems with observational studies than with many other approaches in psychological research, but ethics do need to be carefully thought through and discussed with others before starting a study. The British Psychological Society guidelines see natural observation as being unproblematic, but we need to consider the extent to which we have a right to record the behaviour of others in public social settings, and issues such as anonymity and confidentiality also need to be carefully considered. We are still accountable for what we produce in observational reports.

In conclusion, despite the potential drawbacks, observation will produce rich and exciting results, which may well help to challenge existing assumptions about social life, experience and rules, and to point the way to new developments. Admittedly (and this is true of all methods in psychology, quantitative and qualitative), a lot still depends on who the researcher is, but following the guidelines above should help to minimise the problems of this effect. Of all psychological methods, naturalistic observation is probably potentially the least reactive and the one that is most likely to produce valid results and insights that are very much rooted in 'real life'.

Chapter summary

This chapter has provided a detailed summary of the background and technique of observation as a qualitative research method, with a worked exemplar in depth based on an observation of bus stop queuing. This is followed by a discussion of the advantages and disadvantages of observation as a qualitative research technique.

References

Albert, S. and Kessler, S. (1978) 'Ending social encounters'. *Journal of Experimental Social Psychology*, **14**, 541–53.

Argyle, M. (1987) *The Psychology of Interpersonal Behaviour*. Harmondsworth: Penguin.

Bales, R. F. (1950) *Interaction Process Analysis: A Method for the Study of Small Groups*. Chicago: University of Chicago Press.

Berger, P. L. and Luckmann, T. (1967) *The Social Construction of Reality*. London: Allen Lane.

Cary, M. S. (1978) 'Does civil inattention exist in pedestrian passing?' *Journal of Personality and Social Psychology*, **36**, 1185–93.

Goffman, E. (1963) *Behavior in Public Places*. New York: Free Press.

Langer, E. J. (1978) 'Rethinking the role of thought in social interaction', in J. H. Harvey, W. Ickes and R. F. Kidd (eds) *New Directions in Attribution Research*. New York: Halsted Press.

Latané, B. and Darley, J. M. (1970) *The Unresponsive Bystander: Why Does He Not Help?* New York: Appleton-Century-Crofts.

Mann, L. (1977) 'The effect of stimulus queues on queue-joining behavior'. *Journal of Personality and Social Psychology*, **35**, 437–42.

Marshall, C. and Rossman, G. B. (1989) *Designing Qualitative Research*. London: Sage.

Minuchin, S. (1974) *Families and Family Therapy*. Cambridge, MA: Harvard University Press.

Oxford English Dictionary (1989) 2nd edn. Oxford: Oxford University Press.

Reason, P. and Rowan, J. (eds) (1981) *Human Inquiry: A Sourcebook of New Paradigm Research*. Chichester: Wiley.

Webb, E. J., Campbell, D. T., Schwartz, R. D., Sechrest, L. and Grove, J. B. (1981) *Nonreactive Measures in the Social Sciences*, 2nd edn. Boston: Houghton Mifflin.

Chapter 5

Ethnography

Katherine Runswick-Cole

Introduction

Ethnography is a fascinating, exciting and popular mode of inquiry with the potential to create new forms of research production. The aim of this chapter is to introduce the researcher to some of the methods, issues and dilemmas associated with ethnography. At the end of the chapter, some of these ideas are brought to life through the lens of a research project ('Does Every Child Matter, Post-Blair? The Interconnections of Disabled Childhoods'), with the aim of illustrating some of these debates in practice.

Although ethnography is usually associated with qualitative research, some ethnographers have used both qualitative and quantitative methods; however, this chapter focuses primarily on qualitative approaches. Ethnographic methods most usually rely on 'participant observation', which is sometimes seen as synonymous with ethnography, but methods also include interviews, analysis of written documents and focus groups. Ethnography is essentially a multimethod form of research. Recent technological developments have meant that multimedia methods are increasingly common and web-based methods represent a new direction within ethnography that has opened up a range of approaches, opportunities and challenges for researchers in a media age. Ethnography has a long and somewhat colourful past in the social sciences and, despite its history and current popularity, the theories and practices of the ethnographic method continue to be negotiated, contested and developed by researchers within social sciences and beyond.

Origins of ethnography

Ethnography has its roots within sociology and anthropology. Over the last 40 years, however, ethnography has become a familiar approach within the social sciences and the humanities, and this approach has also been extended to applied areas such as education and medicine (Hammersley 1990). Tedlock (2000) offers a helpful overview of the historical origins of ethnography that she traces back to the late nineteenth century. Yet it is Malinowski's (1922) fieldwork in the Trobriand Islands that it is often cited as the key early ethnographic text (e.g. Atkinson and Hammersley 1994; Tedlock 2000). Tedlock (2000) reminds us that Malinowski did not invent fieldwork but acknowledges his study's distinctiveness because of its detail in documenting every aspect of the social life of the islanders. Moreover, it was Malinowski who first suggested that the ethnographer's role should be to 'grasp the native's point of view, their relation to life and to realise their vision of their world' (1922: 25). Malinowski's call has since been seized upon enthusiastically by generations of ethnographers in the hope that complete immersion in the 'native's' world will enable them to develop social understanding.

Not surprisingly, perhaps, there have also been criticisms of Malinowski's call to 'grasp the native's point of view'. First, the call to 'go native' has been criticised by those who fear that the researcher will take up 'complete membership' of the group or culture they are observing and thereby lose their 'distance' from the research (Adler and Adler 1897, cited in Tedlock 2000: 457). More troubling is the critique that suggests that 'going native' may also carry the risk of moral degeneration (Tedlock 2000). Crucially, the implicit association between 'the native' and 'moral degeneracy' reveals the values of a colonial past evident in the origins of ethnography. One reading of ethnography's history is that ethnography has been discovered, developed and perfected in the 'Global North' in order to tell stories about marginalised populations often in the 'Global South' (Behar 2003). Indeed, Behar (2003: 3) has argued that ethnography has its origins in 'flagrant colonial inequalities'.

Postcolonial researchers, like Behar, challenge the value of ethnographic approaches that objectify the 'native' and regard 'them' as sources for information retrieval (Spivak 1985). These criticisms of the ethnographic method might well have prompted a decline in ethnographic inquiry, but ethnography has not become a relic of its colonial past, rather it has grown in popularity as a method across the social sciences and humanities (Behar 2003). The historical roots of ethnography teach us perhaps that it is important to acknowledge the 'lingering shame' (Behar 2003: 16) associated with ethnography, as it is only by being mindful of its shady past that we are able to take a more egalitarian approach and to decolonise the ethnographic method (Goodley and Runswick-Cole 2011a).

Traditionally, as we have seen, ethnography has focused on 'extraordinary individuals' (Spradley 1979), with the associated dangers that 'minority' and/or 'marginalised' groups have been both exoticised and/or oppressed. However, paradoxical as it may at first seem, a focus on groups about whom little is known or who have been excluded from research in the past can also have emancipatory potential. The focus on minority and/or marginalised groups can open up a space for emancipatory research as there is then potential for different perspectives to be heard (Barnes 1992). For example, whereas in the past research has been conducted 'on' minority groups, an emancipatory approach challenges researchers to work 'with' minority groups. Ethnographic approaches have been used to analyse the everyday experiences of social groups whose agendas and meaning makings have been under-represented in mainstream debates.

For example, in her study reflecting on the experiences of disabled pupils in schools, Vlachou (1997: 3) justifies her ethnographic approach as an opportunity for previously 'hidden voices' to be heard. Another example is the work of Goodley (2000) who employed an ethnographic method in his work with people with the label of learning difficulties. People with the label of learning difficulties have been widely perceived to be unable to be active participants within research. Research studies have often focused instead on the views of proxies, including parents and professionals. By immersing himself in the lives of people with the label of learning difficulties and by employing a mixture of methods to explore their social worlds, Goodley was able to turn up the volume on the voices of a group of people whose voices were not usually heard.

The purpose of ethnographic research is often to 'make the strange familiar', yet ethnographic inquiry is also used to 'render the familiar strange' (Goodley 2002: 4). Ethnographic methods can be used to look again at familiar cultures. By turning the gaze back on to familiar cultures, the opportunity is open to think again about practices within those cultures and to challenge taken-for-granted assumptions about social groups and/or contexts. It is not unusual, for example, for practitioner researchers in educational and medical contexts sometimes to use ethnographic approaches in this way when evaluating practice in their own settings (Hargreaves 1997).

Features of ethnographic research

Whether the aim is to 'make the strange familiar' or to 'render the familiar strange', ethnography requires the researcher to immerse himself or herself in the culture under investigation using a variety of methods. In practical terms, ethnography usually refers to social research that has a number of the following features:

- It explores the nature of social phenomenon through first-hand observation in natural settings (Atkinson and Hammersley 1994).
- Researchers respond to the field rather than entering it with preconceived hypotheses or analytic categories into which they code the data.
- Researchers seek to 'relinquish' their will and to find the 'unexpected stories' (Behar 2003: 16).
- There is detailed exploration of a small number of cases, perhaps only one (Atkinson and Hammersley 1994).
- The analysis explores meaning making and produces 'thick' descriptions (Hammersley 1990).

Typically, some (or all) of the following methods are employed: observation; interviews; focus groups; and multimedia and web-based approaches. It is to an exploration of these methods that we turn in the next section.

(Participant) observation

As we have seen, ethnography is usually associated with 'participant observation' and the terms are sometimes used interchangeably. However, as Atkinson and Hammersley (1994: 248) explain, definitions of 'participant observation' are difficult to 'pin down'. To this end, the distinction is often made between participant and non-participant observation. (see Chapter 4 on Observation). Participant observation is described as the researcher playing 'an established participant role in the scene studied' (Atkinson and Hammersley 1994: 248). An example might be that of a researcher taking on the role of a teaching assistant in a classroom setting, in contrast to a non-participant observer who would not aim to take on an active role. However, Atkinson and Hammersley (1994) show that the simple binary distinction between participant and non-participant observer is not particularly helpful, not least as it implies that the non-participant observer has no role at all, and yet simply by being present, the observer becomes part of the social world they are studying. It might then be more useful to think of the roles of non-participant observer and participant observer as being on a continuum. The researcher's place on the continuum is determined by a number of factors including: the extent to which the researcher is known to those they are studying; what is known about the research and by whom; the activities the researcher adopts within the field and the extent to which the researcher is able to adopt the role of insider or outsider (Atkinson and Hammersley 1994). It may also be possible for the researcher to adopt different places on the continuum at different times and in different contexts when interacting with a group of people but clearly not all the factors which influence the researcher's stance are within their control.

In line with ethnographic principles, observation is an approach 'which gives importance to the interpretation of actions and the contexts in which they occur' (Greig and Taylor 1999: 81). Crucially, it involves a person spending extended periods of time, not one-off encounters, in a setting observing and recording the interactions of group members. It is because of its intensive and long-term character that ethnographic observation provides important insights into the nature of the researcher's relationship with their informants (Christensen and Prout 2002).

As we noted above, participant observation has typically been used as a method to access groups who have 'hidden voices' and so it is often seen as being a particularly relevant method when eliciting information from or about babies and children. Used carefully, participant observation can contribute to an emancipatory approach. If participant observers are able to 'relinquish' themselves in the process (Behar 2003), observers can share part of the agency in the research process with the participant. The opportunity for children to play a dynamic role within participant observation has been welcomed by those who see children as active social agents in their worlds (Christensen and Prout 2002; Clark et al. 2003). Morris (2003) has also argued that 'being with' a child is a key method for understanding their experiences, particularly for children who have complex impairments, and that participant observation often opens up more opportunities for finding out about their views and experiences than other methods.

Interviews

As we see in Chapter 6 (this volume) about interviews, in 1997 Atkinson and Silverman made the claim that we live in an 'interview society'. Interviews are a common part of the day-to-day life of many people in the UK and across the globe. Many of us are familiar with the job interview process but still more people also listen to and/or watch interviews on the television, radio or, indeed, online. Listeners and viewers are familiar with very different interview styles on radio and television. Interview methods are used frequently within qualitative research (Kvale and Brinkman 2009). However, ethnographic interviews can be seen as a distinct category of interview.

Ethnographic interviews are most often used to complement other ethnographic methods. Ethnographic interviews are usually very non-directive; in other words, the interviewer asks open questions and does not begin the interview by telling the participant exactly what they are interested in. Instead, in the spirit of being guided by the participant as expert in their social world, they wait for topics to emerge from the conversation. In order to generate talk, ethnographic interviewers ask general questions, often about everyday interactions and occurrences. So, for example, Bauman and Greenberg Adair (1992: 13) suggest that the ethnographer might ask 'Can you tell me what a typical day might be like?' or 'Can you tell me what happened at the doctors?'. Rich, in-depth ethnographic interviews can elicit responses that create a picture of what it would have been like to be there.

Focus groups

When an interview is carried out with a group of people at the same time, this is often called a focus group. As ethnography focuses on people in their social contexts, focus groups are considered to be a key ethnographic method. Focus groups can provide opportunities for the discussion of complex and contradictory ideas, allowing a variety of views to be explored. However, this exploration of a plurality of perspectives can also mean that focus group research is potentially fraught with difficulties (Crang and Cook 2007). Managing the different personalities and perspectives within the group can be a challenge for the researcher. Getting the balance between having a free-flowing exchange of ideas and 'keeping on track' can also be a source of tension for the researcher who may take on a 'moderator role' of gently guiding the discussion (Cameron 2001). However, it is just these complexities that mean that focus groups can be the sites of production of rich data.

Focus groups have typically been used within two areas of social science: psychotherapy and market research. Focus group meetings in the psychotherapeutic tradition not only offer opportunities for sharing ideas but also for mutual support. Crang and Cook (2007) cite Alcoholics Anonymous as an example of such meetings. However, focus groups are also used for market research when paid consumers are assembled to discuss their reactions to new products (Crang and Cook 2007). Focus groups now have presence beyond social sciences in the UK, in user group consultations and by political parties.

Deciding who will be in the focus group, how many people you will require and where the focus group will be held are key questions for the researcher. There are also issues of whether you want to set up a new group of people or approach an existing group to form the focus group. A new group of people may take time to establish relationships and build trust before a free-flowing conversation can take place. However, approaching an existing group means that the researcher may not be aware of the group's history and ways of working and this may also take time to negotiate. The location, time of day, duration and nature of the group will all impact on whether or not people will be willing to be participants. There is a host of possibilities and challenges to be addressed. Despite the challenges it presents, focus group research remains a popular mode of inquiry, with recent examples including such diverse studies as the use of focus groups to explore 'successful aging' (Reichstadt *et al.* 2007); focus groups to explore migrant workers' experiences (Pratt 2001); and to talk about sex (Frith 2000). Focus groups are now sometimes also conducted online as ethnographers embrace multimedia approaches.

Multimedia methods

As ethnography is essentially a multimethod approach, the rise in new technologies has opened up opportunities for ethnographic researchers including: photographs, mapping, tours and online methods. Multimedia approaches sit well within ethnographic traditions that aim to explore 'hidden voices' as the use of these methods allows the researcher to recognise the different voices or languages of participants (Clark *et al.* 2003). Multimedia approaches offer the opportunity to supplement or even move away from the reliance on the written or spoken word in research production.

The phenomenon of digital technology has meant that there has been an increase in the use of cameras and photographs in research projects. This has particularly been the case in research with young children. There have been a number of studies where children have used cameras to document important places and people in early years settings (Clark *et al.* 2003). In Denmark, studies (e.g. Rasmussen 1999; Clark *et al.* 2003) have involved asking children to take photographs and then using these as the starting point for interviews. Photographs can serve to represent experiences that might not be easily articulated in other ways. At the same time, researchers must remain conscious of the risk that by invading participants' life-worlds through the medium of photography, research is a form of surveillance. Clark *et al.* (2003) in their research with children, point to the irony that the more imaginative the methods become for listening to young children, the greater the possibility of invading their private worlds.

Recently tours, modelling and map-making have all been used by ethnographers to elicit children's views (Clark *et al.* 2003). In early years settings, tours involve young children taking researchers on a guided walk around their preschool setting (Clark *et al.* 2003). Children direct the tour and the methods used to record it, including taking photographs, drawings, maps and audio-recordings. Interestingly, these techniques were not originally developed with children, but were adapted from participatory approaches used in the context of international development, known as *participatory rural appraisal* (PRA) (Chambers 1994). PRA recognises the knowledge and analytical abilities of local people and challenges researchers to reflect on the potentially colonising impact of traditional modes of research production. Mountian *et al.* (2009) offer a convincing, though critical, analysis of the potentials of using visual methodologies to capture the everyday, mundane and ordinary aspects of social life.

As online methods have also gained increasing popularity, Kozinets (2010) has written a comprehensive guide to the conduct of ethnography over the internet – *netography*. The enthusiasm for online methods is fed by the researcher's awareness of the number of eager users interested in being online, browsing the web, writing blogs, engaging in discussions, visiting virtual worlds and using social networking sites.

In principle, netography has many advantages. It offers participants privacy and is convenient, not least because participants don't need to leave home to take part. However, it is still the case that not everybody has a computer at home or even access to a computer, and this means that some groups might be excluded from research. Issues of privacy may arise if participants use shared computers in schools or internet cafés, for example (Stafford *et al.* 2003). *Internet research ethics* (IRE) has emerged as a growing area in social sciences with much discussion of what constitutes ethical research online (Kozinets 2010).

Issues for ethnographers

Clearly ethical debates are not only an issue for online ethnographers. We have already seen that ethnographic research methods have a tendency to produce a colonising discourse – presenting the 'Other' interpreted through the values of the researcher (Denzin and Lincoln 2000). Denzin and Lincoln (2000: 35) argue for a qualitative research ethic that calls for 'collaborative, trusting, non-oppressive relationships between researchers and those studied'. Considering carefully issues of informed consent, deception, privacy and confidentiality are important for all modes of qualitative inquiry. Researchers can seek guidance from a range of ethical codes of practice issued by professional organisations (e.g. British Psychological Society; British Educational Research Association; British Sociological Association). However, the ethical codes themselves can be ambiguous and difficult to interpret so that researchers are often presented with decisions about how to act in an ethical manner (Goodwin *et al.* 2003).

Certainly, the identity of the researcher will impact on the ethics of the research production. In the case of Goodwin *et al.* (2003), it was the researcher's position as an anaesthetic and recovery nurse which enabled her to gain access to the research context. Indeed, 'gaining access' to participants and contexts is a further issue for ethnographic research. Being a member of the group studied may help the researcher to gain access, and the process of 'enculturation' necessary for participant observation may already have taken place. However, being an 'insider' may also add the complex layer of ethical issues including the risk of an abuse of power within pre-existing relationships. 'Outsider' researchers, who wish to study groups of which they are not a member, may have difficulty in accessing research participants and may need to take longer to familiarise themselves with the field and to build relationships with participants.

Researchers often approach 'gatekeepers' (Hammersley and Atkinson 2007) to gain access. However, it is important also to negotiate access with all the people participating in the research. In her research with children, Cocks (2006) explains that while adults were the gatekeepers to children's social worlds and gave informed consent for the children to participate in her research, she also asked permission from the children. Cocks makes a useful distinction between 'consent' which she uses to denote that an adult has given permission for a child to take part in research and 'assent' which she uses to indicate that a child has given permission to take part in research after the researcher has sought permission from the child's parent/carer.

The position of the researcher is also closely tied up with the issues of the status and value of ethnographic research. Ethnographic research produces 'thick' descriptions and these descriptions are described as a co-production – a product of the ethnographer's interaction with participants in the field – rather than an 'objective' record of what really happened. Ethnographic researchers do not attempt to write themselves out of the analysis, rather they tend to offer a reflexive account of their role within it.

However, while what ethnography essentially has to offer is a rich description of the social world, ethnographers also claim that it is possible to use ethnographic data to generate a 'theoretical description' (Hammersley 1990). Hammersley (1990) points to the tension within this claim: on the one hand, descriptions cannot be theories, but on the other hand, all descriptions are informed by theoretical assumptions in the sense that our assumptions play a role in determining our descriptions. The place of theory development within ethnography is closely linked to the methods used to analyse the data generated by ethnographic inquiry. The work of Glaser and Strauss (1967) in developing *grounded theory* is often used to support the analysis of ethnographic data. Grounded theory is used to depict concrete situations and to generate theory, but the distinctive feature of grounded theory is that the researcher derives categories for analysis directly from the observations in the field, not from preconceived theories or hypotheses. Charmaz (2000: 509) claims: 'Grounded theory methods consist of systematic inductive guidelines for collecting and analyzing data to build middle-range theoretical frameworks that explain the collected data.' This description of grounded theory has been disputed by postmodernists and poststructuralists who challenge the subtle positivist tendencies of the 'systematic' method, and by those who question the logic of the claim that is possible to create generalised theories from a particular case (Hammersley 1990).

Despite the questions about the possibilities for theory development within ethnographic research, researchers continue to argue that there is a place for 'analytic ethnography' which asserts the possibilities of theory development within ethnography and strives to create systematic procedures for analysing data (Snow *et al.* 2004).

Research example

In this section, some of the issues raised above are discussed in the context of an ongoing research project funded by the Economic and Social Research Council, 'Does Every Child Matter, Post-Blair? The Interconnections of Disabled Childhoods' (RES-062-23-1138). The aim of the project is to explore the lives of disabled children in the North of England in the light of the policy agenda for children under the umbrella of *Every Child Matters* (DfES 2004). The research team is in the process of listening to disabled children and young people, their parents/carers and professionals to discover what it means to be a disabled child in England in the 2000s. The project employs a variety of ethnographic approaches including: participant and non-participant observation, interviews, focus groups and multimedia methods.

From the start, the colonising tendencies of ethnographic research were acknowledged by the research team. Indeed, we saw an exploration of research with disabled children as a useful place to attempt to deconstruct ethnographic research, not least because disabled children are so often thought of as being extraordinary, vulnerable and passive (Goodley and Runswick-Cole 2011b). We argued, following Fanon (1993: 30), that disabled children should be able to 'write back' within the research process. 'Writing back' promotes the perspective of the minority with the aim that this will expose and challenge the medicalising and pathologising tendencies which underpin so much of the research with, or perhaps more accurately, 'on' disabled children (Goodley and Runswick-Cole 2011b). The research team was mindful of the potential to contribute to further 'othering' of disabled children through the research process. We therefore sought to stress the potential of disabled children.

Despite our commitment to putting children at the centre of the research, as the children were aged between 4 and 16, adults were the gatekeepers to children's participation. This meant that we did not approach children without the consent of their parents/carers, which clearly influenced which of the children could take part. However, following Cocks (2006), we sought the children's assent to taking part in the research and we saw this as an ongoing process. Each time we met with the children and young people we checked that they were happy to continue to take part. This meant paying attention to how the children were behaving and feeling whether they were bored, tired, distracted, comfortable or engaged. We were also careful to try to negotiate times of day and venues that suited the children and their families.

Following Morris (2003), we were clear about the information children should receive before agreeing to take part in research: they should know what questions will be asked; what their parents/staff will be told; if the research has a point and if it will change anything; why they have been picked; what information the researcher already knows about the child and who gave it. We agree with Morris's suggestion that children should know about the researchers' skills/experience.

Crucially for any researcher working with children, we were also clear that although we would not tell other people what the children had said without their permission, if they told us something that meant that we had good reason to believe they were at risk of harm, we would need to pass this on. The issue of anonymity was also treated with care as, for example, the combination of revealing a child's rare impairment label and ethnicity may risk exposing his or her identity.

Participatory ethnographies

Our original research proposal aimed to 'ethnographically explore the lives of disabled childhoods', and we did use a mixture of ethnographic methods, including observation, interviews, focus groups and multimedia methods. However, our attention was also drawn to what we could learn from the ways in which disabled children and young people were already documenting their lives. Several children and young people in the study were using digital photography and video; sometimes they were in the photograph and sometimes they were the photographer or filmmaker. This documentation became what we called 'participatory ethnography' (Goodley and Runswick-Cole 2011a). In addition to spending time with children, and sometimes when this is what they wanted, instead of spending time with them, we drew on their interest in photography and film. We invited children to use photography and film in ways that they enjoyed. Mindful of the need to 'relinquish' control within ethnographic research, we followed the lead of some of the children who were happy to show us their worlds in photography, but were not happy for us to enter them in person. The photographs that children shared were also used as starting points for conversations and following the principles of 'photovoice' (Booth and Booth 2003): narratives drawn from the photos were co-constructed with the children. Extracts from 73247's story (the pseudonym the young person used for himself) are presented below.

The first photo he showed us was of a television showing a picture: 73247 watched a lot of television. In our first meeting he told us he wanted to be an actor in films. He did not want to do Shakespeare or plays or boring stuff like that and in films he thought it is easier to learn your lines, you get to say them again if you go wrong. 73427 did not do drama at school, but he did not see his lack of experience or his short stature as a barrier to being an actor.

The second photo he showed us was of a laptop computer again showing a picture: the computer is an important part of his life. He enjoys surfing the web and using Facebook. He has never been bullied online and says he would never accept friends' requests from people he did not know (although he has had them). All the friends he has online are people he already knows. He thinks that adults worry too much about this kind of stuff.

The third picture he showed us was a Lego model he had built, which was of his local super-market complete with the CCTV on the corner of the building. He spends a lot of his time at home playing with Lego.

Despite the growing popularity of photovoice as a research method, it remains the case that image-based research is often perceived to have a 'lower status' and as being on the 'margins' of qualitative research (Prosser 2000: 134).

Finally, despite Atkinson and Hammersley's (1994) concerns about the limits of 'analytic ethnography', we were aware in our analysis of the possibilities of theory development within ethnography and by visiting and revisiting the data we aimed to follow systematic procedures for analysing data (Snow *et al.* 2004). This generated a range of themes within the research including: violence (Goodley and Runswick-Cole 2011(b)); play (Goodley and Runswick-Cole 2010); leisure (Goodley and Runswick-Cole, under review) and psychologisation in the lives of disabled children (Goodley 2011).

In our analysis of the children and young people's participatory ethnography we were aware of the danger that by offering an analysis of the children's photos we were at the same time fracturing the data (Charmaz 2000) and reducing the potential impact of the powerful images which the children had presented. We paid close attention to the interpretations we, as adults, were bringing to our analysis by being attentive to Titchkosky's (2008) advice 'to watch our watching, to read our readings'. It was not our intention to diminish the voices of children and young people by offering our analysis, but we were aware that simply revealing marginalised voices does not necessarily bring about change.

Chapter summary

Ethnography can be an absorbing, fascinating and potentially emancipatory form of inquiry. Despite the contested nature of the method, ethnography continues to be viewed as an exemplary example of the qualitative approach. The multi-method nature of ethnography opens up opportunities for forms of participation in research that challenge traditional modes of research production and allow participants to shape the research and subsequent analyses. Perhaps the most exciting development in ethnography in recent years is the new opportunities opened up by access to multi-media and digital technologies. The possibilities for ethnographic research now seem endless.

References

Atkinson, P. and Hammersley, M. (1994) 'Ethnography and participant observation', in N. K. Denzin and Y. K. Lincoln (eds) *Handbook of Qualitative Research*. Thousand Oaks, CA: Sage.

Barnes, C. (1992) 'Emancipatory disability research: realistic goal or impossible dream?' Accessed October 18, 2010. www.leeds.ac.uk/disability-studies/.../Barnes/Chapter%202.pdf.

Bauman, L. J. and Greenberg Adair, E. (1992) 'The use of the ethnographic interview to inform questionnaire construction'. *Health, Education, Behaviour*, **19**(9), 9–22.

Behar, R. (2003) 'Ethnography and the book that was lost'. *Ethnography*, **4**, 15–39.

Booth, T. and Booth, W. (2003) 'In the frame: photovoice and mothers with learning difficulties'. *Disability and Society*, **18**(4), 431–42.

Cameron, J. (2001) 'Focusing on the focus group', in J. Hey (ed.) *Qualitative Research Methods in Human Geography*. Oxford: Oxford University Press.

Chambers, R. (1994) 'Origins and practice of participatory rural appraisal'. *World Development*, **22**(7), 953–69.

Charmaz, K. (2000) 'Grounded theory: objectivist and constructivist methods', in N. K. Denzin and Y. S. Lincoln (eds) *Handbook of Qualitative Research*, 2nd edn. London: Sage.

Christensen, P. and Prout, A. (2002) 'Working with ethical symmetry in social research with children'. *Childhood*, **9**(4), 477–97.

Clark, A., McQuail, S. and Moss, P. (2003) *Exploring the Field of Listening to and Consulting with Young Children*. London: DfES.

Cocks, A. (2006) 'The ethical maze: finding an inclusive path towards gaining children's agreement to research participation'. *Childhood*, **13**(2), 247–66.

Crang, I. and Cook, M. (2007) *Doing Ethnographies*. London: Sage.

Denzin, N. K. and Lincoln, Y. S. (2000) 'The discipline and practice of qualitative research', in N. K. Denzin and Y. S. Lincoln (eds) *Handbook of Qualitative Research*, 2nd edn. London: Sage.

DfES (2004) *Every Child Matters: Change for Children*. London: DfES.

Fanon, F. (1993) *Black Skins, White Masks*, 3rd edn. London: Pluto Press.

Frith, H. (2000) 'Focusing on sex: using focus groups in sex research'. *Sexualities*, **3**(3), 275–97.

Glaser, B. G. and Strauss, A. L. (1967) *The Discovery of Grounded Theory: Strategies for Qualitative Research*. New York: Aldine.

Goodley, D. (2000) *Self-advocacy in the Lives of People with Learning Difficulties: The Politics of Resilience*. Maidenhead: Open University Press.

Goodley, D. (2002) *Ethnography Research Design: Qualitative Methods and Approaches*. Sheffield: Department of Educational Studies, Sheffield University.

Goodley, D. (2011) *An Introduction to Disability Studies*. London: Sage.

Goodley, D. and Runswick-Cole, K. (2010) 'Emancipating play: Dis/abled children, development and deconstruction'. *Disability and Society*, **25**(4), 499–512.

Goodley, D. and Runswick-Cole, K. (2011a) 'De-colonizing methodologies: disabled children as research managers and participant ethnographers', in S. Grech and A. Azzopardl (eds) *Communities: A Reader*. Rotterdam: Sense Publishers.

Goodley, D. and Runswick-Cole, K. (2011b) 'The violence of disablism'. *Journal of Sociology of Health and Illness*, **33**, 602–17.

Goodley, D. and Runswick-Cole, K. (under review) 'Doing childhood: disabled children, play and leisure'. *Disability Studies Quarterly*.

Goodwin, D., Pope, C., Mort, M. and Smith, A. (2003) 'Ethics and ethnography: an experiential account'. *Qualitative Health Research*, **13**, 567–77.

Greig, A. and Taylor, J. (1999) *Doing Research with Children*. Thousand Oaks, CA: Sage.

Hammersley, M. (1990) 'What's wrong with ethnography? The myth of theoretical description'. *Sociology*, **24**(4), 597–615.

Hammersley, M. and Atkinson, P. (2007) *Ethnography: Principles in Practice*. New York: Routledge.

Hargreaves, D. (1997) 'In defence of research for evidence-based teaching: a rejoinder to Martyn Hammersley'. *British Educational Research Journal*, **23**(4), 405–20.

Kozinets, R. V. (2010) *Netography: Doing Ethnographic Research Online*. London: Sage.

Kvale, S. and Brinkman, S. (2009) *Interviews: Learning the Craft of Qualitative Research Interviewing*. London: Sage.

Malinowski, B. (1922) *Argonauts of the Western Pacific: An Account of Native Enterprise and Adventure in the Archipelagoes of Melanesian New Guinea*. London: George Routledge and Sons, Ltd.

Morris, J. (2003) 'Including all children: finding out about the experiences of children with communication and/or cognitive impairments'. *Children and Society*, **17**, 337–48.

Mountian, I., Lawthom, R., Kellock, A., Sixsmith, J. A., Duggan, K., Haworth, J. T., Kagan, C. M., Brown, D. P., Griffiths, J., Hawkins, J., Worley, C., Purcell, C. and Siddiquee, A. (2009) 'On utilising a visual methodology: shared reflections and tensions', in P. Reavey (ed.) *Visual Psychologies: Using and Interpreting Images in Qualitative Research*. London: Routledge.

Pratt, G. (2001) 'Studying immigrants in focus groups', in P. Moss (ed.) *Feminist Geography in Practice: Research and Methods*. Oxford: Blackwell.

Prosser, J. (2000) 'The moral maze of ethics', in R. Usher and H. Simons (eds) *Situated Ethics in Educational Research*. London: Routledge.

Rasmussen, K. (1999) 'Om fotografering og fotografi som forskningsstrategi I barndomsforskning'. *Dansk Sociologi*, **1**(10), 63–78.

Reichstadt, J., Depp, C. A., Palinkas, L. A., Folsom, D. P. and Jeste, D. V. (2007) 'Building blocks of successful aging: a focus group study of older adults' perceived contributors to successful aging'. *American Journal of Geriatric Psychiatry*, **15**(3), 194–201.

Snow, D. A., Morrill, C. and Anderson, L. (2004) 'Elaborating analytic ethnography: linking fieldwork and theory'. *Ethnography*, **4**(2), 153–5.

Spivak, G. C. (1985) 'Three women's texts and a critique of imperialism'. *Critical Inquiry*, **12**(1), 243–61.

Spradley, J. (1979) *The Ethnographic Interview*. Orlando, FL: Harcourt.

Stafford, A., Laybourn, A. and Hill, M. (2003) '"Having a say": children and young people talk about consultation'. *Children and Society*, **17**, 361–73.

Tedlock, B. (2000) 'Ethnography and ethnographic representations', in N. K. Denzin and Y. S. Lincoln (eds) *Handbook of Qualitative Research*, 2nd edn. London: Sage.

Titchkosky, T. (2008) *Reading and Writing Disability Differently: The Textured Life of Embodiment.* Toronto: University of Toronto Press.

Vlachou, A. D. (1997) *Struggles for Inclusive Education.* Buckingham: Open University Press.

Chapter 6

Interviewing

Katherine Runswick-Cole

Introduction

We live in an 'interview society' (Atkinson and Silverman 1997). Interviews are everywhere: on the television, on the radio and in the published media, including on the web. It is no surprise, then, that qualitative research interviews can seem very familiar, especially as they can take on a form similar to an everyday conversation. Conversations are a spontaneous exchange of views between two or more people, and, just like a conversation, an 'inter-view' is an 'inter-action' between people (Kvale and Brinkman 2009: 32). However, research interviews usually differ from a day-to-day conversation in several important ways. First, interviews are most often organised in such a way that they focus on a predetermined theme or topic chosen by the researcher. Second, the accounts shared in the interview will be recorded, sometimes by the interviewer taking notes, but more often by voice recording and subsequent transcription of the recording (Potter and Hepburn 2005). Finally, interviews, unlike day-to-day conversations, are analysed and disseminated (Kvale and Brinkman 2009). In addition to choosing the topic for the interview, the interviewer shapes it with questions that determine the nature of the interaction as much as the interview is shaped by participants' answers (Kvale and Brinkman 2009). The seemingly familiar nature of research interviews and the undoubted popularity of interviews as a research method have meant that interviews are seen as relatively easy to carry out. However, they are perhaps more difficult to do well than at first appears (Potter and Hepburn 2005).

This chapter guides the would-be interviewer through the origins and history of interviews as a social science research method. Then it examines different types of qualitative interviews and methods of analysis, and finally considers some of the questions and challenges that qualitative interviewers must address, using examples from an ongoing research project to explore the issues.

Origins of research interviews

The term 'interview' came into use in the seventeenth century (Kvale and Brinkman 2009). Before the term 'social science' was first used in France in the 1790s (Oakley 1998). However, qualitative interviews have been used as a research method for around a hundred years and are associated, in particular, with the Chicago School in sociology in the 1930s and 1940s (Fontana and Frey 2001). Since the 1980s, interviews have become a hot topic for methodological discussion (Kvale and Brinkman 2009) and in 1997 Atkinson and Silverman declared that we live in an 'interview society'.

Technological advances have also increased the popularity of qualitative interviews, not least because the means of recording interviews have expanded and recording devices have become smaller and more convenient to use. The growth of the use of the internet has also created new opportunities for qualitative interviews both in terms of contacting potential interviewees and for carrying out 'virtual interviews' (Madge and O'Connor 2002; Kozinets 2010). As social sciences have increasingly drawn on phenomenology, which focuses on understanding social phenomenon from the point of view of the actor, this has contributed to the popularity of the interview as a research method (Kvale and Brinkman 2009). Interviews, it is claimed, 'give voice to common people, allowing them to freely present their life situations in their own words' (Kvale and Brinkman 2009: 481). Not surprisingly, it seems that qualitative researchers often put 'special faith' in the interviews as 'the prime means of data collection' (Atkinson and Silverman 1997: 304).

Structured, semi-structured and unstructured interviews

Within social sciences, research interviews fall into three categories: unstructured, semi-structured or structured interviews (DiCicco-Bloom and Crabtree 2006). Structured interviews usually involve one person asking another person a list of predetermined questions, with a limited set of response options (Fontana and Frey 2001). The interviewer records the responses according to a code predetermined by the project leader. The interviewer controls the interview with the aim that all the respondents are asked the same questions in the same way (Fontana and Frey 2001). Often the aim of a structured interview is to produce quantitative data and so structured interviews are not the main focus here. Semi-structured and unstructured interviews, on the other hand, are usually used to produce qualitative data and it is to these types of interview that we turn next.

No interview is completely unstructured. This is because the interview topic has been chosen in advance, usually by the researcher (DiCicco-Bloom and Crabtree 2006). However, some researchers, particularly those working with an ethnographic tradition (see Chapter 5), use relatively unstructured interviews in which they allow themselves to be guided by the interviewee and attempt to 'relinquish' control over the interview (Behar 2003). Unstructured interviews are often used alongside other methods including participant observation and researchers use interviews to elicit more information about the behaviours, interactions, rituals or artefacts they have observed (DiCicco-Bloom and Crabtree 2006).

In contrast, semi-structured interviews are sometimes used as the sole data for the project, and unlike unstructured interviews, which are often opportunistic and conducted in the 'field', semi-structured interviews are usually organised to be at a specific time and place, negotiated between the interviewer and interviewee. Semi-structured interviews are shaped by a set of predetermined questions, but the interviewer may ask the questions in any order, leave questions out or introduce new questions in response to what the interviewee has said. Using semi-structured interviews can be a time-consuming business as it usually takes between 30 minutes and several hours to complete one interview, although, as for other interviews, there are no hard and fast rules about how long semi-structured interviews should take.

Analysis

Interviews produce copious amounts of rich and messy data for analysis. It is important to remember that the interviewers' and interviewees' talk should both be included in the analysis (Potter and Wetherell 1994). The quantity of data produced in an interview can be great and requires time for data analysis. Silverman (2001: 823) distinguishes between two types of data analysis: a 'realist' approach and a 'narrative' approach. In the 'realist' approach, the researcher attempts to discover the 'realities' of the experiences of the interviewee. Analysis might involve some form of coding of the data, which is sometimes computer assisted using a programme such as NUDIST or N-VIVO. However, Silverman also describes a 'narrative' approach in which the researcher's analysis of the data is concerned with the stories people tell, rather than seeking the 'truth'. While a 'realist' approach is more attractive to 'social scientists who theorize the world in terms of the impact of (objective) social structures upon (subjective) dispositions' (Silverman 2001: 824), for interviewers who understand the interview as a story co-constructed between interviewee and interviewer the 'realist' approach is clearly limited and a 'narrative' approach is preferred.

However, the place of analysis within a 'narrative approach' is also highly contested. Blumenfeld-Jones (1995: 25) has offered a useful distinction between narrative analysis used by 'those who focus upon the stories of individuals as story with meaning' and analysis of narrative used by 'those who analyse narratives in order to generate themes for further analysis'. This inductive approach has clear links with grounded theory (Glaser and Strauss 1967). However, Polkinghorne (1995) argues that it is unhelpful to offer an analysis of narrative. Polkinghorne claims that the generation of themes for further analysis fractures the data and as a result informants are portrayed less fully.

Yet, as Goodson points out, simply revealing marginalised voices does not necessarily bring about change as 'new stories do not by themselves analyse or address the structures of power' (1995: 95). In addition, analysis can be used to oppose unsympathetic readings of texts that might exclude and oppress marginalised groups (Goodley *et al.* 2004). Stories can be made stronger by being closely analysed and interrogated, and it is often through analysis that the influence of wider society is revealed (Booth and Booth 1998).

Challenges for qualitative research interview

We have already seen that it is important for the researcher to be able to justify the choice of the interview method for their study. At every stage of the study, interviewers meet with questions and challenges that they must address. In the next sections, some of these issues are explored using examples from an ongoing research project funded by the Economic and Social Research

Council, 'Does Every Child Matter, Post-Blair? The Interconnections of Disabled Childhoods' (RES-062-23-1138). The aim of the project is to explore the lives of disabled children in the North of England in the light of the policy agenda for children under the umbrella of *Every Child Matters* (DfES 2004). The research team is in the process of listening to disabled children and young people, their parents/carers and professionals to discover what it means to be a disabled child in England in the 2000s. The project employs a variety of ethnographic approaches (see Chapter 5) including qualitative interviews with children and adults. However, the examples used here are taken from the use of qualitative interviews with mothers of disabled children.

Overuse

As we have seen, interviews are a popular method of qualitative inquiry. However, the popularity of the method has led critics to claim that qualitative researchers rely 'disproportionately' on interviews as a research method (Atkinson and Silverman 1997). The suggestion that the interview method is overused leads Potter and Hepburn (2005: 2) to suggest that 'the ideal would be much less interview research, but much better interview research'. Potter and Hepburn (2005) rightly point out that often in research studies the appropriateness of the interview method is taken for granted, rather than justified explicitly.

The overuse of the interview method was certainly an issue for the project under discussion here. First, the research team were acutely aware of the large amounts of interview data that already exists which have been gathered from disabled children, their parents/carers and professionals, including data collected by members of the research team themselves (Goodley 2007; Runswick-Cole 2007; McLaughlin *et al.* 2008). In fact, it can be argued that mothers of disabled children are an over-researched group given the number of studies that have focused on their experiences (Beresford 1994; Read 2000; McLaughlin *et al.* 2008). Yet, in the ever-changing policy climate for disabled children and their families, the mothers' stories are changing too. Within the project, the aim is to collect the stories in the hope that they might effect positive change for disabled children and their families and the interview method remains a very effective way of collecting narratives, allowing interviewees to tell their stories in their own words.

There is the danger, however, that the predominance of the use of interviews in research relies too heavily on the spoken word as the means of gathering information. Kvale and Brinkman (2009) describe interviews as a method for the 'common people', but in the project we were aware that use of the spoken word alone would exclude some potential participants and, where appropriate, we sought to support the interviews with multimedia approaches (see Chapter 5 for more detail).

Positionality

Just as it is important for a researcher to justify his or her choice of method, it is also important to make explicit the researcher's position within the research, or their 'positionality' as it is sometimes termed within the social sciences. By making clear their positionality, researchers reflect on aspects of their lives that might influence the conduct of their research study; this might include disclosing aspects of their knowledge, values and beliefs. There are, of course, aspects of the interviewer's positionality that can be difficult to conceal including gender, race, class and dis/ability. While it may not be possible or desirable for a researcher to conceal these aspects of their positionality, it is important for the interviewer to be aware of them. Fontana and Frey (2001: 655) ask whether the researcher should 'dress down' to look like the respondents or whether we should dress as representatives of 'our academic cultures'. While Fontana and Frey make some hierarchical assumptions about the 'superordinate' status of the interviewer and 'subordinate' status of interviewee that may not be accurate or helpful, their call to consider how interviewers present themselves to interviewees is worth considering. The practice of the researcher reflecting on the influence of his or her position within research is known as 'reflexivity'. A further key question for the researcher is the extent to which he or she 'reveals' the 'hidden' aspects of his or her positionality to participants. However, Rose (1997) has critiqued researcher reflexivity that is illustrated as 'transparent', describing her own 'failure' to achieve 'transparent reflexivity' as well as offering critiques of such an approach by arguing that it is not always easy for researchers to identify their positionality.

Nevertheless, the positionality of the interviewer plays a decisive factor in the way in which the interview is conducted. Guidelines exist which offer some guidance to the interviewer in terms of conducting ethical interviews (see below) and it is essential for the interviewer to have knowledge of these. However, it is the researcher's knowledge, characteristics, experiences and values that will determine the conduct of the interviews.

Close relationships between interviewers and interviewees have been criticised as the researcher is seen to 'go native' (see Chapter 5) and losing any sense of professional distance (Kvale and Brinkman 2009). The authenticity of the relationship between the interviewer and the participant has also been questioned, as interviewers have been accused of 'faking friendship' (Kvale 2006: 482) and exploiting a sense of rapport in pursuit of the 'data' which may lead participants to disclose information they would rather have left unsaid.

As with all qualitative studies, the positionality of the interviewer in the current study was key. However, we paid particular attention to the positionality of the interviewer in this study because she was also the mother of a disabled child, or an 'insider researcher', a member of the group with whom the research was carried out. This raised questions of whether or not the interviewer should disclose her status and may well have influenced how she was able to develop a rapport with the other mothers. The ways in which these issues were tackled within the study were heavily influenced by feminist approaches to qualitative interviewing.

Feminist approaches

Feminist critiques of the interview method, although not homogeneous, have suggested that what has traditionally been presented is an essentially 'masculine' view of research and 'knowledge' which relies on 'objective' and 'hygienic' methods (Oakley 1981, 1998). While traditional modes of interview production call for 'professional distance', feminists have argued that it is impossible and undesirable for the interviewer to bracket, or put to one side, their emotional responses. On the contrary, emotional responses are welcomed as part of the interview process (Oakley 1981) and are seen as having the potential to release the researcher from the straitjacket of traditional patterns of research production (Kvale and Brinkman 2009). There have been calls for 'passionate scholarship' in which 'conscious partiality' is a 'substitute for the rule of value neutral research' (Oakley 1998: 713). 'In-depth' interviews are seen as a means of listening to respondents, paying attention to the detail and producing 'faithful' analyses (Oakley 1998). Feminists have also encouraged 'reciprocity' within research interviews where there is a process of 'give and take' and self-disclosure on the part of the interviewer is used in order to generate 'thick' data, but also to develop 'collaborative theorizing' with participants (Harrison *et al.* 2001: 324).

However, other feminist researchers have pointed to the potentially exploitative nature of such research interviews where relationships of empathy and trust serve to elicit unguarded confidences and participants risk saying things they later wished they had left unsaid (Burman 1997). The extent to which building trust and rapport with a participant becomes a process of 'faking friendship' (Kvale 2006: 482) is a thorny issue for all researchers.

As a research team, we followed Oakley (1981: 31) who suggests that 'hygienic' research is neither possible nor desirable. We broke some of the 'masculine rules' of interviewing, conducting what Oakley calls 'illegitimate interviews'. This meant that the interviewer (I) did disclose the fact that she was also the mother of a disabled child. There were several occasions when the interviewer gave practical information to the participants, particularly about entitlements to short break facilities or information about other services for children, as the extract below with Roberta (R), a mother, demonstrates:

R: And during the half term I can't take both of mine out together, 'cause I mean they're both crazy in different ways, in inverted commas, and so one will just throw themselves on the floor, the other one will run off, one will just stop and not co-operate. So over half term I don't go anywhere, because I've got both of them. And so I put them in care club for two days, which is always a disaster 'cause Lauren doesn't really cope with it, but I can't cope unless she goes, 'cause I can't have them all week.

I: Well, there might be something, we get this sitting service from the local volunteer bureau, and the other thing that's happened recently is that we got some support from money funded through Aiming High for Disabled Children [AHDC]. The volunteer bureau have used the money to set up a befriending group, so now there's someone who comes once a fortnight for just under two hours. There might be something similar in your area. (At this point, the interviewer and interviewee began to look on the internet for information about AHDC in Roberta's local area.)

There were times in the interviews where roles were 'reversed' as the mothers asked the researcher a series of questions. In one interview, Natalie (N), the mother of a 4-year-old disabled child, asked the interviewer (I), the mother of a 13-year-old disabled child, a series of questions. At this point in the interview it seems roles have been reversed as the interviewer responds to the interviewee's questioning. Natalie was interested in how the interviewer's experiences of parenting had changed over time:

N: I think the thing is, I mean I don't know how it is for you, but even now four and a half years on, it is still a roller coaster, I still have days when it upsets me and days when I think it is fine. And I don't know, I would assume it gets slightly less like this?

I: Yeah, I think it does . . . But yeah, most of the time you're in the fine days, and some days you slip into something else. And the thing is things change and that can sometimes be difficult . . .

N: You know the whole thing about puberty starting and a different kind of place and different challenges . . .

In this extract, the mother of the younger child asks questions of the mother of the older child. There is curiosity on the part of the parent of the younger child about the interviewer's experience of parenting an older child. In the interviewer's response, although there is an element of reciprocity and a willingness to share her parenting experiences with the interviewee, there is also evidence of the researcher 'holding back' as she is ambivalent about whether things get easier as a disabled child grows older. However, even this hesitation could be seen to lead Natalie to talk about her own worries about the onset of puberty.

However, we were also cautious about this approach, so that there were times of self-monitoring when the interviewer 'held back' in talking about her own life. Although, as the extracts above illustrate, the interviewer and the mothers shared some common experiences, it is important to recognise that the experiences of mothers of disabled children are not homogeneous and issues of class, ethnicity, age and the status of the 'academic' researcher all influence the relationship between the interviewer and interviewee (McLaughlin *et al.* 2008).

As a team, we were conscious of trying to avoid the charge that the interviewer was 'faking friendship' in order to elicit 'thick data' which the participants later regretted sharing. We attempted to address this by taking the interviews back to the interviewees, where this was what they wanted, and asking them if they were still happy for us to use what they had said. Although this was one attempt to address the power imbalance between the interviewer and interviewee, we remained mindful of the power imbalances at work in the research relationships.

Voice

Closely linked to the issue of power is the question of voice in qualitative interviews. If the 'data' which results from the research interview is conceived of as a co-production, this raises difficult questions for researchers over whose voice is represented in the subsequent data. Often, researchers wishing to 'give voice' to marginalised groups have chosen interviews as their preferred method of data collection (Goodley 2000). The use of narrative or life history approaches are common among researchers who set out to 'give voice' to groups whose voices are not usually heard. Narrative researchers make claims that through 'in-depth' interviews it is possible to delve into the 'lived experience' of the respondents, thereby generating 'authentic' accounts (see Chapter 9 on narrative). Yet for researchers who accept the interactive nature of the in-depth interview, the value of the narrative is not in its ability to produce an 'objective' account of the social world, but access to a co-construction of 'subjectivity' (Kvale 2006). In the current project, the stories produced were clearly presented as co-constructions between two people, interviewer and interviewee, who were both mothers of disabled children.

Emancipatory interview research

The project also drew heavily on the discipline of disability studies. Disability studies is a relatively new academic discipline and it is interdisciplinary and diverse, drawing on sociology, linguistics, economics, anthropology, politics, history, psychology and cultural studies although in the UK it is rooted in sociology. A key feature of disability research conducted from within disability studies has been a commitment to 'emancipatory' disability research. Barnes (1992) described emancipatory disability research as research 'with' rather than 'on' disabled people. Barnes (1992) was critical of the exclusion that disabled people have experienced in the research process as subjects, not participants in research, and the powerless position this put disabled people in. He argued that disabled people could and should be involved in all stages of the research from the choice of topic for research, method design, data collection and analysis to dissemination.

While researchers within disability studies strive to work within the principles of emancipatory disability research, this is often difficult to achieve at every stage of the research process. In the current project, for example, the project is externally funded by a research council and the research team is made up of university-based researchers. The original bid was written by the research team. However, despite this acknowledgement of the lack of participation by parents/carers and children at the start of the process, the principles underlying the project are participatory as we encouraged the participants to shape the direction and methods used within the research and to comment on and contribute to our findings and analysis. This represents our attempts to address the power imbalance within the research project.

However, following Foucauldian understandings of power relationships (Foucault 1982), we also recognise that power does not flow in one direction. Interviewees have the power to decide whether or not to take part in the project. They are able to withdraw at any time, refuse to answer questions, and certainly shape the nature of the research interview, including time, place, duration and questions answered. Indeed, Miller and Glassner (1997) suggest that the participants' stories can be narratives of resistance of marginalised groups, which offer alternative accounts to those which usually circulate. Issues of power relationships in research are part of the ethical maze (Cocks 2006) facing the interview researcher.

Ethics

Kvale and Brinkman (2009: 62) argue that 'an interview inquiry is a moral enterprise'. As with all qualitative methods, ethical issues necessarily arise because the interview involves delving into people's private lives with the intention of placing these accounts in a public arena (Kvale and Brinkman 2009). Within most areas of the social sciences, it is usual to submit a proposed qualitative project for ethical review before the project can proceed. Within health, education and psychological research there are a number of ethical protocols to which researchers must adhere. The value of submitting a project for ethical review before it can go ahead is that this requires the researcher to think through ethical issues that might arise at every stage of the research project.

As ethical issues can arise at every stage of the research inquiry, it is important to be mindful of ethical issues at each stage of the research. In the first instance the choice of the research topic must have purpose and value. Furthermore, the research design must take into account issues of informed consent and confidentiality, and the participants must be made aware of the possible outcomes of taking part in the study. The appropriateness of the interview method must also be considered, especially given Atkinson and Silverman's (1997) warning against the uncritical overuse of the interview as a research method. Anonymity and confidentiality are key issues for the researcher at the transcription stage, and an ethical inquiry requires that the transcription must also be as close as possible to the conversation that has taken place between the interviewer and interviewee.

Studies can be compromised if the researcher fails to make explicit the way in which the analysis is carried out and whether or not, and to what extent, research participants are able to comment on the analysis. At the stage of reporting the project and disseminating findings, issues of anonymity and confidentiality are key. The impact of the dissemination on individuals or groups of people who have taken part in the study is also an ethical concern for researchers. This was a key ethical concern for our study as at a time of economic crisis and policy flux in services for disabled children we were particularly mindful of how our work might be interpreted and impact on the lives of the families.

The interactive nature of research interviews, combined with the closeness that can develop between interviewer and interviewee, leads Kvale and Brinkman (2009) to point out the dangers in long and repeated interviews on personal topics which may result in a quasi-therapeutic relationship which could make the interviewee vulnerable. Kvale and Brinkman's (2009) concerns could be seen as patronising and paternalistic as they fail to acknowledge the vulnerability of the interviewer in such situations, where both are sharing personal stories. Moreover, some researchers have found that telling their story can be therapeutic for the teller as well as the audience (Atkinson and Silverman 1997). In the current study, different mothers had different reactions to the process of telling their stories. While one mother described it afterwards as 'an ordeal', because it had brought back unhappy memories, another described the interview process as 'uplifting'.

Practicalities

As well as deciding when and where the interview will take place and determining the questions that will shape the interview, the researcher also needs to negotiate the number of times the participant is willing to be interviewed. If the interviews are longitudinal (i.e. they take place over a period of time) the researcher will need to decide on length of the gaps between interviews and negotiate this with the participant. In a longitudinal study, it is common for participants to 'drop out' of a research project. In the current project, as family circumstances changed, some families withdrew from the study.

On a practical note it is, of course, important to have good quality and reliable equipment with which to record the interview. When deciding when and where to conduct an interview, it is useful to think about whether there will be too much background noise, or indeed people who might overhear the conversation. Once the data is recorded it must be carefully looked after in order to ensure the participants' confidentiality and anonymity. Recordings must be destroyed once transcribed and the data analysis is complete. Transcription is an extremely lengthy process and researchers have to decide whether to do the transcription themselves or pay someone else to do it for them – although, of course, not everyone involved in research will have the luxury of choice. The advantages of paying for a transcription service are huge in terms of time saved. However, in the process of transcribing the data some researchers find that they get to know the data better. It allows them to reflect on their role as the interviewer. They are more likely to be able to make sense of indistinct words, and the familiarity with the data gained by doing the transcription yourself can mean that you save time during the analysis process.

In the current study, we did encounter difficulties with voice recordings, usually when there was a lot of background noise, where the mother preferred to be interviewed in a café rather than her own home. This made transcription particularly laborious.

Chapter summary

This chapter has revealed the history and popularity of the qualitative interview as a research method. Despite the popularity of the interview as a qualitative research method, as Potter and Hepburn (2005) suggest, it is difficult to do well. First, the interviewer must consider whether or not an interview is, in fact, the most appropriate method. Second, they must decide: who they want to interview, when and where and for how long and how often. The interviewer must decide how to present themselves to the interviewees and to what extent they intend to disclose aspects of their positionality to the participants in the study. In conducting the interview, the interviewer must decide to what extent they are going to keep a 'professional distance' or whether they are going to become 'passionate' researchers conducting 'illegitimate' interviews (Oakley 1981). The daunting task of analysing large amounts of data also faces the researcher, along with the need to be explicit about the approach to analysis used. Questions of power and ethical considerations permeate every stage of the research process, presenting further challenges for the researcher. Yet, despite the challenges presented by qualitative interview research, interview methods offer the researcher a means of discovering hidden stories, often from marginalised groups, and as such it is no wonder that the qualitative interview remains such a popular method.

References

Atkinson, P. and Silverman, D. (1997) 'Kundera's immortality: the interview society and the invention of the self'. *Qualitative Inquiry*, **3**(3), 304–25.

Barnes, C. (1992) 'Emancipatory disability research: realistic goal or impossible dream?' Available online at: www.leeds.ac.uk/disability-studies/.../Barnes/Chapter%202.pdf.

Behar, R. (2003) 'Ethnography and the book that was lost'. *Ethnography*, **4**, 15–39.

Beresford, B. (1994) *Positively Parents: Caring for a Severely Disabled Child*. London: HMSO.

Blumenfeld-Jones, D. (1995) 'Fidelity as a criterion for practicing and evaluating narrative inquiry', in J. Amos Hatch and R. Wisniewski (eds) *Life History and Narrative*. London: Falmer.

Booth, T. and Booth, W. (1998) *Growing Up with Parents with Learning Difficulties*. London: Routledge.

Burman, E. (1997) 'Minding the gap: positivism, psychology and the politics of the qualitative method'. *Journal of Social Issues*, **58**, 785–801.

Charmaz, C. (2001) 'Grounded theory: objectivist and constructivist methods', in N. Denzin and Y. Lincoln (eds) *Handbook of Qualitative Research*. London: Sage.

Cocks, A. (2006) 'The ethical maze: finding an inclusive path towards gaining children's agreement to research participation'. *Childhood*, **13**(2), 247–66.

DfES (2004) *Every Child Matters: Change for Children*. London: HMSO.

DiCicco-Bloom, B. and Crabtree, B. F. (2006) 'The qualitative research interview'. *Medical Education*, **40**, 314–21.

Fontana, A. and Frey, J. H. (2001) 'The interview: from structured questions to negotiated text', in N. K. Denzin and Y. S. Lincoln (eds) *Handbook of Qualitative Research*, 2nd edn. London: Sage.

Foucault, M. (1982) 'The subject and power', in H. Dreyfus and P. Rabinow (eds) *Michel Foucault: Beyond Structuralism and Hermeneutics*. Brighton: Harvester.

Glaser, B. G. and Strauss, A. L. (1967) *The Discovery of Grounded Theory: Strategies for Qualitative Research*. New York: Aldine.

Goodley, D. (2000) *Self-Advocacy in the Lives of People with Learning Difficulties: The Politics of Resilience*. Maidenhead: Open University Press.

Goodley, D. (2007) 'Becoming rhizomatic parents: Deleuze, Guattari and disabled babies'. *Disability and Society*, **22**(2), 145–60.

Goodley, D., Lawthom, R., Clough, P. and Moore, M. (2004) *Researching Life Stories: Method, Theory and Analyses in a Biographical Age*. London: Routledge Falmer.

Goodson, I. (1995) 'The story so far, personal knowledge and the political', in J. Amos Hatch and R. Wisniewski (eds) *Life History and Narrative*. London: Falmer.

Harrison, J., MacGibbon, L. and Morton, M. (2001) 'Regimes of trustworthiness in qualitative research: rigors of reciprocity'. *Qualitative Inquiry*, **7**(3), 323–45.

Kozinets, R. V. (2010) *Netography: Doing Ethnographic Research Online*. London: Sage.

Kvale, S. (2006) 'Dominance through interviews and dialogues'. *Qualitative Inquiry*, **12**, 480–500.

Kvale, S. and Brinkman, S. (2009) *Interviews: Learning the Craft of Qualitative Research Interviewing*. London: Sage.

Madge, C. and O'Connor, H. (2002) 'On-line with e-mums: exploring the internet as a medium for research'. *Area*, **34**(1), 92–102.

McLaughlin, J., Goodley, D., Clavering, E. and Fisher, P. (2008) *Families Raising Disabled Children: Enabling Care and Social Justice*. Basingstoke: Palgrave Macmillan.

Miller, J. and Glassner, B. (1997) 'The "inside" and the "outside": finding realities in interviews', in D. Silverman (ed.) *Qualitative Research: Theory, Method and Practice*. London: Sage.

Oakley, A. (1981) 'Interviewing women: a contradiction in terms', in H. Roberts (ed.) *Doing Feminist Research*. London: Routledge and Kegan Paul.

Oakley, A. (1998) 'Gender, methodology and people's ways of knowing: some problems with feminism and the paradigm debate in social sciences'. *Sociology*, **32**, 707–31.

Polkinghorne, D. E. (1995) 'Narrative configuration in qualitative analysis', in J. A. Hatch and R. Wisniewski (eds) *Life History and Narrative*. London: Falmer Press.

Potter, J. and Hepburn, A. (2005) 'Qualitative interviews in psychology: problems and possibilities'. *Qualitative Research in Psychology*, **2**, 1–27.

Potter, J. and Wetherell, M. (1994) *Discourse and Social Psychology*. London: Sage.

Read, J. (2000) *Listening to Mothers*. Maidenhead: Open University Press.

Rose, G. (1997) 'Situating knowledges: positionality, reflexivities and other tactics'. *Progress in Human Geography*, **21**(3), 305–32.

Runswick-Cole, K. (2007) '"The Tribunal was the most stressful thing: more stressful than my son's diagnosis or behaviour": the experiences of families who go to the Special Educational Needs and Disability Tribunal (SENDIST)'. *Disability and Society*, **22**(3), 315–28.

Silverman, D. (2001) 'Analyzing talk and text', in N. K. Denzin and Y. S. Lincoln (eds) *Handbook of Qualitative Research*, 2nd edn. London: Sage.

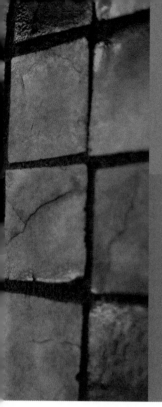

Chapter 7

The repertory grid and its possibilities

Carol Tindall

Introduction

Kelly was a psychotherapist interested in facilitating individual change. It was from this position and experiential base that he developed his theory, in the sociocultural milieu of the USA in the 1950s. The unique idiosyncratic individual is at the heart of Kelly's (1955) *personal construct theory* (PCT). He emphasises that it is our individual experiencing which forms the basis of our personal reality. PCT is phenomenological with an individual ontology. It focuses on how things (phenomena), particularly ourselves and other people, appear to us and are understood by us; in Kelly's terms, how we personally construe ourselves, others and the world which we inhabit.

Some brief and necessarily selective background to PCT is required as the methods of PCT are firmly grounded in the ontological base of the theory, although 'they [PCT methods] are still sometimes applied as if they were standardised, objective tests, perhaps reflecting the divorce of techniques from their theoretical basis' (Walker and Winter 2007: 460). Our reality, according to Kelly, is continually created via the meanings we attach to our experiencing. We are understood as meaning makers. Kelly's person is an adventurer actively engaged in exploring their social world, forever in process, striving to understand themselves, others and what is going on around them. His interest was in how people know rather than what they know, the processes involved in this individual sense making, which for Kelly are rooted in the meanings we attach to our experiences. He proposed that each of us develops our highly individual personal frameworks of meaning based on processing our understanding of experiencing – this he termed our construing. It is our construing, our meaning making, that is influential, not the actual experiences themselves. Our construing is continuous; we are constantly engaged in meaning making and modifying our constructs, much of which goes on almost beyond our awareness. Construing is experiencing at all levels of awareness, thoughts, feelings and actions, in personal harmony.

It is this dynamic building up and simultaneous ongoing search for personal meaning that is our reality, our basis for understanding the world, including ourselves. Kelly emphasised our sense of agency, rather than the ways we might be structured by our biology, our early years' experiences or social processes. We are not merely expressions of our genetic inheritance, our unconscious drives, nor performers of the social ideologies of our time – we make choices:

> People are neither prisoners of their environment nor victims of their biographies but active individuals struggling to make sense of their experiencing and acting in accordance with the meaning they impose on those experiences.
>
> (Kelly 1955: 15)

Our current reality is just that, according to Kelly – current, open to personal reconstruction. The philosophical basis of PCT, 'constructive alternativism', makes this potential for reconstruction clear by acknowledging that we can always understand things differently, and that we alter our construing in an attempt to improve our ability to anticipate: 'even the most obvious occurrences in daily life might appear utterly transformed if we were inventive enough to construe them differently' (Kelly 1986: 1). It therefore follows that each individual's subjective reality is personal to them and thus different from others. This championing of personally constructed multiple realities, open to change, positions PCT as a relativist theory.

Our understanding is, according to Kelly, constructed by recognising the similarities and differences in our experiencing. Our meaning making is assumed to be based on idiosyncratic opposites or bipolar constructs. Similarity can only be fully understood in the context of difference. Each bipolar construct gains its meaning from both poles, that is, each pole qualifies the meaning attached to the other. For example, if one person uses a construct of dull-creative while another uses dull-suggestive, we know that these people are experiencing others differently and have therefore constructed different realities. Our constructions of meanings become fine tuned, richer, more nuanced as we gain a greater variety of experiences. In this way we actively engage in creating a framework of understanding of ourselves, others and events of all sorts, based on the sense we impose on the experiences we encounter.

Our frameworks are theorised by Kelly as being hierarchically linked; core constructs are central to our meaning making, to our concept of self. They are our value system and it is these which we use to impose personal order on our lives. Each core construct subsumes a cluster of subordinate constructs, which in turn subsumes more subordinate constructs and so on. This active framework, which has its roots in our personal history of sense making, is simultaneously used as the lens through which we interpret current activity and also anticipate what is likely to happen next. Our personal frameworks, if they are serving us well, enable us to choose appropriate actions from the range of actions we believe are available to us. Our choice is informed by our anticipation of those actions offering us the greatest possibility for learning and extending ourselves.

Essentially, our personal network of constructs is our current narrative of what seems to be going on, which gains its validity by testing out its utility in our lifeworld. If our very personal understanding of what is going on chimes with others' understandings and enables us to interact effectively, then it is useful and therefore valid – if not, we need to readjust or reconstrue. Kelly, ever the pragmatist, emphasised the importance of the personal utility of our constructs. Essentially – do they work for us? This internally located system of experientially based constructs that is constantly being validated and fine tuned symbolises a self that is meaning-based, fluid and changeable, a person with agency, theories and plans, with echoes here again of relativism.

I am interested to see that since the first edition of this book in 1994, a variety of authors have explored potential links between Kelly's theory of personal construction and social constructionist principles. This was always an enticing liaison, although fraught with dilemmas, the most fundamental being the individual ontology of Kelly versus the social ontology of constructionism. PCT, it is claimed, has the potential to begin to dissolve this dualism, although this potential has not been realised and still remains in 2010 'a division left unresolved' (Burkitt 1996: 71). From a constructionist perspective we are all constructs of our cultural and historical context, we are ourselves embedded meaning makers. As Billig (1987) suggests, what we think of as the private sphere of the mind is in fact an internalised version of the public sphere of society.

This fits very neatly with PCT. Although Kelly's focus was very much on the private sphere, he emphasised that our personal understandings arise from joint social action. Indeed, even our sense of self is seen as relational, constructed by our understanding of others' views of us (Bannister 1983). We anticipate and choose to act based on our understanding of others' constructions, a meshing together in a social context of each person's construct system, to enable individual understanding and inform choice of action. Clearly any system that is learned via social interaction can never be entirely personal (Butt 2001); the individual and their social world are inextricably intertwined. Aspects of context are implicitly present in PCT and many (Salmon 1990; Chiari and Nuzzo 1996; Mascolo *et al.* 1997; Butt 2001) have emphasised the embeddedness of construing. Clearly our individual constructs arise from the social world in which we immerse ourselves; it is this which offers us possibilities. As Walker and Winter suggest: 'we are enmeshed within a cultural decision matrix which at the same time presents choices and limits the extent of the choices available' (2007: 456). Just as our idiosyncratic constructs arise from our social contexts, so too are they validated within our contexts. The social reality that surrounds us is our testing ground. Thus, we are firmly embedded active creators of our own personal meaning. However, we should remember that Kelly's interest was in the individual decision maker, caught up in the structures and ideologies of their social worlds, not the structures themselves.

It is the experiential and lifelong active learning basis of PCT, the constant enriching of our understandings or reconstruing, that gives us the grounding for our idiosyncrasy. We do not necessarily buy into the current social values and discourses that surround us. We filter and reconstrue them in ways that make particular sense to us by actively engaging in exploring and understanding our lifeworld.

It is also true that even within the same sociocultural context and time frame, there are myriad cultures and settings in which we immerse ourselves, which impact on our construing. We can imagine that the person attempting to live a sustainable life on a small UK island, for example, is engaged in a set of very different experiences from those of a London city banker. Each too is likely to have developed different understandings, via their individual history of sense making, through which to make meaning of their experiences, which will further personalise their reality. It is this individuality that was important to Kelly. However, we clearly invest our individuality in our social networks, constantly interacting, both influencing and being influenced by others within our networks – we are indeed social beings. Butt (2001) makes a very convincing argument for PCT to be elaborated as a social psychology: 'one which emphasizes the primacy of interaction and social practices' (p. 76). He also claims that Kelly offers a postmodern understanding of self as a fictional and provisional construction (p. 86).

The repertory grid

Kelly's individual is a unique system of experientially based constructions potentially open to change, there is no notion in PCT of an essential self. Kelly developed a whole set of phenomenologically based qualitative research methods to enable access and revelation of each person's idiosyncratic personal frameworks. Pope (2003) suggests that making these constructs explicit, available for exploration and reflection, is the first step in opening up the possibility of change. Here I intend to focus on the potential for qualitative exploration that the repertory grid offers. For information on PCT's other methods, see Fransella (2003) and Tindall (1994). Grids offer the potential to reveal the ways in which people understand and engage with their personal worlds, and importantly the implications of their idiosyncratic sense making. For researchers, grids offer an opportunity to glance into aspects of people's personal worlds, as revealed by the grid. Repertory grids (rep grids) that offer a different way of doing phenomenological enquiry remain marginal within social psychology, rarely appearing in texts such as this, which is why this level of detail about how to create a grid is necessary here. However, their utility and potential are evidenced by the array of contexts within which they seem to have proved useful to practitioners: for example, exercise and sport settings (Gucciardi and Gordon 2009); educational psychology (Higgins *et al.* 2009); clinical settings (Neimeyer and Winter 2006); the Probation Service (Macrae and Andrew 2000); CAMHS (Moran *et al.* 2009); and Smith's (1990) case study work using rep grids to explore his participant's changing sense of self during transition to motherhood. For a comprehensive summary of the variety of contexts within which PCT has recently been used, see Walker and Winter (2007: 463–7).

All PCT methods reflect phenomenological principles; the subjectivity of the participant is key to the research. Our aim as researchers is to gain an insider's perspective. Kelly was very clear that if you wanted to understand someone, then you must be curious about them, ask them about themselves, for each of us is our own expert. It is we as researchers who are the naïve explorers in the participant's world, aiming to do our best to understand. In order to gain an authentic participant voice we must involve ourselves in the lifeworld of our participants, empathise with them, get to know their story, explore their social worlds through their frameworks. Higgins *et al.* support the rep grid's ability to offer this, claiming 'that PCP allows me [an educational psychologist] to hear the pupil's voice' (2009: 7). Research is understood as a formalised version of everyday construing. Both participant and researcher are engaged in a collaborative mutual exploration to access and represent aspects of the participant's reality, ideally driven by the participant's need to understand, but it is likely that the research question may well also be part of the researcher's reality. The subjectivity of the participant and researcher is acknowledged as central to the research process, as is the opportunity that the ongoing process offers both for new understandings. However, we must bear in mind that the completed research is a construction, a partial representation of the participant's current reality, and needs to be judged on its utility, its fitness for purpose, whatever the stated purpose, and is of course open to reconstruction.

The research process of negotiating a repertory grid

I want to take the opportunity here to emphasise the rep grid's humanist grounding: 'PCP is basically a humanist theory . . . with an emphasis on free choice and the creation of personal meaning' (Raskin 2002: 5). Used in the Kellyan, humanist sense, the participant is in charge. It is the person doing the construing (not the researcher) who is at the heart of the meaning making used to develop the grid, thus shifting the power dynamic somewhat. The researcher is of course responsible for the research process within which the participant makes choices and takes responsibility for providing the personal information used to create the grid. If our aim is to access part of the participant's world, to hear their voice, then it is they who need to provide the content of the grid and we as researchers who need to facilitate their ability and willingness to provide authentic content.

Initially I will introduce three ways in which the grid might be used, outline the tasks involved in developing useful grids and highlight the grid's potential for unexpected revelation. For more detail of the variety of ways in which the rep grid might be used, see Walker and Winter (2007). Each of the options here provides the opportunity of constructing a repertory grid to reveal in part either your own construing of an aspect of your reality if you choose to work alone, or the opportunity to focus on shared or joint understandings if you choose to work with someone else. Each of these grid variations may be seen as ways of structuring conversations, either with yourself or with others, and are interpretations, not neutral reflections of reality (Jankowicz 2003).

First, you may use the grid to focus on yourself, on how you experience an aspect of your own life; such a focus on self is unfortunately a relatively rare opportunity in psychology but is very much in keeping with Kelly's focus on reflexivity. Alternatively, you may facilitate someone else interested in exploring an aspect of their reality to develop a grid. Whoever completes the grid is required to reflect on their own experiencing with the intention of gaining insight and thus increasing self-awareness, which offers the potential to facilitate change.

You may prefer to focus on the extent of your understanding of someone you have a need to understand for personal or professional reasons; i.e. your ability to empathise, to connect with another's reality. This involves your participant constructing a repertory grid to reveal their current understanding of a mutually agreed topic. Their grid is then offered to you in skeleton form to complete 'as if' you were them. The extent to which you are able to understand their understanding is revealed once the grids are combined. Our ability to understand, although not necessarily agree with, the way an event or context is experienced by someone else, facilitates more effective interaction with that person.

Third, you may want to focus on agreement, to explore the extent to which your construction of a negotiated aspect of a personal or professional relationship agrees with your participant's. This involves you both in a process of collaboration to produce a skeleton grid which you jointly consider appropriate to the topic of exploration. Then you each complete the grid separately from your own perspective, revealing, once the grids are combined, the extent to which your current understanding of the topic matches theirs. Specifically you are exploring the particular areas and extent of agreement between your view and your participant's view of your jointly selected topic. Areas of agreement and discord will be highlighted during the analysis, thus opening up problem-solving potential.

Caution

There is often the assumption that PCT methods operate at a superficial, known level. This indeed may be the case. It depends to some extent, although not entirely, on the level at which you and/or your participant choose to work. Anyone completing the grid needs to be aware of the potential it has for making explicit personal links and patterns between constructs and elements. Such revelations of idiosyncratic understandings offer new insights and thus potential for change; often the very reason for completing it and indeed an absolute strength of the grid. However, simultaneously they may be disturbing. Both you and your participant need to be aware of the possibility of such revelations. As Salmon and Claire (1984: 203) made clear: 'Grids offer access to living material, to the very terms in which people experience and engage with their own personal worlds . . . enable the elicitation of hitherto unverbalized levels of construing, and reveal the complex intuitive ramifications involved in making human sense.' As with any research it is essential that you gain the fully informed consent of your participant, that is, they must know of the possibility of revelations in order to give informed consent.

Generating a repertory grid

Initially, you need to identify a current personally relevant area of interest. Next, you need to think about a specific research aim or question, either alone or, if you have elected to explore understanding or agreement, you need to negotiate a topic and research aim of mutual interest with your participant. The topic and research aim will usually be driven, in true Kellyan spirit, by personal or professional curiosity and arise from experience.

Having decided on your research aim, you then need to choose elements which reflect your topic area. If your research aim is something to do with your current roles, then the elements will be your roles. Elements are 'items of experience', according to Thomas and Harri-Augstein (1985: 99); they are anything that gives rise to construing. They can be people, aspects of work, leisure activities, television programmes, holidays, cultures, social activities, restaurants, etc. Your element sample needs to vary on dimensions relevant to the topic and the participant/s in order to develop the most illuminating grid. Your aim when choosing your elements is to allow the most useful grid to be generated. Inadequate elements limit the grid's possibilities. Elements should be representative of your topic, relevant to your research aim and known reasonably well. For example, if I am interested in my construing of friends, then my elements need to represent my range of friends and friend possibilities in my life: someone who is a well-established friend; a relatively 'new' friend; someone who was a friend but is no longer; friends from different contexts of my life; someone who has the potential to be a friend but who is currently marginal; maybe a friend I find tricky and another I find easy, and so on. If I am interested in how I understand myself in comparison with how I understand my friends, I must also include myself as an element.

If you choose to work with someone else to explore your level of understanding of that person then you must explain to them how to generate the grid. The topic selected for exploration needs to be of mutual interest and because you both need a good understanding of the elements chosen by the participant there is some collaboration involved. If you are interested in exploring your degree of agreement with your participant, maybe as a mentor/mentee, for example, elements need to be jointly negotiated.

Structuring the grid around a range of elements that clearly represent the topic area and are personal to whoever is generating the grid provides the greatest possibility of developing a grid which offers new understandings. It is rather like ensuring that your interview topics have the potential to generate rich informative material of the topic being explored. I suggest using about ten elements, more than ten can become unwieldy and fewer than six reduces possibilities. For examples of ranges of elements for all three grid variations see Tindall (1998). In order to build the grid, the chosen elements need to be written across the page (see Figure 7.1).

Your next task is to make explicit some of the current understandings of the topic by using the chosen elements to elicit constructs. This is done by choosing any three of the ten elements, either randomly or systematically, and asking how two of these elements are the same and different from the third. The identified similarity, whether positive or negative, is written on the left of the grid and the identified difference on the right. The language used to identify construct

ELEMENTS

Similarity pole	Interesting	Own	Ideal	Quirky	Dodgy	Mundane	Dislike	Difference pole
Secure together								Subject to outside forces
Equalish								One dominant
Separate lives								United
Embrace change								Traditional values
Loosely bonded								Bonded through children
Trust and loyalty								Fabrications
Supportive								Dismissive (not really present)
Habit holds them together								Commitment holds them together
Home-based living								More transient living
Closed to each other								Open and accepting

Figure 7.1 Ali's grid (Ali is introduced in the worked example on p. 109)

poles will be idiosyncratic. Participants should be encouraged to represent their meanings as individually and as clearly as they can. Metaphors and phrases are often more meaningful than single word labels. Accessing constructs is often managed by writing each element on a separate card, shuffling the cards and choosing the top three to work with. Used cards are returned to the pack, reshuffled and the next top three chosen, and so on. The purpose here is to reveal the participant's current bipolar constructs and the process continues until the participant runs out of constructs. Ideally, you will have 20 or so constructs to work with. These may be whittled down to between 10 and 15 at a later stage (see Figure 7.1).

If you are exploring understanding, your participant accesses their constructs using the method outlined above and adds them to their grid. If you are exploring agreement, there is a need to jointly develop constructs. In reality it seems to be more effective if each of you identifies your own constructs using the jointly chosen elements and then come together to negotiate which to include, ensuring that both of you contribute as equally as possible. At the end of this stage you should have a skeleton grid with elements and constructs identified, as in Figure 7.1.

Next, each element needs to be located on each construct using an ordinal scale of 1–5. A 1 indicates that the element is experienced as very like the similarity end of the bipolar construct. A 5 indicates that the element is experienced as very like the difference end of the construct. A rating of 3 may indicate that the element being considered is experienced as neutral on that construct, or fluctuating, sometimes like the identified similarity and at other times like the identified difference. In this way all of the elements are positioned in relative terms on each of the constructs, but the numbers carry no inherent meaning. They are not test scores used to compare across grids; they simply add shades of meaning to the relationships between elements and constructs as currently understood by the participant. If you are exploring understanding, then you use your participant's skeleton grid and complete the ratings that you expect they have given. If you are exploring agreement, however, you take the jointly developed grid and each complete the rating separately as yourselves.

It is at this stage in the process that you may find that some of the constructs are not applicable to some of the elements. The best way to deal with this is to refine the grid. You may decide to change an element or, much more likely, change a construct. For example, the grid shown in Figure 7.3 (p. 110) initially included relationship elements Ideal and Exciting, which attracted very similar ratings from all participants. Therefore, Exciting was deleted as it was not adding greater meaning to the grid, although it is interesting to note that for all these participants their ideal relationship is also one that is seen as exciting. Equally, constructs are refined at this point and any that are too similar need looking at. The elements in the grid shown in Figure 7.3 attracted constructs *Traditional parenting/Shared parenting* and *Couple not well connected/ Couple well connected* which were very similarly rated across elements. During the negotiation between the participant and myself it was decided that the *Connected* construct contained more useful information about how relationships are understood; therefore this is the one that was kept. Modifications such as these during data collection are very much part of the qualitative process. When making such changes it is necessary to remember that the research aim is always the focus, or alternatively you may choose to modify your aim. The purpose is to develop the most authentic and illuminating grid, which in the example below offers participants understandings of couple relationships.

Analysis

Analysis is a focus on patterns of meaning evident in the grid that are relevant to the research aim, not a search for all possible meanings. Grid analysis is also a relatively open part of the research process, one which allows the participant to explore their current understanding of their area of interest by analysing construct patterns. Alternatively, they may choose to explore how they understand the grid elements in relation to one another by comparing element patterns, or their interest may be in the associations between elements and constructs. All are possible.

Before patterns of understanding and agreement between you and your participant can be identified, the grids need to be combined. Take a blank grid, divide each square diagonally and include both sets of ratings in the divided square. Use different colour pens, one for each of you. See Figure 7.2 for an illustration of part of a combined grid. If you are interested in exploring understanding or agreement with someone and need more detail than I present here of how to generate and analyse joint grids, please see Tindall (1998).

Analysis is an ongoing integral part of the research process. Understandings are evident from the outset, from the choice of topic, through to the specific aim, to which elements and constructs are chosen and discarded, and beyond to how readily constructs are verbalised and used. As our interest is in the participant's understanding, it is initially for them to analyse and gain their own understanding of the grid.

Conversational exploration

This exploration can be the most useful aspect of the analysis. Use your reflexive awareness, or encourage your participant to use theirs, to explore grid revelations by conducting a critical conversation with yourself about what the grid has illuminated. Are you aware of any omissions? What are the implications of associations revealed? Are there many surprises? It may be a good idea to discuss grid revelations with a trusted friend. Remember if you do that you are dealing with two different ways of experiencing what is going on. To increase self-awareness, remain open to their views rather than impose your own reality on them or accept their reality as more useful than yours.

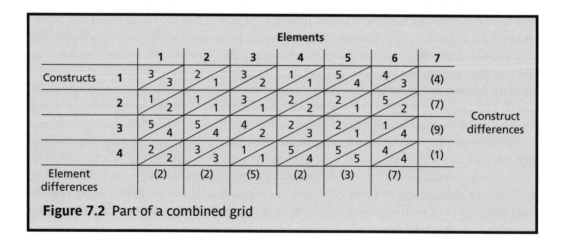

Figure 7.2 Part of a combined grid

The critical, exploratory conversation needs sensitive handling for the understanding and agreement options, as you are dealing with your participant's reality as well as your own understandings. Encourage your participant to comment on meanings and patterns apparent to them from their own grid and the degree of understanding/agreement that you have achieved, which is apparent from the combined grid. If your participant does not verbalise obvious connections made explicit by the grids, it is not necessarily your role to voice them. Emergent implications may be sensitively checked out with the participant, but do be aware of the potential for harm. The grid may make explicit associations that the participant chooses not to acknowledge at this time with you.

A worked example

I worked with two women who were interested, as I was, in focusing on understandings of personal rather than work settings. After much discussion the three of us, Ali, Lexis and Eva, decided to explore our construing of couple relationships. I followed their interest enthusiastically. Participants, including myself, were keen to take time to reflect on and gain some illumination of our understandings of couple relationships. I also felt the need to re-engage with the experience of working up a grid with participants.

I talked to participants about the key aspects of the rep grid, highlighting that it was their understandings using their own language that we were attempting to access. Each was also cautioned about the potential for surprise understandings to be revealed. I showed them Alex's rep grid (Tindall 1994: 80) as an example of a completed grid highlighting the revelations which emerged for Alex. We began by separately developing some mini grids around relationships to ground ourselves in the process and focus on intimate relationships. Between us we negotiated a potentially representative range of couple relationship elements. These were: Interesting, Own, Ideal, Quirky, Dodgy, Mundane, Dislike (see Figure 7.1). We each then had to individually identify known relationships which for us were, Mundane, Quirky, Dodgy, etc. Interestingly, when participants were deciding which relationships to identify with each element all asked about the possibility of using fictitious couples as elements. This is absolutely fine as it is the participant's understandings we are aiming to reveal – whether the relationships are real or fictitious is not important. What is important is that participants have a relatively detailed view of the relationship, real or fictitious.

Together we developed our individual grids, that is, we were all in the same room but completed our own grids quite separately from each other. Grids were constructed with enthusiasm, thoughtful moments and much laughter. Constructs initially flowed very readily in response to the card method described above, and more haltingly latterly; each of us writing our constructs on our own grids. These were not spoken of by any of us during the development of our grids, although each of us later shared our completed grids.

My reading of construct choices suggests a different underlying value for understanding relationships for each participant. Ali used constructs such as: *Secure together–More subject to outside forces; Trust and loyalty–Fabrications; Steady–Volatile; Support each other–Dismissive of each other, not really present; Together due to habit–Together due to commitment.* These constructs illustrated for me at least an underlying value of support and companionship. Lexis identified the following constructs: *Rely on each other–Independent of each other; Mundane, dull–Make an*

Similarity	Interesting	Own	Ideal	Quirky	Dodgy	Mundane	Dislike	Difference
Peaceful	4	4	4	4	5	1	2	Some conflict
Have fun	1	3	3	3	4	2	5	Seem distant
Not well connected	5	4	5	5	1	4	1	Strong connection
Enthusiastic life	1	1	1	1	4	2	5	Switched off
Egalitarian	4	2	1	2	4	2	5	One-sided
Fun to be with	1	1	1	2	4	5	5	Hard work
Joint agreements	2	1	1	1	3	2	5	One dictates
Loyal	2	2	1	1	4	1	5	Undermine each other
Open and accepting	2	2	1	1	4	4	4	Tad rigid
Risk taking	4	2	1	4	4	5	5	Cautious
Talk about emotions	1	4	1	4	4	1	5	Functional communication

ELEMENTS

Figure 7.3 Eva's grid illustration

effort in the relationship; Fun couple–'Nice' couple; Alive and engaged in relationship–Lacking energy; Closed to each other–open and accepting; Stuck–Future plans. Lexis herself during completion of the grid spontaneously identified that many of her constructs are to do with the liveliness she sees within the couple and whether each is seen as actively engaged in the relationship or merely present. Eva's example included here (see Figure 7.3) suggests to me an underlying value of equality as an important aspect of her understanding of couples.

Analysis

The completed grid is a partial representation, according to PCT, of Eva's current experiencing of couple relationships. Bearing in mind that the research aim is to explore Eva's understandings of couple relationships, our first interest must be in constructs (grid rows). My reading of Eva's set of constructs, developed for this purpose at this time and with me, is that many are aspects of relationship equality. It may be that equality is an important value for Eva, one that she is alert to. Looking at associations between constructs, it seems that Eva experiences all those couples viewed as *Open and accepting* to also be *Loyal* and *Fun to be with*; the corollary being that couples viewed as being a *Tad rigid* also *Undermine each other* and for Eva are experienced as *Hard work*. This implies that Eva may use these constructs in combination. For example, Eva may assume that a 'new' couple she finds *Fun to be with* is also *Loyal* and *Open*, whereas a couple she experiences as *Hard work* is more likely to be understood as *Rigid* and *Undermining of each other*.

According to Kelly, these understandings are what Eva has gained from her experiences of couple relationships, both directly and indirectly, and this association of understandings will in turn affect her experiencing of relationships around her, including her own. Interestingly, the couple she identified as *Mundane* fail to follow this pattern as they are seen as *Hard work*, *Somewhat rigid*, yet *Loyal*. A mirror image association evident in Eva's grid is found between *Have fun–Seem distant* and *Not well connected–Strongly connected*. If we swap *Seem distant–Have fun*, there is a good but not exact match with *Not well connected–Strongly connected*, suggesting that Eva sees *Strongly connected* couples as ones that *Have fun*, and conversely couples seen as *Not well connected, Seem distant* to Eva. Another interesting construct association for me is the one between *Egalitarian–One-sided* and *Risk takers–Cautious*. The only exceptions to the use of this association are the two couples identified as Quirky and Mundane, all other couples who are experienced as *Egalitarian* are understood to be *Risk takers*, while the couples viewed as *Cautious* are understood to be *One-sided*. There are numerous patterns within the grid which are potentially worthy of elaboration with Eva, via conversational exploration. However, such explorations need to be guided by Eva's reading of her grid.

Eva might have been interested in comparing her view of her own relationship with her view of other couples in her grid. In this case she would focus on analysing patterns across elements (grid columns). We can see that her view of her Own relationship is not too distant from what she regards as her Ideal, the greatest difference being that she views her Own relationship as involving largely *Functional communication*, whereas her ideal couple would *Talk about emotions*. Her Own relationship and the one she finds Interesting are also reasonably close. There are similarities too between her Own relationship and the one she identified as Dodgy, specifically on the constructs *Talk about emotions–Functional communication*, *Have fun–Seem distant* and *Peaceful–Some conflict*. There is a difference of at least two points on the five-point scale on all other constructs, the greatest differences being on *Not well connected–Strongly connected* and *Enthusiastic–Switched off*.

To fully explore the personal implications of the understandings of couple relationships revealed here, we would need to know a little more about Eva. One of the most effective ways to do this is to use the grid content as a basis for a detailed exploration of Eva's current views of couple relationships. This would need sensitive handling and Eva would need to be assured that the exploration would be guided by her reading of the grid and the level of disclosure would be entirely her choice; in line with Kelly's view of participants being experts on their own lives and that meanings should not be imposed by outsiders. However, these are not easy, clear-cut decisions to make. The purpose of the conversational exploration, which is rather like an interview using the grid as the starting point, is always to extend understanding of the participant's world. When working alongside participants, we must be mindful that it is their personal understandings that are being discussed and be sensitive to and respectful of their reactions. We must tune in to their responses and be guided by them as we are explorers within their reality.

Evaluation

The repertory grid puts the participant centre stage – our interest is in their subjectivity, the sense they make of their world. Participant reading of the grid is of primary value, rather than outsider or theoretical understandings. In reality, as is evident from the numerous practitioner papers cited, practitioners such as teachers, probation officers and therapists also analyse or provide a reading of the grid. The main purpose, however, to the extent this is possible, is to externalise the participant's current understanding, sometimes solely to gain insight, or more often to use the insight as a basis for intervention, sometimes involving professionals.

A specific strength of the grid is its ability to highlight the implications of individual understandings in ways that an interview never can. Examples of surprise revelations abound in the literature. For instance, when Barbara Thompson (1975), a nursery school teacher, analysed her own grid she was able to see that her need for a tidy classroom was inhibiting the children's creativity which she was keen to facilitate. Gaining this information about how she used her constructs enabled her to offer a classroom that invited creativity. Alex (Tindall 1994) was also astonished to see that he had construed himself as very similar to someone that he had 'no respect for'. Salmon (1995) – using the Salmon line which is a variation of the grid – demonstrated how pupils and their teacher had completely different understandings of the purpose of design and technology; the pupils understanding the classroom as a mini production unit while the teacher believed it be a space for collaborative creativity. Macrae and Andrew (2000: 37), also claim that PCT understandings have enabled them to see how they might 'reconcile the need to develop effective noncollusive ways of engaging with violent men, with the feminist analysis of domestic violence'.

Can we assume that the understandings gleaned from the grid are authentic? This is in part to do with the ethical tensions inherent throughout the dynamic of the research process. I agree with Willig's (2005) notion of the qualitative research process as an adventure, one which intrinsically involves many dilemma-laden decisions. Working phenomenologically, venturing into personal meanings sometimes not yet acknowledged or articulated by participants, needs sensitive handling. The authenticity of the participant's voice may well be undermined by a researcher's lack of sensitivity around ethical issues and by the censoring that the participant engages in during completion of the grid. Ethical issues are never absolutes that can be easily dealt with via a checklist but ever-present aspects of the research process (see Chapter 14).

We are working with language which does not have the capacity to authentically convey the richness and nuances of personal experience. Nor can we assume that the same term is understood similarly by participants and those working with them. An assumption of PCT which also has an effect on the authenticity of the meanings revealed is that our understandings are bipolar. Participants are required to identify idiosyncratic opposites in order to complete the grid; they are forced to think in terms of opposites. These key aspects of the grid process potentially diminish the authenticity of the participant's voice.

What of the authenticity of readers other than the participant? A common mistake we make as readers is to believe that the grid offers a complete and general picture of participant reality, rather than one that is partial and specific to the grid topic, and due to the constant enriching of understanding, one that is also transient. Readers bring their own subjectivity to their reading, informed by their personal, theoretical and possibly professional frameworks. There is much debate about our ability to bracket our own understandings (Finlay 2008) when attempting to understand others on their own terms, and indeed whether bracketing (if achievable) is desirable. If we are constantly engaged in construing, as Kelly claims, then it is inevitable that we bring our own reading to the grid. How else can we understand other than through our own frameworks, no matter how self-aware we may be? Just as participants complete the grid for a particular purpose, so each reader, professional or otherwise, will read the grid according to their own agenda/s. We must therefore make our agenda, our part in the research, including the analysis, transparent by including reflexive commentary. See Finlay (2008) and Chapter 1 of this text for consideration of how bracketing intertwines with reflexivity. Such an account of subjectivity does not give permission to make claims that cannot be grounded in grid content unless they are identified as speculative.

Kelly's focus on the interior world of the individual neglects the way we are situated in particular sociopolitical contexts at specific times that structure possibilities for all of us. Many, including Kelly, have emphasised the social nature of personal construing (see Introduction), but the ontological gap between personal and social constructionism continues to be too vast to be successfully negotiated. Interestingly, for each of the three individually developed grids mentioned above, I was able to identify a different major underlying theme or discourse! Ali's seemed to me to be based on the ideology of support and companionship, Lexis' on active engagement in the relationship, and Eva's on equality. There is no doubt that the powerful external forces within which we are located affect our experiencing and the 'decisions' we make through life. In Smail's words:

> Rather than being . . . autonomous agents . . . we are in fact infinitessimal social atoms caught in a vast and complex web of power. . . . Not only can we not choose our place in society, but neither can we select our personal experience, decide how to feel about it, nor determine the quality of our relationships through 'acts of will'.
>
> (Smail 1996: 124)

Writers such as Wendy Stainton-Rogers, Carolyn Kagan, David Smail and Frank Furedi make clear from their different positions how our location within networks of power both facilitate and limit possibilities for us all and leave some without access to resources that the many take for granted.

It is evident that systems within which we are located both facilitate and limit personal possibilities and thus our experiencing. Two examples from very different cultures illustrate how our personal lives are structured by the systems within which we are located. First, there is no doubt that the excessive working hours culture in the UK, common in recent years, impacts in serious ways on people's experiences of and contribution to relationships beyond work (Lewis and Campbell 2007). We have yet to see the effects on personal lives of the current (2010) recession, with the inevitable job uncertainty and compulsory redundancies for some. These UK examples demonstrate the power that the political and economic systems have to structure personal lives. A very different example comes from San Cristobel, Ecuador, where I spent some weeks in 2008. What I observed, which surprised me, was young fathers taking care of children before and after school and being actively involved in all aspects of family life. On talking to couples about this, all identified the fact that there were eight men to each woman on the island, and both women and men agreed that this seemingly naturally occurring imbalance affected their relationships.

Chapter summary

In this chapter I emphasise the humanist principles within which PCT and the rep grid are grounded. I use a worked example (with variations) to demonstrate the range of possibilities the rep grid offers to reveal the idiosyncratic meanings that people continuously develop and make use of to construct their reality, framed by the possibilities offered by their sociocultural and political contexts.

References

Bannister, D. (1983) 'Self in personal construct theory', in J. R. Adams-Webber and J. C. Mancuso (eds) *Applications of Personal Construct Theory*. Toronto: Academic Press.

Billig, M. (1987) *Arguing and Thinking: A Rhetorical Approach to Social Psychology*. Cambridge: Cambridge University Press.

Burkitt, I. (1996) 'Social and personal constructs: a division left unresolved'. *Theory and Psychology*, **6**(1), 71–7.

Butt, T. W. (2001) 'Social action and personal constructs', *Theory and Psychology*, **11**(1), 75–95.

Chiari, G. and Nuzzo, M. L. (1996) 'Psychological constructivisms: a metatheoretical differentiation'. *Journal of Constructivist Psychology*, **9**, 163–84.

Finlay, L. (2008) 'A dance between the reduction and reflexivity: explicating the phenomenological psychological attitude'. *Journal of Phenomenological Psychology*, **39**(1), 1–32.

Fransella, F. (ed.) (2003) *International Handbook of Personal Construct Psychology*. Chichester: Wiley.

Gucciardi, D. F. and Gordon, S. (2009) 'Construing the athlete and exerciser: research and applied perspectives from personal construct psychology'. *Journal of Applied Sport Psychology*, **21**(1), 17–33.

Higgins, F., Leahy, C., Mlewa, D., Pike, J., Sharkey, H. and Webster, K. (2009) 'Personal construct psychology in Cardiff Educational Psychology Service'. Cardiff: Cardiff: Educational Psychology Service.

Jankowicz, D. (2003) *The Easy Guide to Repertory Grids*. London: Wiley.

Kelly, G. A. (1955) *The Psychology of Personal Constructs, Volumes 1 and 2*. New York: Norton (reprinted by Routledge, 1991).

Kelly, G. A. (1986) *A Brief Introduction to Personal Construct Theory*. London: Centre for Personal Construct Psychology.

Lewis, J. and Campbell, M. (2007) 'UK work/family balance policies and gender equality, 1997–2005'. *Social Politics*, **14**(1), 4–30.

Macrae, R. and Andrew, M. (2000) 'The use of personal construct theory in work with men who abuse women partners'. *Probation Journal*, **47**(1), 30–8.

Mascolo, M., Craig Bray, L. and Neimeyer, R. A. (1997) 'The construction of meaning and action in development and psychotherapy: an epigenetic approach', in G. J. Neimeyer and R. A. Neimeyer (eds) *Advances in Personal Construct Psychology*. Greenwich, CT: JAI Press.

Moran, H., Pathak, N. and Sharma, N. (2009) 'The mystery of the well-attended group: A model of personal construct therapy for adolescent self-harm and depression in a community CAMHS service'. *Counselling Psychology Quarterly*, **22**(4), 347–59.

Neimeyer, R. A. and Winter, D. A. (2006) 'To be or not to be: personal constructions of the suicidal choice', in E. Thomas (ed.) *Cognition and Suicide: Theory, Research and Therapy*. Washington, DC: American Psychological Association.

Pope, M. (2003) 'Construing teaching and teacher education worldwide', in F. Fransella (ed.) *International Handbook of Personal Construct Psychology*. Chichester: Wiley.

Raskin, J. D. (2002) 'Contructivism in psychology: personal construct psychology, radical constructivism, and social constructionism'. *American Communication Journal*, **5**(3), 1–25.

Salmon, P. (1990) 'Kelly then and now'. Paper presented at the Second British Conference on Personal Construct Psychology, York, UK.

Salmon, P. (1995) *Psychology in the Classroom: Reconstructing Teachers and Learners*. London: Cassell.

Salmon, P. and Claire, H. (1984) *Classroom Collaboration*. London: Routledge and Kegan.

Smail, D. (1996) *How to Survive Without Psychotherapy*. London: Constable.

Smith, J. A. (1990) 'Transforming identities: a repertory grid case-study of the transition to motherhood'. *British Journal of Medical Psychology*, **63**, 239–53.

Thomas, L. F. and Harri-Augstein, E. S. (1985) *Self Organised Learning: Foundations of a Conversational Science for Psychology*. London: Routledge.

Thompson, B. (1975) 'Nursery teachers' perceptions of their pupils: an exploratory study', in J. M. Whitehead (ed.) *Personality and Learning, Vol. 1*. London: Hodder & Stoughton.

Tindall, C. (1994) 'Personal construct approaches', in P. Banister, E. Burman, I. Parker, M. Taylor and C. Tindall, *Qualitative Methods in Psychology: A Research Guide*. Milton Keynes: Open University Press.

Tindall, C. (1998) 'Glances into personal worlds: the construction and analysis of repertory grids', in D. Miell and M. Wetherell (eds) *Doing Social Psychology*. London: Sage.

Walker, B. M. and Winter, D. A. (2007) 'The elaboration of personal construct psychology'. *Annual Review of Psychology*, **58**, 453–77.

Willig, C. (2005) *Introducing Qualitative Research in Psychology: Adventures in Theory and Method*. Maidenhead: Open University Press.

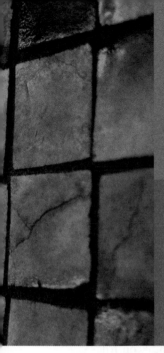

Chapter **8**

Psychosocial analysis

Ian Parker

Introduction

A 'psychosocial analysis' of text as part of the emerging tradition of work in 'psychosocial studies' adds a new dimension to studies of talk and text in discursive psychology. The new dimension it claims to address is the dimension of the 'subject' and it promises an approach to 'subjectivity' that answers some of the criticisms of discourse analysis made from within mainstream psychology as well as criticisms levelled by humanist opponents of laboratory-experimental approaches in the discipline. This chapter reviews the background to the new interest in the 'subject' in psychosocial studies and the role of psychoanalytic theory in describing subjectivity in research. The stance to research taken by two different psychoanalytic approaches is described, and a critical evaluation is provided, along with a critical evaluation of the place of psychoanalytic theory in this new turn to discourse-analytic work.

The return of the subject

The rise of interest in qualitative research in psychology in the last quarter century has been characterised by a concern with *language*. The 'turn to language' in the new paradigm revolution arguments in the 1970s emphasised that the 'accounts' that people give of their actions should be taken seriously, and that these accounts were woven into the 'roles' and 'rules' that structured the little social worlds that human beings inhabit (Harré and Secord 1972; Harré 2004). Language for these new paradigm researchers was the medium through which human subjects reflexively describe and perform who they are for others, and the term 'subject' was thus reclaimed from psychology. The argument was that mainstream laboratory-experimental paradigm psychology treated people as if they were objects, and deception was routinely used in that old paradigm because it was only after the 'subject's' attention was distracted that the experimenter would be able to detect the relationship between independent and dependent variables.

The new paradigm, which argued that for scientific purposes we should treat people as if they were human beings, brought back a more nuanced philosophical conception of the human 'subject' as a creative agent making sense of the world and able to describe that world to researchers. Unlike studies relying on introspection in the earliest years of psychology, however, the new paradigm saw this creative sense-making as already being a public activity through which the human being accounts to others through a shared language. It was the task of the new paradigm researcher in the turn to language to access and value that shared language, to puzzle with subjects as participants in the research about what was going on; and this was done in a number of different settings ranging from schoolrooms to football terraces (Marsh *et al.* 1974; Morgan *et al.* 1979).

The turn to language was given another twist in the turn to *discourse*, and many discourse analysts who worked in the new paradigm tradition also valued the creative activity of the subjects they interviewed. However, there was a shift of attention now to the forms of language as such rather than what the subject made of those forms, and many analysts argued that these forms of language operated independently of the conscious intentions of speakers in conversations and interviews or authors of written texts. These forms of language were sometimes termed 'interpretative repertoires', which acknowledges the creative engagement with discourse of each subject drawing upon them (e.g. Potter and Wetherell 1987), and sometimes termed 'discourses' (e.g. Parker 1992). Discourse analysis developed as a sensitivity to language which attended to the way people constructed their accounts and drew upon different interpretative repertoires, the functions these constructions served and the variability between different constructions and different repertoires. Sometimes also they focused on the way that speaking positions were constructed for subjects, on the functions of discourses in maintaining or resisting power and the contradiction between discourses (e.g. Wetherell and Potter 1992). While one tradition drew on studies of scientific knowledge and preferred to side-step questions about 'humanism' – that is the claim that human beings are the consciously aware locus of action – the other, drawing on structuralist and 'post-structuralist' debates around the work of the historian and philosopher Michel Foucault (1979, 1981), argued that we should take an 'anti-humanist' stance (Parker 2002; Hook 2007). To say that one is 'anti-humanist' means that already existing social and discursive conditions for action are taken seriously; they are the 'conditions of possibility' for things to be said by individuals in different cultures at different points in history.

The different approaches to discourse did not discount human agency, but they were more insistent than the first 'new paradigm' researchers that a search for individual intentions or cognitive paraphernalia inside the head of speakers as an explanation for what was happening in discourse was mistaken (Nikander 1995). Discourse analysis studied *discourse*, not what we imagine to lie beneath it, and speculation about what the individual subject meant by what they were doing would, many discourse analysts argued, get mired in the worst of old paradigm positivist psychology (Edwards and Potter 1992). Laboratory-experimental psychology, they argued, was asking the wrong questions about the inside of the 'subject', and a different notion of subjectivity in language, in discourse, was needed that refused to reduce explanation to the level of the individual. In retrospect, it could now be argued that the turn to language and turn to discourse were already 'psychosocial' approaches, and it is possible now to do discourse analysis under this broad new umbrella term (e.g. Frosh and Saville-Young 2008). However, there was still a key question that haunted the new approaches, one that was asked of them by psychologists and by humanist researchers who wanted to know what people were really thinking when they used language; 'What is the nature of the subject?' Old paradigm psychologists (e.g. Morgan 1996) and new humanist critics of laboratory-experimental psychology (e.g. Reason and Rowan 1981) demanded that the discourse analysts elaborate an alternative model of the subject that would satisfy them.

One alternative was eventually provided by researchers who had preferred 'thematic analysis' to 'discourse analysis', and a description of 'themes' in an interview or written text appeared to them to be more meaningful or, what was more important, it was meaningful to the speaker or author. Thematic analysis did not develop so much as a reaction to the 'anti-humanism' as a simpler more accessible way of doing discourse analysis – it is not – but it did open the way to a more commonsensical view of subjectivity, one that is closer to humanism (cf. Braun and Clarke 2006). Out of this work emerged 'interpretative phenomenological analysis' which boldly claimed that it could indeed answer the question posed by psychologists, that it could disclose the intentions of speakers (e.g. Smith *et al.* 2009). It was a simple answer, and after all the pressure and prevarication it fitted the bill perfectly, and has been successful in psychology for precisely this reason. However, another more complex answer to the question of the subject which now underpins 'psychosocial' studies has been provided from within discourse analysis, and that answer, which draws on psychoanalytic ideas, is the focus of this chapter.

The role of psychoanalysis in psychosocial research

It should be pointed out that psychoanalysis is something of a poisoned chalice to those looking for an alternative in psychology, and especially for discourse analysts. This is because, although Freud's approach and that of his followers has been marginalised in psychology over the years, even to the point where some critics see it as 'the repressed other of psychology', and perhaps even radical as an alternative to the mainstream of the discipline for this reason, the approach is still very problematic for those looking for something genuinely different. Many early psychologists saw psychoanalysis as part of psychology. Theories about child development through an 'Oedipal' complex of personality structures based on points of fixation at different stages and of pathology resulting from unconscious sexual conflict are usually concerned with what is going on inside each individual rather than with changing social contexts. It is for this reason that psychoanalysis is seen as an approach sleeping with the enemy – as part of psychology – by many feminists who would otherwise be sympathetic to varieties of discourse analysis (e.g. Wilkinson and Kitzinger 1995). This has to be kept in mind when we are considering the value of psychoanalysis as a source of alternative models of the 'subject' and 'subjectivity' for discourse analysis.

One of the advantages of the psychoanalytic 'psychosocial' approach to studies of discourse, and in social research generally, which gives it an edge over the more simplistic phenomenological approaches, is that it appears to answer the question of subjectivity in a much more comprehensive way than mainstream psychology (e.g. Clarke and Hoggett 2009). Not only is there an answer to the question about what is going on inside the object of research, that is the research subject who is participating in an interview, for example, but there is an attempt to account for what is happening for the researcher as subject. In fact, there is an attention to the interweaving of the subjectivity of researcher and participant. This focus on subjectivity has become the hallmark of the version of psychoanalysis currently most popular in psychosocial studies. However, the picture is a little more complicated and we need to explore two quite different versions of psychoanalysis that are being brought into play now in this alternative strand of psychological research.

The first approach that we can for shorthand purposes term the 'Kleinian' approach has its origins, as the term suggests, in the work of Melanie Klein (1986) who came to Britain in the late 1920s and whose work became one of the mainstays of what is sometimes known as the 'British tradition' in psychoanalysis. One of the distinctive aspects of her psychoanalytic approach in clinical work, an aspect that has now been emphasised in psychosocial studies, is that she assumes that there is unconscious communication between the patient and the analyst. Unconscious feelings of anxiety or anger, for example, may be transmitted from patient to analyst, even though the patient may not consciously be aware of what they are doing, and the feeling can then have an effect on the unconscious of the analyst, who can attend to what is happening because they have undergone psychoanalysis themselves and they undergo supervision of their clinical work. The transmission comprises a moment of 'projection' as the feeling is put into the analyst by the patient and 'identification' as the analyst absorbs it; the term 'projective identification' thus describes the process as a whole. Just as the patient lives their relationship with their analyst through 'transference' – which describes how the patient relates to the analyst at some unconscious level as if they were a significant figure from the past – so the analyst, in this Kleinian version of psychoanalysis, is assumed to respond to that transference with what is called 'countertransference' (Parker 2010a).

In research the stakes of this approach are immense, and the notion of 'countertransference' is used by Kleinian 'psychosocial' analysts to make sense of what they might feel when they are conducting, transcribing or interpreting interview material, or approaching any other kind of text. There is therefore not merely an understanding of the subject as interviewee brought into the equation, but also an understanding of the subject as interviewer. The idea of 'free association' is borrowed from psychoanalysis where it is used to describe how the patient attempts to speak to their analyst about whatever comes into their head, however irrelevant, ridiculous or unpleasant, and this forms the basis of a 'free associative narrative interview' method in which the researcher free associates to the transcript after the interview (Hollway and Jefferson 2000). For example, studies concerned with fear of crime include interviews with participants that interpret the responses of this individual as a 'defended subject' who replays in the relationship with the researcher key underlying anxieties that structure their life (Hollway and Jefferson 2001, 2005).

The second approach has its origins in the psychoanalytic theory of Jacques Lacan (2006), which is much better known as a clinical practice and conceptual framework outside the English-speaking world, particularly in continental Europe and Latin America (Roudinesco 1990). Lacan argued against the reduction of psychoanalytic phenomena to the level of individual psychology, and against an appeal to unconscious fantasy as if it was something that pre-existed and operated beneath language (Parker 2003). The processes that many psychoanalysts believed to be wired in to child development, including an understanding of sexual difference and Oedipal relationships to the parents were seen instead as being an effect of the entry of the subject into language, into discourse. One can perhaps see the appeal of this version of psychoanalysis to some discourse analysts, for the 'subject' in this approach is first and foremost a subject of language, and the unconscious is understood to be the discourse of the Other (Lacan 2006). An even more radical aspect of the approach is the argument by some Lacanian psychoanalysts that the phenomena that appear in the clinic, on the couch as the patient speaks to the analyst, are specific to that particular setting. This is, in effect, a strong version of a social constructionist argument which states that different contexts produce different forms of reality for those involved. For example, one study takes one paragraph of an interview with a member of a guerrilla group in Mexico and then elaborates a detailed analysis over the course of the book in order to explain key Lacanian concepts and to illuminate how the discourse employed in the interview is working; how it is constructed, how it functions and what variability there is within it (Pavón Cuéllar 2010).

When this approach is brought into social research, then, there need to be some modifications of the framework – Lacanians will not be willing to treat everyday interaction or a research interview as being like psychoanalysis – but there are quite specific concepts in this version of psychoanalysis that can be put to work instead. Rather than appealing to quite specific clinical phenomena like 'free association' and 'transference', Lacanian psychoanalytic researchers make use of Lacan's distinctive approach to language and to discourse, an approach which he then elaborates in a particular way for clinical work (Parker 2005a). This is an approach to language that includes an attention to a phenomenon first noted by Freud which is the 'retroactive' nature of discourse, in which the significance of one element only becomes clear later on, after the event. It also includes a theory of language in contemporary society as composed of four 'discourses', some of which have classic psychoanalytic reference points – of the 'master', 'university', 'analyst' and 'hysteric' – but which are concerned with the construction of different forms of social relation and positions for the speaking subject (Lacan 2007).

Negotiating an example

The example extract to illustrate some key points is from an unusual interview, and it forces us to tackle questions about the conditions in which interviews take place. It is tempting to imagine that a research interview – in which a psychologist, say, asks questions of a participant who may or may not be paid to take part – can simply build rapport and understanding, but the precise conditions in which one speaks invites, incites, makes possible certain kinds of account (Parker 2005b). Some discourse analysts have concluded that it is therefore better to take stretches of naturally-occurring conversation or para-verbal displays of emotion (e.g. Hepburn 2004), but even then we need to ask what is natural about each specific kind of interaction. An interview, even the interview included here, produces an intense relationship in which the interviewer attempts to make sense of what is going on, and it is in these conditions that they may experience things that they imagine are coming from the interviewee. In this case, in line with the research focus of most interviews, we will focus on the way the interviewer might be attempting to extract information, good 'data'.

This interview is from about mid-way of a film, *The Negotiator* (Gray 1998), in which 'Chris' (the interviewer) has been brought in at the request of 'Danny' who has taken hostages. Danny, who is a hostage negotiator himself, has specifically asked for Chris to be the negotiator because he believes that because Chris comes from outside the district he is less likely to be tangled in the corruption and murder scandal that Danny has been framed for. Chris is therefore positioned as an ostensibly neutral research interviewer keen to know what is going on, and Danny is in the position of an interviewee anxious for their own account to be taken seriously. Here, Chris arrives, and in the opening conversation by phone with Danny aims to establish some rapport, to mark a position from which to negotiate. Danny asks Chris what he does in his spare time:

Chris: I read a lot of books you know. I er I watch a lot of old movies you know. AMC. You got satellite? They show those old westerns.

Danny: Westerns huh. I like comedies myself. I did like Shane though.

Chris: Shane. That's a good one. But I'd have picked one where the hero *lives* at the end you know, like Rio Bravo or er Red River.

Danny: I think you're talking about the wrong movie there Chris you know. Shane *lives*. At the end of it he's riding off and that kid er Brandon=

Chris: =Brandon de Wilde=

Danny: =de Wilde is calling his name 'Shane, come back Shane'.

Chris: Well Danny, I'm sorry to have to be the one to tell you this, but Shane *died*.

Danny: You never see Shane *dead*. That's an assumption.

Chris: No. It's a common mistake you see. In the final shot you see him slumped over on his horse. He doesn't look back because he can't. Shane's *dead*.

Danny: He's slumped because he's shot, not because he's *dead*.

Chris: Well I guess you think that Butch and Sundance live too. Although you never see them dead, they're entirely surrounded.

Danny: Oh, so now you're some kind of history buff.

Chris: Yeah, I generally read histories and biographies.

Let us approach this extract first through the optic of Kleinian psychosocial analysis. The first thing to be noted is the way that Danny assumes the position of interviewer, asking Chris what he does in his spare time, and this move enables him to assert his similarity with Chris – they are both negotiators – and perhaps some competition with him. There is therefore a kind of rapport which perhaps is underpinned by unconscious rivalry, and this kind of 'identification' would signal to the analyst that perhaps the interviewee was anxious about their own position, and perhaps also about other things.

The second notable aspect is the topic of 'Shane' that Danny introduces, and the dispute between the two over whether Shane lives or not. A Kleinian psychosocial analysis would notice that the motif of Shane being called to by the 'kid' introduces a relationship into the interview that may signal something about the way the interviewee is experiencing the relationship with the interviewer. This brings the psychoanalytic notion of 'transference' into the equation, though it would be too far-fetched in such a brief extract to speculate about other issues that Danny may be bringing from his own past into the interaction with Chris.

The third aspect that would interest this kind of analyst may be the way Chris asserts his authority as interviewer toward the end of the extract, reminding Danny that he is interested in 'histories and biographies', the very stuff of psychosocial research interviews. This would serve to bring Danny back into line, positioned as the one who answers the questions, and we could perhaps see signs of 'projective identification' in which the interviewer responds to unconscious communication, in this case anxiety and rivalry, on the part of his interviewee.

A Lacanian psychosocial analysis would take a different tack, preferring to stay with the actual text, noticing, first, that the exchange between the two is framed by a certain kind of discourse, that of the Western (a motif introduced into the conversation by Danny) which then makes sense of the relationship as one involving a killer and Chris as a stranger in town brought in to clean things up.

Second, the question of whether Shane lived or died would be seen as one which reiterates the stakes of the interview. This reiteration of a key underlying question could be seen as something like transference in classic psychoanalytic terms, but for the Lacanian analyst what would be more relevant would be the way that this 'transference' was operating through a repetition of 'signifiers' – terms like 'death' and 'killer' that operated as the condition of possibility for this interview to take place.

Third, the analyst would notice that there is a battle of position here, but would focus on the way it seems to revolve around the place of knowledge and a relation that each of the participants has in relation to knowledge. As in every interview, the interviewer is keen to discover what the interviewee knows, and the interviewee often assumes that the research interviewer knows something more than them. In this case, Chris asserts his knowledge of the film *Shane*, knowledge that Danny also takes to be about 'history' – 'so now you're some kind of history buff'; a useful theoretical frame for this is to see Chris positioned within what Lacan calls the 'discourse of the master' and Danny in the rebellious 'discourse of the hysteric' who tries to turn the tables and question those in control. These brief suggestions are drawn from a more detailed Lacanian analysis of the text (Parker 2010b).

Advantages and disadvantages of the approach

There are some attractions of the psychoanalytic approach in general that we can briefly note before turning to what each of the specific Kleinian and Lacanian approaches have to offer.

The first advantage is that psychoanalysis provides a host of alternative concepts for describing subjectivity that are quite different from mainstream psychology, either of laboratory-experimental psychology that is dominant inside the discipline or of the commonsensical everyday uses of psychological language in the outside world. Rather than reducing explanation to the different kinds of 'personality' that define types of individual, for example, the notion of 'subject' itself is a richer more inclusive concept. It includes what is conscious and what is hidden to individuals as they reflect upon themselves in different forms of language (Branney 2008).

In this way, psychoanalysis potentially opens up possibilities for questioning dominant forms of self-understanding and treating these as forms of ideology. Just as some currents in discourse analysis treated forms of language as maintaining or resisting forms of power, so psychoanalysis can help us unravel the way we become attached to those forms of power or resistance at a deeper level, in a way that is, unbeknownst to us, harmful and self-sabotaging. The concern with contradiction at the level of the subject – contradiction between consciousness and the unconscious, and contradiction within the unconscious itself – is a fruitful way of interpreting the world because the insight interpretation brings may also lead to social change.

Kleinian analysis of the experience of anxiety and the communication of this anxiety to the researcher through the mechanism of 'projective identification' therefore draws attention not only to the power of dominant representations of social relationships, but also, at the same time, shows that there is a deeper level of connection between human beings. Distress at alienating social conditions is a sign that every human subject would like to be free of this distress and that they see a relationship with other human beings as a way of managing or evading it. This is the rationale for arguments in the Kleinian tradition that despite its rather gloomy picture of unconscious fantasy there is a redemptive aspect to the approach which makes psychoanalysis as a form of therapy worthwhile, and which can also inspire the researcher to facilitate a deeper understanding of social issues (Rustin 1982).

Lacanian analysis also embeds its descriptions in forms of discourse, and even though it does use the same basic psychoanalytic vocabulary as the Kleinians – unconscious, repression, fantasy, and so on – it is also primarily concerned with possibilities for change. Here we have to bear in mind that there is a historical dimension to the analysis we give of any piece of text, and that the psychoanalytic concepts which we use are applicable in certain kinds of culture where the nuclear family is still dominant and at a point in history where there is a peculiar kind of alienation suffered by human beings separated from others. The Lacanian dimension of the 'Other' in this way opens up a universal dimension of human experience for all those who use language as well as attending to the particularity of each speaking subject (Hook 2008).

Turning to disadvantages, we will say a little bit about what is problematic about each of the two approaches, and then, in the chapter summary, look at some other ways of approaching psychoanalysis in psychological research.

The first thing that should be noticed about the methodological approach taken in Kleinian psychosocial analysis is that key motifs that are borrowed from psychoanalysis as such are transformed in the research relationship (Frosh and Baraitser 2008). In the case of 'free associative interviewing', for example, it is now the analyst who free associates rather than the interviewee, and it is only the strong belief in the phenomenon of 'countertransference' that enables the researcher to believe that their own free associations could reveal anything meaningful. In fact, it often turns out that it is only because the researcher claims to 'feel' something about what is happening in the interview that it is taken seriously. What the actual interviewee feels is beside the point. There is therefore a retreat from the position that was argued for many years by discourse analysts, which was that we needed to read the text of the interview itself very closely and base our judgments about what was going on only on the text. The psychosocial researcher undercuts this position by insisting that only they can understand some aspects of the interview because they were there at the time. It is then difficult for the reader of the report to challenge an interpretation; instead they must believe what the researcher thinks they have felt about what happened (Burman 2008).

A second, related problem is that the ethics of the research relationship is seriously compromised because the Kleinian researcher bases interpretations on their experience of the interview which they are not willing to share with the interviewee (Parker 2005b). This point concerning ethics is quite different from the argument made by discourse analysts before the emergence of psychosocial research. For discourse analysts, it was not relevant to share the interpretation of a piece of text with its author – whether the text was of a published media text or of an interview transcript – because their analysis concerned forms of language – interpretative repertoires or discourses – rather than the intentions of the author. The inclusion of the authors in the process of interpretation was proposed by some discourse analysts interested in action research, but this methodological step was made for political reasons, not because it was unethical not to do otherwise (e.g. Parker 2004). In the case of Kleinian psychosocial research, however, there is a strong belief that the deep unconscious motivations of the author are important and the rather ethically dubious argument is sometimes made that psychoanalytic interpretations should not be shared with the author for, it is said, 'ethical reasons' (Hollway and Jefferson 2000). The idea is that such interpretation may be disturbing, be misunderstood or painful to hear. Unlike the practice of Kleinian psychoanalysis, then, in which the most extreme and bizarre interpretations, including interpretations about transference are given to the patient, in this version of the approach in psychosocial research we are told that for 'ethical reasons' interpretations should not be disclosed. (This ethical problem is one reason why I have not in this chapter included an actual interview and interpreted what research participants said.)

This brings us to a third problem, which is that psychoanalysis operates as a form of enclosed expert knowledge which only the initiated researcher is allowed to employ, and they then share their understanding and application of that knowledge with readers who are often not in the position to evaluate it, based on their 'subjects' who are not even told everything about what is going on (Gellner 1985). This approach returns us to exactly the kind of problems of deception and scientific expertise in the laboratory-experimental tradition that the new paradigm and then discourse analysis objected to. The research subjects are reduced once again to being treated as objects. In order to take Kleinian psychosocial studies seriously, one has to suspend disbelief and buy into the series of claims that are made about the nature of the subject, the role of unconscious fantasy, the repetition of relationships through transference and the role of 'projective identification' in communicating things to the analyst who is expert enough to be able to pick them up by attending to their own 'countertransference'. Again, we should note that this kind of 'communication' model was exactly what was criticised by advocates of the turn to language and discourse analysis (Easthope 1990). Furthermore, this all has to be taken seriously by readers of the research reports even though they know that the psychosocial researcher has not actually necessarily undergone psychoanalysis themselves.

In the case of the Lacanian approach, there is a particular problem of 'expertise' that needs to be tackled, even though Lacanians claim to be very concerned with the status of knowledge within what they term the 'discourse of the university', one in which those who think they know impart their accumulated wisdom to those who do not (Lacan 2007). The problem is that Lacan himself wrote and gave public seminars that are quite mystifying to the uninitiated, and this mystification is then often relayed to the Lacanians and their audience in academic settings. The approach is supposed to be so radically different from mainstream psychology and commonsense that it then, deliberately it seems, makes no sense to anyone. This problem is compounded by the fact that Lacan often mischaracterised those he was attacking and citing so that this version of psychoanalysis operates as a hermetically enclosed system which seems to have no real regard for the truth (Billig 2006).

A second problem concerns the notion of 'truth' that Lacan operates with, one that departs from any criterion of good analysis that a psychological researcher would be happy with. Here, even though Lacanians argue for a strict distinction between the clinic as the site for psychoanalytic phenomena like 'transference' and even for the 'unconscious' and the outside world, we come up against a limit to the application of any kind of psychoanalysis outside the clinic as a means of bringing about social change (Parker 2011). The problem is that 'truth' for Lacanians is a process of speaking – that one is articulating as patient something crucial about oneself to the analyst as Other and hearing oneself say it – not an empirically verifiable fact of some kind. Because there is nothing of this kind occurring when a social researcher as psychosocial analyst is reading a piece of transcript, it is difficult to claim that there is 'truth' in the Lacanian sense of the term. The criteria that one would use in analysis are not applicable in social research, and so it is difficult to know what criteria one should adopt instead (cf. Parker 2005b).

A third problem is that the Lacanian psychosocial analyst is thereby caught in an irresolvable performative contradiction in which they have to appear to be giving a valid interpretation of the material when their theoretical framework actually forbids them from doing so in the first place. As with many other forms of psychoanalysis (but with the exception of the Kleinians, for example), interpretation in the clinic is not seen as something that is delivered by the psycho-analyst in order to enlighten or educate the patient. This is precisely why Lacanians are suspicious of the 'discourse of the university', and they are particularly concerned that this discourse might come to structure and so sabotage psychoanalysis. Interpretation is something that is made by the patient, which is why Lacan used the term 'analysand' to refer to them, the 'analysand' is the one who analyses, while the analyst catalyses and facilitates the analysis. To give an 'interpretation' of a piece of text therefore risks indulging in the worst of analytic practice as Lacanians would see it, and is to adopt what they call the position of a 'metalanguage' which pretends to be completely separate from and superior to what is being spoken about (Lacan 2006).

Chapter summary

Is there a way out of the problems that psychoanalysis seems to have created for itself, a way out that would take forward the debates over the nature of language that discourse analysis opened up and which psychosocial studies promised to provide a solution to? There are two options that would, in different ways, remain faithful to the new paradigm and discursive revolutions. Both entail taking seriously the discourse-analytic concerns with construction, function and variability, or alternatively and in a slightly different key more in tune with the work of Foucault, with the constitution of subjectivity, power and contradiction. Both entail treating psychoanalysis as a 'topic' as well as a 'resource'.

The first option is to be found in detailed studies of Freud's own writings which resituate the process of 'repression' in *language*, in the dialogical process by which Freud identified certain issues and turned away from others. The argument here is that repression should not be seen as something happening inside the head of the speaker, not seen as happening inside the heads of Freud's patients, for example, but that attention to certain things in conversation always requires that we 'disattend' to others. There are signs in Freud's own case studies of things that his patients, and Freud himself, would rather not speak about, and one can analyse his texts to show how it is that conversation of a particular type creates what we then think of as 'the unconscious' (Billig 1999). The implication for social research concerned with other kinds of text is that what we take to be 'repressed' or 'unconscious' material should be traced to the conversational process by which unwelcome ideas are pushed aside. Humour then becomes one site in which veiled reference to these ideas is made and there is a sense of transgression, as if something was being released from repression (Billig 2005).

A second option would be to examine why psychoanalytic ways of interpreting 'repression' and the 'unconscious' are so popular today, and here psychoanalysis would itself be treated as a kind of *discourse*. Rather than take all of the phenomena that psychoanalysis refers to for granted, these phenomena would be seen as elements of 'psychoanalytic discourse' that has come to pervade popular commonsensical psychological forms of explanation, fuelling the 'psychologisation' of contemporary neoliberal culture (Parker 1997). In this way of approaching the question, psychoanalysis would be treated as part of the problem rather than as part of the solution. However, by the same token, the very power of psychoanalysis to inform the way that people talk about and understand themselves and others would be the reason why it needs to be taken seriously. Psychoanalytic explanation may therefore be relevant to understand subjectivity at this point in history whether people like it or not, and the paradox is that psychoanalysis then becomes useful as an account of the subject because it explains the hold its own discourse has on people who both like and dislike it in equal measure (Parker 2009).

If these arguments are right, then we cannot avoid a psychosocial analysis. For all of the problems in the way it uses psychoanalysis, it needs to be engaged with and argued with. We cannot avoid it any more than we can avoid discourse, any more than we can avoid using language to share and debate with each other about what we think psychology is about.

References

Billig, M. (1999) *Freudian Repression: Conversation Creating the Unconscious*. Cambridge: Cambridge University Press.

Billig, M. (2005) *Laughter and Ridicule: Towards a Social Critique of Humour*. London: Sage.

Billig, M. (2006) 'Lacan's misuse of psychology: evidence, rhetoric and the mirror stage'. *Theory, Culture and Society*, **23**(4), 1–26.

Branney, P. (2008) 'Subjectivity, not personality: combining discourse analysis and psychoanalysis'. *Social and Personality Compass*, **2**(2), 574–90.

Braun, V. and Clarke, V. (2006) 'Using thematic analysis in psychology'. *Qualitative Research in Psychology*, **3**, 77–101.

Burman, E. (2008) 'Resisting the deradicalization of psychosocial analyses'. *Psychoanalysis, Culture and Society*, **13**, 374–8.

Clarke, S. and Hoggett, P. (eds) (2009) *Researching Beneath the Surface: Psycho-Social Research Methods in Practice*. London: Karnac.

Easthope, A. (1990) '"I gotta use words when I talk to you": deconstructing the theory of communication', in I. Parker and J. Shotter (eds) *Deconstructing Social Psychology*. London: Routledge.

Edwards, D. and Potter, J. (1992) *Discursive Psychology*. London: Sage.

Foucault, M. (1979) *Discipline and Punish: The Birth of the Prison*. Harmondsworth: Penguin.

Foucault, M. (1981) *The History of Sexuality, Vol. I: An Introduction*. Harmondsworth: Pelican.

Frosh, S. and Baraitser, L. (2008) 'Psychoanalysis and psychosocial studies'. *Psychoanalysis, Culture and Society*, **13**, 346–65.

Frosh, S. and Saville-Young, L. (2008) 'Psychoanalytic approaches to qualitative psychology', in C. Willig and W. Stainton Rogers (eds) *The Sage Handbook of Qualitative Research in Psychology*. London: Sage.

Gellner, E. (1985) *The Psychoanalytic Movement, or The Coming of Unreason*. London: Paladin.

Gray, F. G. (dir.) (1998) *The Negotiator*. Hollywood, CA: Warner Brothers.

Harré, R. (2004) 'Staking our claim for qualitative psychology as science'. *Qualitative Research in Psychology*, **1**, 3–14.

Harré, R. and Secord, P. F. (1972) *The Explanation of Social Behaviour*. Oxford: Blackwell.

Hepburn, A. (2004) 'Crying: notes on description, transcription, and interaction'. *Research on Language and Social Interaction*, **37**(3), 251–90.

Hollway, W. and Jefferson, T. (2000) *Doing Qualitative Research Differently: Free Association, Narrative and the Interview Method*. London: Sage.

Hollway, W. and Jefferson, T. (2001) 'Free association, narrative analysis and the defended subject: the case of Ivy'. *Narrative Inquiry*, **11**(1), 103–22.

Hollway, W. and Jefferson, T. (2005) 'Panic and perjury: a psychosocial exploration of agency'. *British Journal of Social Psychology*, **44**, 147–63.

Hook, D. (2007) *Foucault, Psychology and the Analytics of Power*. London: Palgrave.

Hook, D. (2008) 'Absolute other: Lacan's "big Other" as adjunct to critical psychological analysis?' *Social and Personality Psychology Compass*, **2**(1), 51–73.

Klein, M. (1986) *The Selected Melanie Klein* (ed. J. Mitchell). Harmondsworth: Penguin.

Lacan, J. (2006) *Écrits: The First Complete Edition in English*. New York: Norton.

Lacan, J. (2007) *The Other Side of Psychoanalysis: The Seminar of Jacques Lacan, Book XVII*. New York: Norton.

Marsh, P., Rosser, E. and Harré, R. (1974) *The Rules of Disorder*. London: Routledge and Kegan Paul.

Morgan, J., O'Neill, C. and Harré, R. (1979) *Nicknames: Their Origins and Social Consequences*. London: Routledge and Kegan Paul.

Morgan, M. (1996) 'Qualitative research: a package deal?' *The Psychologist*, **9**(1), 31–2.

Nikander, P. (1995) 'The turn to the text: the critical potential of discursive social psychology'. *Nordiske Udkast*, **2**, 3–15.

Parker, I. (1992) *Discourse Dynamics: Critical Analysis for Social and Individual Psychology*. London: Routledge.

Parker, I. (1997) *Psychoanalytic Culture: Psychoanalytic Discourse in Western Society*. London: Sage.

Parker, I. (2002) *Critical Discursive Psychology*. London: Palgrave.

Parker, I. (2003) 'Jacques Lacan, barred psychologist'. *Theory and Psychology*, **13**(1), 95–115.

Parker, I. (2004) 'Discursive practice: analysis, context and action in critical research'. *International Journal of Critical Psychology*, **10**, 150–73.

Parker, I. (2005a) 'Lacanian discourse analysis in psychology: seven theoretical elements'. *Theory and Psychology*, **15**, 163–82.

Parker, I. (2005b) *Qualitative Psychology: Introducing Radical Research*. Maidenhead: Open University Press.

Parker, I. (2009) *Psychoanalytic Mythologies*. London: Anthem.

Parker, I. (2010a) 'The place of transference in psychosocial research'. *Journal of Theoretical and Philosophical Psychology*, **30**(1), 17–31.

Parker, I. (2010b) 'Psychosocial studies: Lacanian discourse analysis negotiating interview text'. *Psychoanalysis, Culture and Society*, **15**, 156–72.

Parker, I. (2011) *Lacanian Psychoanalysis: Revolutions in Subjectivity*. London: Routledge.

Pavón Cuéllar, D. (2010) *From the Conscious Interior to an Exterior Unconscious*. London: Karnac.

Potter, J. and Wetherell, M. (1987) *Discourse and Social Psychology: Beyond Attitudes and Behaviour*. London: Sage.

Reason, P. and Rowan, J. (eds) (1981) *Human Inquiry: A Sourcebook of New Paradigm Research*. Chichester: Wiley.

Roudinesco, E. (1990) *Jacques Lacan and Co.: A History of Psychoanalysis in France, 1925–1985*. London: Free Association Books.

Rustin, M. (1982) 'A socialist consideration of Kleinian psychoanalysis'. *New Left Review*, **131**, 71–96.

Smith, J., Flowers, P. and Larkin, M. (2009) *Interpretative Phenomenological Analysis: Theory, Method and Research*. London: Sage.

Wetherell, M. and Potter, J. (1992) *Mapping the Language of Racism: Discourse and the Legitimation of Exploitation*. Hemel Hempstead: Harvester Wheatsheaf.

Wilkinson, S. and Kitzinger, C. (eds) (1995) *Feminism and Discourse*. London: Sage.

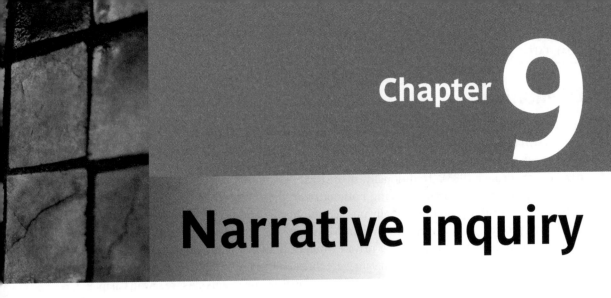

Chapter 9

Narrative inquiry

Dan Goodley

Introduction

Narrative inquiry engages with the storied character of psychological and cultural life. Such an approach is especially relevant in a contemporary age of postmodernity: a biographical age in which cultural, social and psychological narratives are being imagined, produced and consumed (Hardt and Negri 2000). While modernity was characterised by an entrancement with grand overarching narratives of societal progress, such as science, socialism and capitalism (Lyotard 1979), the postmodern citizen finds herself engulfed by a plethora of narratives aided, not least, by technological advances of the internet (Lash 2001). Hardt and Negri (2004) suggest that we live in a time of the multitude: an epoch where stories are shared within seconds from one side of the globe to another; where potentially an infinite number of perspectives can be generated around a single issue, and perhaps through which the sharing of narratives can empower and provide alliances between people in ways that cross national, class, race, income and age boundaries. Narratives of psychology, personhood and identity fascinate and drive our interactions with others. Facebook and blogs allow snippets of information, brief tales of everyday life and arguments and viewpoints to be immediately shared between one another. We live in a culture saturated by and fascinated with storytelling. The story is the chosen methodology of the presentation of the self. When narratives are used to make sense of our selves and the selves of others, then stories are productive: narrative constitutes the self. Rather than viewing accounts as ways of describing the self, narratives mould a sense of self. And behind any story is a place and time: a spatial and temporal background that shapes the ways in which a self is made and a story is told. Narrative inquiry not only provides access to psychological and cultural lives but also gives the words for these psychologies and cultures to be lived.

Orientations

Narrative and storytelling have occupied a fascinating position within psychology. Stories have been drawn upon as key resources in the development of theories and concepts in, for example, psychoanalysis (Bocock 1976), social psychology (Nicholson 1928; Allport 1947), and cognitive psychology (Bruner 1983). Traditionally, mainstream positivistic psychology researchers have criticised qualitative research for being nothing more than 'anecdotal'. The story is, for these self-styled scientists, the quintessentially unscientific, invalid and deeply subjective datum of the qualitative project. Such a view, for Wright Mills (1970: 21), misses the point and power of narrative to examine two key concepts: 'private troubles' of individuals that occur in our relationships with others (often when our own values are threatened); and 'public issues' of organisations and institutions (that often arise as a crisis of institutional arrangements). As we saw in Chapter 3, interpretivist approaches to the study of disability add necessary human flesh to the material bones of structural arguments. Narratives capture private troubles while exposing public issues. In this chapter, our task is twofold:

- to ask what narrative can provide us with in terms of insight and knowledge about psychological and social worlds (do stories allow us to access private troubles and public issues?)
- to outline the kinds of criteria that should be adopted in assessing the quality of narrative inquiry (what makes for a good piece of narrative inquiry?).

Narrative inquiry has become increasingly prominent in psychological research as a means to capture the relationships between the self and others; private and public and self and society. For this chapter I want to draw attention to three narrative forms that provide insight into what we might term the 'sociological social psychological' potential of stories (Hollway 2007). This orientation towards psychology views the individual (and the story they tell) as firmly located in and contributing to their sociological background (the foundations of any narrative). Following my contribution to Chapter 3, I will draw examples from the field of critical disability studies. The first approach, exemplified by Goodley et al. (2004), presents four stories, two of them engaged with disability. These might be viewed as examples of *analytical narratives*.

The account of Gerry O'Toole, for example, is the story of a man with the label of intellectual disabilities who reflects on his life in which his entrance into the dependency of human services and the welfare system was prevented through the promotion of resilience growing up in an inclusive community and family. His account, written from the perspective of a researcher, aims to expose some of the disabling consequences of living in disability space and contexts. Gerry, as the main character, deconstructs the typical character of 'learning disabled service user' because he stands outside this position through his meaningful location in the local community, church, working men's club and local pub football team. This is an account of the psychology of inclusion via avoidance of the usual disabling diagnoses and interventions.

The collection and telling of stories can also embrace imaginative techniques and strategies, such as on-the-go autoethnographies which aim to story the mundane day-to-day experiences of living an ordinary life in a marginalising and hostile community (Angrosino 1994). These kinds of stories attend and analyse the ways in which self and subjectivity are always intimately connected to encounters with the outside world. The collection by Langness and Levine (1986) of various narratives written about and with people with intellectual disabilities demonstrates the reflexive qualities of stories, encouraging the reader to view notions of 'incompetence' and 'handicap' as relational entities, open to change. Such work has fundamentally changed views about the ma(r)kings of intellectual disabilities: exploding the certainties of clinical and statistically based diagnostic processes (Angrosino 1994: 27) and allowing for difference conceptions of the nature of humanity that exist in spite of these diagnoses (Bogdan and Taylor 1976: 20).

The second narrative form, epitomised in the collection edited by Atkinson and Williams (1990), is a powerful anthology of prose, poems, life stories, artwork and pictures by people with the label of intellectual disabilities. These might be viewed as examples of *creative narratives*. Such work is fundamentally important when one considers that much research in the area of intellectual disabilities is 'written about them. We make documentaries about them, on and on, ad nauseum . . . this serves, at least implicitly, to accentuate the difference between them and us' (Stanovich and Stanovich 1979: 83). The contributors to Atkinson and Williams (1990) can be viewed as examples of what Sparkes and Smith (2002) define as ontological narratives – that define who they are – that derive and are intimately connected to intersubjective webs of relationality that highlight public, cultural and institutional narratives. These accounts may also be made up, or reflective of, epic dramas such as capitalism–communism; nature versus civility; progress, industrialisation and enlightenment (Sparkes and Smith 2002). They are crucial because of their emic/insider quality but also because, as Atkinson and Williams (1990: 21) put it, they shift the burden of problems away from the individual on to the society that imposes them. Through their first person testimony, life stories demand researchers to ensure that people emerge with dignity intact (Walker 1981), accounts which contrast markedly with medicalised descriptions of disabled people who are portrayed as helpless, involuntary victims of genetic adversity or the degenerated shells of individuals who might have been (Langness and Levine 1986).

Thinking back to Chapter 3, creative narratives engage with radical humanist and interpretivist positions, rather than functionalist accounts. At their most basic, creative narratives not only recognise and prompt dialogue about difference but show that disability does not finalise a person's option to live in productive ways. Stories ask unsettling questions rather than claiming final answers. Burke (2009) views this as the crucial contribution of novels: to open up various perspectival positions around private and public issues and to offer meticulous anatomies of the human condition. Narrative remains crucial to the development of disability studies because writing the (disabled) subject into the ongoing discourse necessitates a certain exercise of power to construct that subject in some form, to give her shape, and to breathe life into her in ways that might be unknown (Ghai 2002).

The creative narrative is often a risky narrative, but it allows others to think about the kinds of self and subjectivity demanded by particular discourses and institutions of society. Linton (1998) sees this as a crucial role of the liberal arts: to offer active, creative and narrative voices that articulate alternative discourses of and about disability. Smith and Sparks (2004) tease out a number metaphors that were used by men they interviewed who had experienced spinal cord injuries (SCI). Metaphors included fighting but acceptance; incompleteness; choking and suffocating bodies and crumbling blackness. Within the same accounts they also found other metaphors including feeling reborn, up and down, chaotic and a new disabled identity. They argue that these metaphors allowed the men to break out from pathologising ideas about their bodies while also allowing space to feel and think of their new embodied situations (see also Sparkes and Smith 2002). Indeed, associated with this, Sparkes and Smith (2003) found that time was a strong narrative component in the talk of these men. Time was spoken of in terms of discipline (filling time with meaningful words and deeds), ontological security (when one could live towards a future), the link between the materiality of the body and the past, present and future and the freezing of time associated with the moment of acquiring an injury. Smith and Sparkes (2004) consider the ways in which these accounts emerge as characteristics of being disciplined and dominated bodies. Talk is inevitably tied to the discursive powers of the re-habilitative treatments and professionalisation they were experiencing. What emerges from these in-depth studies of a group of men with SCI is the impossibility of separating the ontology of an organically changed body from the omnipotent discourses of in/ability that are inscribed upon these bodies. The complexity of the accounts provided by the men said so much about the use of language and meaning in constituting the bodies the men lived with.

The third narrative form, demonstrated by Potts and Fido (1991), is the *historical narrative*. This text, a narrative research project of the accounts of an institution (The Park) by people with intellectual disabilities, captures perfectly the historical underpinnings of the constitution of the psychology of segregation and oppression:

> When some people dream it is surprising how real and life-like their dreams can be. So much so that we expect to wake up one morning to find them come true and as true as they appeared. I remember experiencing something like this myself some years ago. I was in the general hospital at the time, recovering from diphtheria. It was Christmas Eve and as I slept I dreamed that on Christmas morning when I received my presents, amongst them was a box of dominoes with the coloured spots and on receiving them and having looked through the rest of my presents, I had put my dominoes under my pillow. The first thing I did on awakening on Christmas morning was to look under my pillow only to be disappointed to find that the box of dominoes was not there.
>
> (Ernest, who died in the The Park 1989; quoted in Potts and Fido 1991: 92)

Accounts not only tell of rejection and disappointment but also of resilience and resistance. These are accounts of survivors (Potts and Fido 1991: 130).

> Nobody can help being backward. It's not our fault. Why should people mock people? It isn't their fault they're like that. Some staff thought they were clever but they weren't. They were there to help us, not put us down.
>
> (Grace, Potts and Fido 1991: 133)

> Staff were looking see, keeping their eye on them to see if they were up to mischief.
>
> (Margaret, Potts and Fido 1991: 41)

Texts such as these have been crucial in developing disability studies' sensitivity to the dialectic relationship between human resilience and damaging environments. Narrative histories remind us of the loss that disabled people may suffer – not of ability but a loss of a normal life. Reeve (2008) cites a disabled woman who looks back with sadness at the various treatments she went through in early childhood 'to walk'. Beresford and Wilson (2002) similarly recall the grief of mental heath survivors – not mourning a loss of normality but of wasted time spent in service systems trying to 'get better'. Olkin (2009) describes the need for many disabled people to have the opportunity to narrate their experiences of health and welfare systems that in actuality were abusive and traumatic. Loss and adjustment might relate less to impairment and more to dealing with the lost time spent attempting to conform to the ubiquitous demands of normalising society.

A narrative interview

Mindful of the overview of narrative inquiry described above, we turn now to a narrative of a mother – Angelina – which was collected as part of a British research project funded by the Economic and Social Research Council (RES – 062-23-1138; http//www.rihsc.mmu.ac.uk/postblairproject/): 'Does Every Child Matter, Post-Blair?: The Interconnections of Disabled Childhoods'. We aim to understand what it means to be a disabled child growing up in England. The study was based in the North of England and ran from September 2008 to April 2011. The participants include disabled children aged 4 to 16, their parents/carers and professionals who work with disabled children, including teachers, third sector workers, health workers and social workers. The story for this chapter, however, was gathered from one of the interviews with 20 parents/carers of disabled children and ethnographic research on the community lives of disabled children. The interviews were open-ended and covered a range of issues including families' experiences of health, social care, education and leisure. Children had a range of impairment labels including autism, cerebral palsy, developmental disability, Down syndrome, achondroplasia, profound and multiple learning disability and epilepsy. Our ethnography involved one of the research team (Katherine Runswick-Cole) attending children's birthday parties, bowling, shopping with families. She was also invited to impairment-specific leisure activities, including an autism-specific social club, parent groups, and user consultation meetings set up by local authorities, services and professionals to access the views of families. A few of the families taking part in the interviews were also involved in the ethnography, but the latter was extended to include different children and their families. The ethnography for the project is described by Katherine Runswick-Cole in Chapter 5 of this book. In this chapter we explore the potential of narrative inquiry specifically to ask how it can help us make sense of the experiences of disabled children and their families. The narrative presented in this story draws upon one interview between a researcher (Katherine) and a narrator (Angelina):

- Narrators were accessed via parent groups and other voluntary organisations.
- Narrators were contacted either by phone, email or post.
- On narrators expressing interest in being involved, then participant information sheet and consent forms were sent out via email or post.
- On receiving consent forms back an initial meeting was held, usually in the narrator's home, to get to know a little about one another.
- First interview explored the narrator's life experiences and perspectives on parenting a disabled child.

LIVERPOOL JOHN MOORES UNIVERSITY
LEARNING SERVICES

- Two more interviews were held over an 18-month period which allowed the research team to track any changes in the family's life.
- Interviews were transcribed verbatim.
- Parents were given the option to review copies of all transcripts.
- In some cases, interviews were brought together and a narrative written by either Dan, Katherine or both of us as a collaborative.
- Narrators were given the option of reviewing and, if required, editing the narrative.

The narrative interview of Katherine with Angelina can be characterised in a number of ways. First, the interviews were semi-structured with an emphasis on the narrator guiding the interview. Second, the researcher had a number of interests and research questions in mind. Broadly speaking, the main research question guiding the interview was: What is it like to grow up as a disabled child in contemporary Britain? Other supplementary questions include: How have social policies around disability improved the lives of disabled children and their families? To what extent are families able to access community, education and social care settings? Third, the researcher approached the interview with an explicit ontology and positionality: that of being a mother of a disabled child and a researcher committed to disability studies. This information was shared with the narrators and, to varying extents would undoubtedly influence the interviews. 'Outing oneself' in this way was important. To hold back about this information could be perceived by participants, were they to find out later, as a lack of honesty and openness on the part of the researcher. A problem with being explicit with one's own position relates to the possibility that some narrators have felt they were speaking to an expert and thus worried about how and what they should say. In contrast, a key benefit of this approach was found in the common ground of one parent talking to another parent (of a disabled child). Whatever the pros and cons:

> Narrative activity becomes a tool for collaboratively reflecting upon specific situations and their place in the general scheme of life. . . . the content and direction that narrative framings take are contingent upon the narrative input of other interlocutors, who provide, elicit, criticise, refute and draw inferences from facets of the unfolding account. In these exchanges, narrative becomes an interactional achievement and interlocutors become co-authors.
>
> (Ochs and Capps 2001: 2–3)

Angelina did not want to co-write the story presented below. We have experience of writing alone and collaboratively (Goodley *et al.* 2004). In this case Katherine shaped Angelina's story. The aim was to write a story between 1000 and 1500 words in length. Words were cut and pasted directly from the interview transcript. The chronology of events in the narrative directly reflected when they were presented in the interview. Names of individuals and places were changed or erased. A number of anecdotes were chosen to reflect different events around: diagnosis; parent–professional and parent–parent encounters; experiences of childcare and early years education. Undergirding this decision making were practical concerns around word count, readability and clarity. In addition, other less direct concerns were at play, to which we will return in the latter section of the chapter.

A narrative – Angelina's story – 'Diagnosis, (m)others and parenting a disabled daughter'

Shall I just ramble on? I'm good at rambling. In fact I'm a bit of sucker for people doing research, you know, people in the street, it will only take five minutes and half an hour later I say I'm actually not that interested in your soap or your dusters. But research about disabled children is important, because it really annoys me how much time and effort parents spend fighting and arguing and wasting their valuable resources, their physical and mental energy quite often money as well, fighting for things that should just be there. Quite often fighting for things they are legally entitled to but can't access because, for example, when a tribunal makes an idiotic decision. And all this happens at a time when the child needs most of all the energy of its parents, particularly the primary carer who is also going to be the one doing all the fighting. Anything that can change systems, sometimes it's a bit of case law or a real change in legislation, but it is research that can make a difference.

I had a slightly bumpy pregnancy with Charlotte. I was induced at 36 weeks and she was born weighing 4 pounds 11 ounces. It was obvious straight away that she had a heart problem, but it was a fairly minor one and doesn't really cause her many problems. She was our first child and she was a profoundly unhappy baby. She didn't sleep. She didn't even sleep in the car or buggy like most babies. Eight-hour journeys, she was still awake, still screaming. The first six weeks is all very much of a haze.

As a baby she was very prone to infections, prone to getting a blocked nose, getting ear infections having lots of antibiotics so we had lots of hospital visits. Even when she was born it was obvious things weren't quite right, but nobody told me that. But by about six months it was clear. So I went to the GP and said, 'This is not quite right. I don't know why it's not quite right, I don't know what it is that is not quite right, but it's not right.' Quite often it is the mother, the first one saying there is something not quite right. Mothers can't necessarily put the words to it, certainly can't give the necessary medical terminology for it, just 'it's not right'. But it can be really hard for professionals to hear what the mother is saying, to acknowledge it, to think they're right and then to actually do something about it. It is astonishing they don't take parents seriously because parents don't want things to be wrong with their children. It quite often takes months, sometimes years, sometimes longer for someone to say 'oh yes' or for somebody to spot it themselves and, of course, they think they've spotted it first but the mother's been saying it for years.

So it's all there, something not quite right, but other people didn't want it to be or thought it is better for the mother to bond with the baby before you tell them. At six months the GP referred us to our local assessment centre. At that point Charlotte had the two-day assessment. We had the diagnosis of global developmental delay which is a bleep, bleep, bleep useless diagnosis! It is incomprehensible, it doesn't mean anything and even now if you look it up on the internet there's very little that you can get your head round. It means 'we don't know if they'll walk or talk, to be able to live independently, but we can make some guesses'. It took a couple of years for me to understand what developmental delay really meant. I kind of thought developmental delay means development is delayed but it will stop being delayed, she'll catch up, therefore no problem. I couldn't make the mental leap. I'd thought of Charlotte as not being as disabled as somebody with Down's syndrome, I couldn't quite get my head round that.

But once we got that diagnosis, we then had the support of being able to join the playgroup . We met other parents and other children and that was a much safer environment and you didn't have the pretentiousness of all these mothers. I'm quite prejudiced against a lot of mothers these days. We'd had friends from the National Childbirth Trust support group [*large charity organisation in the UK that offers parenting classes and other forms of support to expectant and new parents*] who'd all had babies at around the same time but that support became fairly useless fairly quickly as it was obvious at a year that their babies were beginning to talk and walk and Charlotte still couldn't hold anything in her hands. She couldn't sit unaided and she was still being miserable and I was still being miserable. The NCT was all these people endlessly going on about how wonderful it was that their baby was doing X, Y and Z which has nothing to do with what the mother does! It is so heavily programmed into babies, you have to really deprive a child to stop them sitting, crawling, standing, walking, climbing, being able to use their hands, basically stick them in a playpen with no toys, but even then they'll still be doing quite a lot of things. It was really uncomfortable being in that environment. One of the people I think I would have been very close to but her child was a very, very early walker. At nine months wasn't just walking but climbing, getting up onto window sills, and my child was still just lying there not doing anything. It was hard at parent and toddler things for the same reasons because Charlotte didn't really do anything and she was hard work. Some babies are happy and smiley and respond and look at you. A lot of women will happily respond to that, but not to a child that is doing very little. New mothers, even nowadays, still have very little experience of disability so don't know how to talk with other mothers of disabled children. Obviously in some ways it is even worse now because there are more tests available now. I've met parents of children with Down's syndrome who've been asked by strangers in the street, 'Why didn't you have the test? Why didn't you get rid of your child?'

I went back to work part-time when Charlotte was 11 months or a year old. That was for my sanity as much as anything else and Charlotte went to a childminder. The childminder was extremely experienced but found Charlotte very difficult because she was so miserable and the other kids didn't want to go in a double buggy with her because she was so miserable. The childminder said a number of years later that Charlotte was the first child that she'd ever had when she'd seriously thought about saying to a mother, 'I'm sorry. I just can't cope with her!' In some ways it was quite encouraging to hear that. Over the years though, it has been quite a consistent thing with people having problems with her but not telling you until much later. When your child starts something new, nursery or school, and they're struggling, why don't they tell you? Why don't they tell you quite early on? Why do they wait years or a term and then say, 'Oh, the first few weeks were dreadful and we really were wondering how to deal with this.' But they didn't talk to me about it. They were pretending everything is fine. It is one of the weirdest things I've come across – the ability of people to be deceptive.

Evaluating narrative inquiry

Angelina's story captures the three narrative forms described at the start of this chapter. Her story is *analytical* in the sense that it allows us to (re)consider what it means to be a parent of a disabled child and in a culture that continues to devalue children so labelled. Her account is also *creative*: it places her as an expert on her parenting and a cultural commentator on the relationships, institutions and discourses that impinge upon her family. She is in many ways our educator, our access into the complexities of family life, disability, childhood and culture. To some extents her account is *historical* – it says something temporally and spatially – about the 'here and now' of parenting a disabled child. Her account also raises some important questions around epistemology (How do we know what we know?), ontology (What do we know?) and methodology (How do we study knowledge?). Let us now address some of these questions.

Narrative as cultural artefact

A text has the potential to open up the world to reveal the sociohistorical horizon which functions as a background to the narrative (Corradi 1991: 109). Narratives constitute an 'excellent discloser of underlying sociostructural relations' (Bertaux 1981: 36). Indeed, as we considered above, Sparkes and Smith (2002) suggest that narratives might be made up of epic dramas. Scott-Hill (2002) suggests that a narrative approach deploys a version of culture that emphasises fluid boundaries between individuals and between the collective and wider social system. Angelina's narrative reveals much about the social and cultural world. Burke (2009) suggests that texts can capture the cultural *Zeitgeist*, act as cultural vents and referents, as they provide metaphors and capture contours of social life.

In reading Angelina's story it is possible to tease out a number of analytical themes – each in their own way cultural artefacts – that provide insights into the discourses, meanings and practices that congregate around disabled children and their families. First, we gain some access into the complex and at times conflicting parental experiences of the *diagnostic process* (McLaughlin *et al.* 2008). While professionals undoubtedly hold the cards when it comes to providing official diagnoses and classifications of impairment, the technologisation of knowledge permits parents to engage, at the very least, in gathering research and information from the internet. In certain ways, then, mothers like Angelina are consumers of knowledge *and* knowledgeable consumers. Second, and related, writ large in the story is the issue of *parent–professional boundaries*. Parents fighting with other potentially more powerful others, such as professionals, is a recurring theme (Goodley and Runswick Cole 2010a). For Angelina the definition of global developmental delay was, quite simply, lacking in descriptive validity. Third, we are drawn to the dominance of *developmentalism* around children's progression and the meeting of milestones. Angelina emotionally recalls the impact of other mothers' ranking their own children's development in her perception of Charlotte. This tyranny of developmentalism permeates all children's lives but takes on particular meaning in relation to those (disabled) children who fail to match the norm (Goodley and Runswick-Cole 2010b). Angelina expresses a rather ambivalent relationship with development – feeling excluded by other mothers' discussions of milestones but critical of educational professionals who failed to identify Charlotte's developmental lag.

Narrative as a tool of deconstruction

If stories reflect the cultures in which they are told, then narratives also shape the cultural worlds that they inhabit. As the contributions to Sarbin and Kitsuse (1994) demonstrate, narrative forms shape the sense of what it means to live, to know and how to feel. Angelina's account is a creative narrative encounter with disability. She questions the kinds of cultural discourses that exist around disability, suggesting that disability remains a difficult topic to broach. Narrative might disturb dominant discourses. Indeed, in other work with parents of disabled children McLaughlin *et al.* (2008: xx) found that the very experience of parenting a disabled child offered opportunities for revisioning disability:

> Kay, a trained doctor, found that having a disabled child impacted hugely on her own work. Facing disabling barriers with her child had made her look again at how she worked with her patients;

'actually being able to sit and take time with people to understand what their problems are. I really started to enjoy that'.

(McLaughlin et al. 2008: xx)

If there were a magic pill, that could 'cure' Roberto of his disabilities, I'm not at all sure that I'd want him to have it. His disabilities are part of him. If you took them away, Roberto would no longer be Roberto. He wouldn't be my child any more . . . if I had another child like Roberto I wouldn't change that neither.

(Helen, mother, McLaughlin et al. 2008: xx)

Narratives may be used in resistant ways in order to challenge dominant discourses that exist around particular objects and subjects. Indeed, as Allport (1947: 40) observed, it is possible to trace social progress in relation to the deployment of vivid stories of personal experience. The historical, creative and analytical elements of story can combine to shift thinking. Angelina's text asks us to think about our ontological preoccupations and existing schema in relation to families, parenting, children and disability. This comes at an interesting time as existing or established knowledge are increasingly being destabilised by a proliferation of disability narratives through media such as the Web. Lash (2001) suggests that the Web offers a flattening of life: opening up and potentially democraticising knowledge.

Narrative as humane text

The writing of a life story, history or biography represents narrators and the object or subject of those narratives in potentially productive ways. Walker (1981: 148) decries the ways in which qualitative analysis fragments and breaks up the accounts of informants: 'Rarely do people emerge from our studies as people and with their dignity intact. Worse still the report may read as though the evaluator was the most intelligent person present.' The presentation of self in a narrative can be a source of enormous pride for narrators, particularly people whose stories have been ignored or stifled. Angrosino (1994: 24) suggests that autobiographies are best interpreted as extended metaphors of self: 'Even persons with conditions that interfere with their ability to construct conventionally coherent narratives nevertheless sustain images and can communicate those images to others of the same culture but using culturally recognisable metaphorical forms.' Perhaps one of the strongest qualities of Angelina's narratives is that we get to hear *her* account, get a glimpse into some aspects of *her life* and, in some small way, are encouraged to emphathise with *her*. Narrative inquiry extends ethical considerations – normally framed in terms of consent, anonymity and withdrawal – to encompass considerations such as making research represent our informants in humane, dignified and authentic ways.

Narrative as methodology

Narrative inquiry calls on us to think critically about the criteria that we use, generally, to judge qualitative research and, specifically, the use of stories. Clearly, we require different gauges to those normally (and normatively) associated with positivistic and quantitative research (see Table 9.1).

Table 9.1 Contrasting criteria for evaluating narrative and non-narrative research

Functionalism/positivism	Interpretivism/radical humanist
Measurement	Narrative
Objectivist	Subjectivist
Validity	Authenticity
Reliability	Specificity
Generalisation	Context-dependent
Representation	Immersion
Fact	Fiction
A distal researcher	A proximal researcher
Deontological ethics	Consequentialist ethics

Drawing on the criteria in the right-hand column of Table 9.1 permits us to ask a number of methodological questions about the narrative project. First, *authenticity*: does a narrative speak with an authentic voice? I would hope the narrative is authentic in the sense that it fairly conveys the words of Angelina. That many of the words are taken verbatim from the transcript would support this view. However, how authentic it appears or feels to the reader – as an account of a mother of disabled child – is less clear.

Second, *specificity*: to what extent does the narrative capture the particularities of one life at a given time and place? Clearly, aspects of spatiality and temporality are captured by the frozen text. The role of a parent group, the impact of a medic's approach to diagnosis, the reactions of an early years practitioner are salient examples of cultural life.

Third, *immersion*: does the story convey some of the richness of a given social context? While only a specific and context-dependent snapshot of one narrator's life, the ensuing analyses reveal the rich potential for insight into the lives of many similar others.

Fourth, *subjectivity*: does the story capture some of the subjective experiences of one narrator that may well be of relevance to similar others? I would argue that the narrative depicts some of Angelina's ontological concerns. The story is not simply descriptive, it is also evaluative in the sense that some of Angelina's preoccupations and reactions are conveyed.

Fifth, *fiction*: to what extent is Angela's account a good story? While making no claims to its literary worth this question demands us to think carefully about the characters, form, plotline and composition of our stories (see Clough's contribution to Goodley *et al.* 2004).

Sixth, *proximity*: how was the researcher involved in the writing of the story?

While above we have described a mechanistic approach to the writing of a narrative, we should acknowledge too that a researcher's ethical, theoretical and political commitments inevitably inform the writing process. Angelina's story of diagnosis captures its complex and conflicting nature rather than focusing on what is wrong with Angelina's daughter. The story is an interpretive tale of diagnosis rather than a functionalist account. The adoption of this epistemological stance means that we at the very least do not contribute (further) to Angelina's experience of rejection by others and, instead, represent her in ways that depict some of her dealings with other people. In this sense, then, narrative inquiry rejects a deontological approach to research ethics (which pursues research regardless of its consequences) and sits more easily with a consequentialist stance where we constantly reflect upon the impact of our research on the people we work with and the possible perceptions we engender of their lives.

Chapter summary

Narrative inquiry highlights debates of theory, methodology and analysis that recur in literature associated with qualitative research. At the heart of all these questions and criteria lies the practice of reflexivity. Narrative inquiry demands particular kinds of questions to be asked by the researcher. The quality of a narrative might be judged in terms of its creative, analytical and historical possibilities. Rather than asking questions of research about stories, perhaps we can ask questions of story about research. To what extent does qualitative research produce rich stories that convey private troubles and public issues? To what extent can narrative inquiry convey the human qualities of our participants alongside the theoretical and practical lessons that they provide for us?

References

Allport, G. W. (1947) *The Use of Personal Documents in Psychological Science*. New York: Social Science Research Council.

Angrosino, M. (1994) 'On the bus with Vonnie Lee: explorations in life history and metaphor'. *Journal of Contemporary Ethnography*, **23**, 14–28.

Atkinson, D. and Williams, F. (eds) (1990) *'Know Me As I Am': An Anthology of Prose, Poetry and Art by People with Learning Difficulties*. Ashford: Hodder and Stoughton in association with the Open University and MENCAP.

Beresford, P. and Wilson, A. (2002) 'Madness, distress and postmodernity: putting the record straight', in M. Corker and T. Shakespeare (eds) *Disability and Postmodernity*. London: Cassell.

Bertaux, D. (ed.) (1981) *Biography and Society: The Life History Approach in the Social Sciences*. Beverly Hills, CA: Sage.

Bocock, R. (1976) *Freud and Modern Society*. London: Van Nostrand Reinhold.

Bogdan, R. and Taylor, S. (1976) 'The judged not the judges: an insider's view of mental retardation'. *American Psychologist*, **31**, 47–52.

Bruner, J. (1983) *In Search of Mind: Essays in Autobiography*. New York: Harper and Row.

Burke, L. (2009) 'Novels and the problem of life itself: the role of literary discourse in contemporary bioethical debate'. Paper presented at the Disability Research Forum, Manchester Metropolitan University, 20 January.

Corradi, C. (1991) 'Text, context and individual meaning: rethinking life stories in a hermeneutical frame'. *Discourse and Society*, **2**(1), 105–18.

Ghai, A. (2002) 'Disabled women: an excluded agenda for Indian feminism'. *Hypatia: A Journal of Feminist Philosophy*, **17**(3), 49–66.

Goodley, D., Lawthom, R., Clough, P. and Moore, M. (2004) *Researching Life Stories: Method, Theory and Analyses in a Biographical Age.* London: Routledge Falmer Press.

Goodley, D. and Runswick-Cole, K. (2010a) 'Parents, disabled children and their allies', in L. O'Dell and S. Leverett (eds) *Working with Children and Young People: Co-constructing Practice.* London: Palgrave.

Goodley, D. and Runswick-Cole, K. (2010b) 'Emancipating play: dis/abled children, development and deconstruction'. *Disability and Society*, **25**(4), 499–512.

Hardt, M. and Negri, A. (2000) *Empire.* Cambridge, MA: Harvard University Press.

Hardt, M. and Negri, A. (2004) *Multitude: War and Democracy in the Age of Empire.* London: Penguin.

Hollway, W. (2007) 'Self', in W. Hollway, H. Lucy and A. Phoenix (eds) *Social Psychology Matters.* Maidenhead: Open University Press.

Langness, L. L. and Levine, H. G. (eds) (1986) *Culture and Retardation.* Dordrecht: Reidel.

Lash, S. (2001) 'Technological forms of life'. *Theory, Culture and Society*, **18**(1), 105–20.

Linton, S. (1998) *Claiming Disability: Knowledge and Identity.* New York: New York University Press.

Lyotard, J.-F. (1979) *The Postmodern Condition: A Report on Knowledge.* Manchester: Manchester University Press.

McLaughlin, J., Goodley, D., Clavering, E., Tregaskis, C. and Fisher, P. (2008) *Families with Disabled Children: Values of Enabling Care and Social Justice.* London: Palgrave Macmillan.

Nicholson, H. (1928) *The Development of Biography.* New York: Harcourt Brace.

Ochs, E. and Capps, L. (2001) *Living Narrative.* Cambridge, MA: Harvard University Press.

Olkin, R. (2009) *Women with Physical Disabilities Who Want to Leave their Partners: A Feminist and Disability-affirmative Perspective.* San Francisco: California School of Professional Psychology and Through the Looking Glass, Co.

Potts, M. and Fido, R. (1991) *A Fit Person to Be Removed: Personal Accounts of Life in a Mental Deficiency Institution.* Plymouth: Northcote House.

Reeve, D. (2008) 'Negotiating disability in everyday life: the experience of psycho-emotional disablism'. Unpublished PhD thesis. Lancaster.

Sarbin, T. R. and Kitsuse, J. I. (eds) (1994) *Constructing the Social.* London: Sage.

Scott-Hill, M. (2002) 'Policy, politics and the silencing of "voice"', *Policy and Politics*, **30**(3), 397–409.

Smith, B. and Sparkes, A. (2004) 'Men, sport, spinal injury and narrative: an analysis of metaphors and narrative types'. *Disability and Society*, **19**(6), 613–26.

Sparkes, A. C. and Smith, B. (2002) 'Sport, spinal cord injuries, embodied masculinities, and narrative identity dilemmas'. *Men and Masculinities*, **4**(3), 258–85.

Sparkes, A. C. and Smith, B. (2003) 'Men, sport, spinal cord injury and narrative time'. *Qualitative Research*, **3**(3), 295–320.

Stanovich, K. E. and Stanovich, P. J. (1979) 'Speaking for themselves: a bibliography of writings by mentally handicapped individuals'. *Mental Retardation*, **17**(2), 83–6.

Taylor, S. J. and Bogdan, R. (1984) *Introduction to Qualitative Research Methods: The Search for Meanings*, 2nd edn. New York: Wiley.

Walker, R. (1981) 'On the uses of fiction in educational research', in D. Smetherham (ed.) *Practising Evaluation*. Driffield: Nafferton.

Wright Mills, C. (1970) *The Sociological Imagination*. Oxford: Oxford University Press.

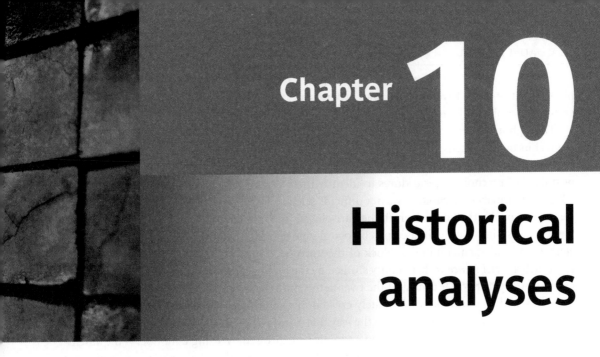

Chapter 10

Historical analyses

Geoff Bunn

Introduction

This chapter has two related aims. First, it sets out the argument as to why historical analyses are a necessary part of psychology. This argument rests on the claim that psychological knowledge and practice must be understood historically. Second, it demonstrates the plausibility of this claim by showing how a psychological entity that was once thought to be a timeless feature of nature is better conceptualised as a socially constructed product of discourse, that is, as a historically situated effect of power.

'Psychology cannot attain the certainty and exactness of the physical sciences,' argued American psychologist James McKeen Cattell, 'unless it rests on a foundation of experiment and measurement' (1890: 373). Although Cattell's vision no doubt still inspires some psychologists, many have emphatically rejected it. Not only has it been argued that the epistemological assumptions underpinning psychological experimentation and measurement are either flawed or remain untested (Danziger 1990a; Michell 1997, 2000), but the foundationalist assumption has itself also been subjected to extensive criticism (Brown and Stenner 2009). Perhaps the most widely repudiated feature of Cattell's statement though is his assertion that psychology should aspire to the status of a physical science. The problem with this ambition can be stated quite simply. Psychology cannot attain the certainty and exactness of the physical sciences precisely because the objects of its enquiries are not physical entities. Whereas objects in the physical sciences often have a precise date of discovery, this is not so for psychology's objects of knowledge. Because psychology's objects are historically situated products of discourse, they are therefore qualitatively different kinds of things to those studied by the physical sciences. A neuron is a physical entity (not a psychological one), whereas a 'nervous breakdown' is a psychological state whose material correlates are unimportant to its phenomenology.

Throughout its history, psychology has often erroneously assumed that psychological objects are real in the same sense that natural objects are real. Despite the fact that the search for psychological universals – 'core mental attributes shared by humans everywhere' – is 'a foundational postulate' of psychology, procedures to identify them remain obscure (Norenzayan and Heine 2005). What makes psychology such a difficult science is that its categories are neither stable, elemental, axiomatic, nor universal; they are elusive 'moving targets' (Hacking 2007). Whereas 'hysteria' was a historically situated psychological state of being, 'hydrogen' is a naturally occurring element, a fundamental building block of the universe. Contrast, for example, a psychological term such as *intelligence* with an entity studied by the biological sciences, *adenosine triphosphate* (ATP). Intelligence was for most of the twentieth century conceptualised as something that has always existed; a natural kind ultimately created by evolutionary processes working on genes. But intelligence was not discovered in the way that X-rays or penicillin were discovered: it is not a *natural kind* of thing. Intelligence can certainly be expressed by a single number – the 'intelligence quotient, IQ' – but that number has no external referent other than to the intelligence test itself. Furthermore, a bewildering number of different operational definitions of intelligence have plagued its study since the term's entry into psychological discourse in the early twentieth century. Intelligence tests are themselves always changing, requiring recalibration every few years in order to ensure that the mean population IQ remains defined at 100 (Gregory 2004: 57). Historical work (e.g. Carson 2007) has shown that intelligence is a radically modern concept. Only God was considered to be intelligent prior to the nineteenth century (in the omniscient sense of 'knowing everything'). At the turn of the twentieth century, a constellation of practical, political and intellectual forces rendered intelligence into a meaningful psychological entity (Danziger 1997: Ch. 5). The twentieth century's meritocratic-biological concept of intelligence came about as a result of the statutory requirement to provide universal education to all children from the 1880s onwards. Educational politics, in other words, is built into the very concept of intelligence – at least as it was understood by psychology in the twentieth century.

Whereas intelligence is a moving target, ATP on the other hand has long been considered to be stabilised knowledge. Discovered in 1929 by Karl Lohmann, the molecule's structure and properties are well known and uncontroversial. Involved in photosynthesis and respiration, ATP is 'the key substance, the general currency in energy conversions within living organisms' (Maruyama 1991: 145). It is a precursor molecule for nucleic acid synthesis and also acts as a neurotransmitter. The complex processes whereby ATP transfers energy (the 'citric acid cycle') were worked out by Hans Krebs in 1937. In 1953 Krebs was awarded a Nobel Prize for his path-breaking work in biology. Even now, over a century since Cattell's optimistic proclamation, psychology has yet to formulate any system, framework, model or theory that approaches the stability, complexity and indeed facticity of the Krebs Cycle.

It is unlikely there will ever be a Nobel Prize in psychology. Psychology has no units of measurement of its own (Trendler 2009),[1] nor has it any scientific laws to speak of, even in the experiment-dominated field of memory research (Roediger 2008). Psychology possesses an

---

[1] Although Clark Hull in his *Principles of Behavior* (1943) proposed the *wat* and the *pav* as measures of 'reaction potential' and 'inhibition' respectively.

inescapable reflexivity that doesn't trouble those sciences that study naturally occurring objects. As Graham Richards (2010: 7) puts it: 'Whereas in orthodox sciences there is always some external object of enquiry – rocks, electrons, DNA, stars – existing as essentially unchanging in the non-human world . . . this is not so for psychology.' Unlike biology students, psychology students do not spend their undergraduate years learning fundamental facts simply because every statement about human nature, however apparently 'fundamental', remains contentious. Whereas biology textbooks communicate established facts, psychology textbooks focus on socialising students into the need for evidence in accounts of generating psychological knowledge (Smyth 2004: 527). Despite having a 'low epistemological profile' compared to common sense, psychology nevertheless possesses knowledge, but it is a knowledge that cannot be regarded as foundational in the way the physical sciences understand the term. Psychology has no essential universal category or any concept of equivalent status to those of electromagnetism, the periodic table of the elements, or the living cell, for example. Indeed, psychology has yet to agree as to what would count as the sort of knowledge it could be unified around. The very level of analysis is itself a problematic issue. Should a unified science of the mind be assembled around the neuron, evolutionary theory, or discourse (see Derksen 2005)?

Psychology's pioneering researchers are less likely to be remembered today because of their reputed discovery of universal truths as they are because their work expresses something interesting about the historical period in which it was formulated. Hugely influential in his own day, William McDougall (1871–1938), for example, was the most celebrated British psychologist of the first half of the twentieth century. Yet today 'he has virtually disappeared from view. What made him significant at the time no longer seems important' (Thomson 2006: 55). The work that McDougall laboured over for a lifetime has vanished like tears in rain.

What role, then, could there be for the historian of psychology? The argument proposed here is that historical analysis becomes vital once it is accepted that psychological knowledge is produced in and through history. Unlike natural objects which can exist in an isolated pure state outside of human culture and society, psychological categories are made possible by a network of related discursive terms, itself a reflection of a particular human society and culture at a certain point in time. 'The human being is not the eternal basis of human history and human culture,' according to Nikolas Rose (1996: 22) 'but a historical and cultural artifact'. It is therefore impossible, argues Roger Smith, 'to write linear histories of global notions of what a person is' (2007: 57). The essential historicity of psychology's subject matter (not to mention the knowledge it has about that subject matter) means that the study of history must play a key role within psychology.

In this chapter I take up Peter Lamont's (2007) proposal to apply discursive psychology to the history of psychology. My aim in this chapter is to analyse the historical emergence of a psychological object in order to expose the conditions of its possibility; to 'deontologise' it. My ambition is to show that an entity which was once taken to have a solid biological foundation – a 'natural kind' – is better understood as 'a historical and cultural artifact'; that is, as the product of a particular moment in history, a 'human kind' (Martin and Sugarman 2001).

Historical analysis and discourse

Implicit within Michel Foucault's proposal to treat discourses 'as practices that systematically form the objects of which they speak' (Foucault 1972: 49) is the recognition that their analysis must take account of *power, objects, techniques* and *language*. If we further accept that discourses transmit meaning regardless of their conceptual consistency, then it follows that we must also acknowledge the *antagonisms* inherent in any discourse as well as its structuring *themes*. If we finally add that all discourses have both a local and immediate *context* as well as a presence in *history*, then we now have virtually all the elements necessary to undertake an 'archaeology of knowledge' in the human sciences.

Discursive psychology is a radically anti-foundationalist approach to psychological knowledge. One of its aims is to challenge the idea that psychological capacities, talents, abilities and qualities are somehow *natural* and therefore ultimately rooted in biology. Discursive psychology argues that there is a fundamental irreducible ontological difference between a *natural kind* of thing (such as sodium chloride, say, or gravity) and a *human kind* of thing (such as the taste of salt, or the experience of weightlessness; Brinkmann 2005). It is therefore extremely sceptical of attempts to reduce the richness and complexity of psychological life to genes, neurochemicals, hormones, personality traits, cognitive structures, and so on. For example, despite the fact that there is no valid evidence for its biological coherence (Corcos 1997), the (racist) concept of 'race' is nevertheless widely believed to be a biologically based natural kind. The term is better understood as a politico-administrative category, as a human kind (Tate and Audette 2001). One only has to think of the aristocracy or unemployment to realise that just because something is socially constructed does not mean that its existence is questionable and that it therefore has no deleterious social consequences.

A historical approach to psychological categories is necessary precisely because its categories are not empirical discoveries; they are historical constructs that have effects (Smith 2005). To give a few examples: emotions are sociocultural constructs whose articulation and experience depend upon particular forms of life and culture (Lutz 1988; Dixon 2003); psychology followed – it did not lead – the conceptual shift from nineteenth-century conceptions of 'character' to the twentieth century's preoccupation with 'personality' (Susman 1984); the puzzle as to whether memory is best conceptualised as working *like a computer* or *like a compost heap* is one that can only be solved ethically, not through the accumulation of empirical data (Randall 2007). In short, whereas it is valid to isolate natural kinds reductively in the controlled environment of the laboratory, this is not so for human kinds or psychological categories. Psychological objects may well come to have a life of their own subsequent to their entry into psychological discourse but that original emergence is a historical and political process. What complicates our understanding of the processes of knowledge generation in psychology is the fact that the operations and procedures used to study psychological objects must be a part of the story of their construction. Psychology's intrinsic reflexivity, in other words, renders a historical understanding of its knowledge necessary. Brown and Stenner (2009: 5) propose replacing the mechanistic ambition to 'attempt to replicate and reproduce the psychological under narrow, laboratory-like conditions' with what they call a 'second order psychology': the following of human experience 'through the myriad of forms that it takes, including the forms mediated by scientific psychology itself'.

One aim of discursive psychology is therefore to challenge all those reductionistic claims that try to essentialise 'human nature' or to base psychological categories on some sort of prior foundational substrate (Brown and Stenner 2009). It does not claim that there are no psychological concepts, or that these are mere social constructs, but rather that psychological qualities are created by – and have effects on – specific historical, social, cultural and political conditions

(Danziger 1993). If we want to understand 'human nature' (note the scare quotes) we have to analyse it in terms of these structures. Ultimately an attempt to understand how psychological capacities are constructed, discursive psychology is an attempt to recognise the close relationship between the ontological status of the objects under investigation and the epistemological procedures designed to investigate them. As Brown and Stenner (2009: 5) argue, the psychological as subject matter 'is ultimately not separable from the forms of knowledge that take it as their object, and these forms of knowledge are in turn inseparable from the forms of social order in which they are implicated'. The purpose of historical analysis is therefore to understand the historical conditions that make psychological categories possible in the first place. This opens up an explicit and indeed necessary role for historical work within psychology (Richards 1987; Danziger 1994, 1996; Smith 1998).

The discovery of *Homo criminalis*

In this chapter I adopt a discursive approach to historical analysis by examining the history of the idea of the 'born criminal' (*Homo criminalis*).[2] A 'distinct category of social perception and analysis' (Wiener 1990: 15), *Homo criminalis* dominated discussions of criminality for nearly half a century from the mid-1870s (see Fink 1938). 'Criminal Man' was conceptualised by nineteenth-century European and North American criminologists as a 'relic of a vanished race, a prehistoric savage living amidst the very flower of European civilization' (Lombroso 1876, quoted in Gibson and Rafter 2006: 24). As the nineteenth century progressed, characterisations of deviance and crime in effect moved from moral to natural categories, eventually appearing more a matter of biology than rationality (Wiener 1990: 229). By the early twentieth century, the explanation of crime in terms of moral weakness had been replaced by scientific, bureaucratic and literary discourses that privileged naturalistic explanations. 'Crime,' as the Italian criminologist Cesare Lombroso (1835–1909) wrote, 'appears to be a naturalistic phenomenon . . . We are governed by silent laws which never cease to operate and which rule society with more authority than the laws inscribed in our statute books' (Lombroso 1887, quoted in Gould 1981: 124). Yet the emphasis on naturalistic causality led to an increase, not a decrease, in the opportunities for governance – the targeting of the criminal's body and mind by mechanisms of regulation and control whose ultimate goal was the maintenance of the social order (Dean 1999).

Objects

The central focus of discourse analysis is the psychological object. The object in question could be an emotion such as *guilt* or *shame*, for example (Demos 1988); or it could be an archaic disorder like *hysteria* (Scull 2009); or it could be a cognitive category like *memory* (Draaisma 2000; Danziger 2008). *Kinds of people* can also be analysed, whether socially valued ('the genius', 'the mother', 'the hero') or reviled (the 'alcoholic', the 'bogus asylum seeker', the 'single mum'; Rose 1991). The first question to be asked therefore is: 'Does the discourse feature a legitimate subject,

---

[2] Because the approach taken here (POTLATCH: Power, Objects, Techniques, Language, Antagonisms, Themes, Context, History) draws inspiration from the work of a variety of psychological discourse analytic approaches including that of Burman *et al.* (1996), Parker (1992), Potter and Wetherell (1987) and Willig (2001), it follows that this method of discourse analysis can be applied not only to historical texts but also to contemporary ones.

a valued citizen?' Or 'Does the discourse feature a devalued unpopular threat to the moral order (an "abject subject" or an illegitimate "Other")?'

Homo criminalis was a heterogeneous tapestry of concepts that wove empirical data together with the wisdom of folklore and tied the utopian dream of a crime-free state to an imaginative use of scientific technique. Constructed as a pernicious risk to society, the 'born criminal' was most definitely a despised subject. To a not inconsiderable degree, Criminal Man was the object around which the discipline of criminology was assembled. This abject figure, Lombroso concluded, was 'an atavistic being who reproduces in his person the ferocious instincts of primitive humanity and the inferior animals' (Lombroso 1911: xiv). Lombroso considered his 'discovery' to be a cousin of 'Neanderthal Man' (whose existence had been publicly announced in 1857), a throwback to an earlier phase of evolution. Such criminals bore extensive signs of their degeneration on their bodies – ape-like stigmata – which the expert eye was reputedly able to read like a book (Davie 2006: 10).

Themes

Discursive work often begins with the description of themes. Essentially this section is about asking what the main ideas are that are being communicated. What is the relationship between words and images? Why was one particular image chosen as opposed to a different one? Two broad themes circulate around Criminal Man: the theme of empirically knowable hereditary defect; and the theme of moral depravity which must be appropriately controlled.

Whereas criminal texts dating from the early nineteenth century were dominated primarily by words – particularly those uttered by criminals themselves – those published towards the end of the century commonly featured statistical tables, anthropometric measures, photographs of body parts and illustrations of tattoos (Rafter 2006). Such devices performed important rhetorical functions. The illustrations in Henry Boies' *Prisoners and Paupers* (1893), for example, consisted of: photographs of immigrants at Ellis Island ('Typical Russian Jews'; 'A Group of Italians'); deformed 'incorrigibles' at Elmira Reformatory; Roman statues, and a painting of a statesman. Criminology has been appropriately described as 'an intertextual bricolage', a jumble of disparate elements drawn from various disciplines all devoted to persuading the reader that criminality was a part of nature (Leps 1992: 44). Different types of evidence appealed to different audiences. The visual and verbal languages of criminal anthropology in effect rendered the criminal body into an easily cognisable entity (Rafter 1997: 113). Criminal anthropology thus conveyed information 'efficiently, powerfully, and pleasurably' (Rafter 2006: 159). With its habitual use of photographs of criminals and their skulls, illustrations of tattoos and so on, criminal anthropology had enormous visual authority. Both graphic and narrative forms of persuasion gave it great popular appeal compared to dry academic texts in other disciplines. The science wove together images of class, race and gender with commonplace understandings of deviance to create an enterprise that possessed incredible epistemological power.

From our vantage point it is important to note that although Lombroso may well have been the most vocal enthusiast for Criminal Man, the concept was already immanent in a range of early to mid-nineteenth-century projects (Davie 2006). While Lombroso was undertaking his celebrated study of Guiseppe Villella's anomalous skull – the event that produced 'the totem, the fetish of criminal anthropology' according to Lombroso himself (Gibson 2006: 139) – Dr. J. Bruce

Thomson, Resident Surgeon of the General Prison for Scotland at Perth, was arguing that crime was 'bred in the bone' and noting 'the ugliness and deformities of criminals, their undersize and weight, and other evidences of degeneration' (Thomson 1870). 'On the border-land of Lunacy lie the criminal populations,' he suggested. The criminal class was marked by peculiar hereditary physical and mental characteristics which were allied to disorders of the mind. This class had '*locale* and a community of their own' in the cities: 'in the midst of foul air and filthy lairs they associate and propagate a criminal population' where they degenerated 'into a set of demi-civilized savages'. Born into crime, 'as well as reared, nurtured, and instructed in it', their criminal habits became 'a new force, a second nature, superinduced upon their original moral depravity'.

History

To situate a psychological object in history is to expose the ideological processes that work towards its ontologisation. The subject's symbolic identity 'is always historically determined' argues Slavoj Žižek (1997/2007), 'dependent upon a specific ideological constellation'. Psychological discourse analysis proposes that all psychological objects have an inherent historicity; a period in time when they come into existence through the intricate workings of culture and society. What then was the historical background to the discourse of Criminal Man? At the start of the nineteenth century the criminal had been little more than 'a pale phantom, used to adjust the penalty determined by the judge for the crime' (Foucault 1988: 127–8). By 1900 a diverse array of intellectual, scientific, practical, social and political developments had combined to create an empirical discipline devoted to systematically analysing the personological causes of crime (Leps 1992).

Cesare Lombroso's *L'uomo delinquente* of 1876 assimilated a number of threads of European thinking about crime into the single figure of the 'born or instinctual criminal'. He would later assert that this simple concept had come to him in 'a flash of inspiration'. But despite this obscurantist claim, it is clear that the concept was anticipated in a variety of nineteenth-century enterprises including statistics, public health, phrenology, evolutionary thought, degeneration theory and penal policy (Garland 2007). Two years before Lombroso's famous 'revelation', the Victorian alienist Henry Maudsley had written:

> All persons who have made criminals their study recognise a distinct criminal class of beings, who herd together in our large cities in a thieves' quarter, giving themselves up to intemperance, rioting in debauchery, without regard to marriage ties or the bars of consanguinity, and propagating a criminal population of degenerate beings . . . this criminal class constitutes a degenerate or morbid variety of mankind, marked by peculiar low physical and mental characteristics.
>
> (Maudsley 1874, quoted in Leps 1992: 29)

As early as 1856, the great Victorian urban investigator and social critic Henry Mayhew had divided society into two races, 'the wanderers and the settlers':

> There is a large class, so to speak, who belong to a criminal race, living in particular districts of society . . . these people have bred, until at last you have persons who come into the world as criminals, and go out as criminals, and they know nothing else.
>
> (Mayhew 1856, quoted in Pick 1989: 183)

Market traders, pickpockets, street performers, prostitutes, sailors and such like together formed a group characterised by 'a greater development of the animal than of the intellectual or moral nature of man ... distinguished for their high cheek-bones and protruding jaws' (Mayhew 1851, quoted in Wiener 1990: 31).

Another important catalyst for the emergence of criminology's psychobiological concept of inherent criminality was the popular science of phrenology, the art of reading character from the contours of the skull (Cooter 1984; Van Wyhe 2004; Rafter 2005; Davie 2006: Ch. 1). The subject's founder, Franz Josef Gall, left a collection of skulls and plaster casts consisting of '103 famous men, 69 criminals, 67 mental patients, 35 pathological cases and 25 exotics (non-European races)'. (Hagner 2003: 200). As one leading exponent put it in 1836, the science 'explains and proves the fact of some individuals being naturally more prone to crime than others' (de Giustino 1975: 146). Emphasising observation and reasoning about empirical facts rather than divine revelation, phrenology catalysed one of the most radical reorientations of ideas about crime and punishment in the western tradition (Rafter 2005: 65–6).

Context

Discursive psychology disputes the separation of a psychological object from its context, maintaining instead that the object is created in and by these contextual frameworks. All psychological categories emerge in a specific sociopolitical environment, and it is the analyst's task to determine whether the wider context involves education, industry, the military or other practical enterprises (Rose 1991). All projects that conceptualise psychological categories in order to pursue pragmatic objectives are potentially implicated in their construction. It follows that an analysis of psychological discourse must attend not only to the object under consideration but also to those empirical procedures and practical techniques designed to manipulate and nurture them in line with political ambitions.

Criminology – a term apparently first coined in 1883 – emerged as the systematic study of the peculiar biological abnormalities of Criminal Man (Rafter 1997: 128). The new science of criminology had been made possible by transformations in an array of enterprises ranging from statistics, prison reform and psychiatry (Wetzell 2000: 17). Although all ended up as components of modern criminology, at the time 'they were discrete forms of knowledge, undertaken for a variety of different purposes, and forming elements within a variety of different discourses, none of which corresponded exactly with the criminological project that was subsequently formed' (Garland 2007: 18). Only when a form of inquiry emerged that centred upon the criminal could these various enterprises be drawn together under the umbrella of a specialist discipline. That criminology and the criminal emerged together was a fact recognised by contemporary observers. The Scottish psychiatrist T. S. Clouston in 1894 wondered what 'anatomical, physiological, and psychological signs are there to distinguish this criminal and his cortex?' He concluded: 'If there are no such signs then there is no such branch of science as criminal anthropology' (Clouston 1894: 218).

Another contextual factor in the rise of *Homo criminalis* was the concept of *degeneration*. Fears about moral and physical decline were expressed in both scientific and literary texts following the formulation of the second law of thermodynamics in 1851 and the publication of Darwin's *Origin of Species* in 1859. The discovery of the entropic cosmos focused minds on the loss of human energies and the dissipation of vigour (Wiener 1990: 173). Richard Dugdale's (1877) best-seller *The Jukes: A Study in Crime, Pauperism, Disease and Heredity* became a synonym for degeneracy on both sides of the Atlantic (Rafter 1997: 38). Novelists such as Oscar Wilde, Robert Louis Stevenson and particularly Bram Stoker all shared a fascination with degeneration and the physiognomy of criminality. In Stevenson's *The Strange Case of Dr. Jekyll and Mr. Hyde* (1886), a Victorian gentleman scientist regresses to an ape-like primitive. In Rudyard Kipling's short story 'The Mark of the Beast' (1890), an Englishman in India defiles a Hindu temple and regresses to a wolf-like state (Clausson 2005). The future earth is imagined to be populated by two degenerate humanoid races in H. G. Wells's *The Time Machine* (1894), one lacking the power of reason, the other devoid of vitality.

Antagonisms

Discourses can exhibit ambivalences, binary oppositions and straightforward contradictions. It is also instructive to attend to the 'ideological dilemmas' (Billig 1988) that structure any psychological discourse. In many cases a positive assertion will only make sense if it is underpinned by a hidden negative contrast. In the case of Criminal Man it is clear that although scientists and novelists shared a fascination with biological criminality, the novelists often criticised many of criminal anthropology's organising concepts. Contrary to the class-based elitist axioms of positivist criminology, for example, Bram Stoker's Count Dracula was a degenerate aristocrat. Stevenson's Dr Jekyll was a respectable middle-class physician who harboured a beast within.

Lombroso's concepts did not meet with universal acceptance. In 1889, French criminologists attacked Lombrosoian doctrine for its determinism, proposing instead to account for criminality with the concept of the 'social milieu' (Nye 1976). Other challenges to the 'Italian School' questioned the reality of cranial anomalies, the dubious statistical data and the lack of criminality in women. Criminal anthropology's detractors generally either took a sociological approach – the socialist Turati asserting that 'bourgeois Society is the biggest criminal' – or they downgraded the importance of biology by pointing to the existence of habitual or occasional criminals. Charles Féré, the author of *Degeneration and Criminality* (1895), blamed the genesis of crime on a combination of inferior physiology and immorality. Colajanni, the author of *Criminal Sociology* (1889), made the compelling criticism that Lombroso and his followers had failed to find a single trait that was absolutely exclusive to delinquents.

In 1892, in a measured article warning of the dangers of over-interpreting criminal statistics, the Rev. W. D. Morrison expressed a sceptical note about Lombroso's theory of the born criminal (Morrison 1892): 'Whatever may be the ultimate fate of Lombroso's theory, he has unquestionably succeeded in calling attention to the fact that a larger proportion of anomalies is to be found among the criminal population than among ordinary members of the community.' A 'debilitated body', after all, had 'a tendency to produce a perverted mind'. But instead of regarding criminal stigmata as signs of an inherent degeneration, Morrison proffered a sociological theory, suggesting that such marks might predispose their possessor to a life of crime simply as a result of social prejudice, a dearth of employment opportunities and an embittered sensibility. The presence of physical anomalies among offenders was neither evidence of their mental capacities nor support for the existence of a criminal type. Physical abnormalities were rather 'proof of a fact apparent everywhere, that the physically anomalous and incapable are less adapted to fight the battle of life, and are accordingly more likely to come into collision with the law' (Morrison 1892: 506, 508).

One of the most striking contradictions of criminological discourse concerned the way the female offender was understood. 'The primitive woman was rarely a murderess,' Lombroso and Ferrero claimed, 'but she was always a prostitute, and such she remained until semi-civilised epochs' (quoted in Hurley 1996: 98). By the late nineteenth century, prostitution had come to be regarded as the quintessential social evil, surpassing drunkenness, blasphemy and adultery in the state's dossier of the undesirable (Laqueur 1990: 230). 'Women criminals are almost always homely, if not repulsive,' Mantegazza claimed. 'Many are masculine; have a large, ill-shaped mouth; small eyes; large, pointed nose, distant from the mouth; ears extended and irregularly planted' (quoted in Kellor 1900: 531). According to Lombroso and Ferrero, not only was the prostitute's foot 'shorter and narrower than in normals', but it was also 'shorter proportionately to the hand'. The 'greater weight among prostitutes' was 'confirmed by the notorious fact of the obesity of those who grow old in their vile trade, and who become positive monsters of adipose tissue' (quoted in Kellor 1900: 530).

Within criminological discourse, the prostitute was an emblem of the inherent depravity of all women. But unlike their male counterparts, female offenders often did not exhibit the visible stigmata of criminality: 'It is incontestable that female offenders seem almost normal when compared to the male criminal, with his wealth of anomalous features.' Lombroso was puzzled by this. It was an undoubted fact, he wrote, 'that atavistically [the female] is nearer to her origin than the male, and ought consequently to abound more in anomalies'. And yet 'an extensive study of criminal women has shown us that all the degenerative signs . . . are lessened in them; they seem to escape . . . from the atavistic laws of degeneration' (Wolfgang 1972: 255).

> This absence of ill-favouredness and want of typical criminal characteristics will militate with many against our contention that prostitutes are after all equivalents of criminals and possess the same qualities in an exaggerated form. But in addition to the fact that true female criminals are much less ugly than their male companions, we have in prostitutes women of great youth, in whom the *beauté du diable*, with its freshness, plumpness, and absence of wrinkles, disguises and conceals the betraying anomalies.
>
> (Lombroso and Ferrero 1895: 100–1)

Lombroso's claim was asymmetrical. Whereas the anomalies of male criminals were visible for all to see, those of female criminals were hidden within the mysterious space of the female body.

Techniques

How an object is conceptualised determines the procedures that can be used to nurture or contain it, depending on the desired outcome. What are people doing to themselves? What are people doing to others? Is there an invitation to endorse, buy or consume something? Above all, attending to technique allows the analysis to proceed towards a focus on power.

Criminology's power rested to some extent on measurement devices which symbolised expertise and scientific precision. Scientific instruments were not just expressions of the extension of the criminological gaze into hitherto unseen spaces; they were tools for the fashioning of a scientific identity for criminal anthropology. These specialised techniques for reading the body furnished criminal anthropology with a 'corporeal literacy that made possible an exegesis and a diagnosis' (Horn 2006: 321). An ability to manipulate scientific instruments and to gather data systematically was a crucial aspect of the construction and maintenance of scientific authority (Horn 2003: 26). A well-appointed laboratory, for example, might have listed among its stock the following instruments: baristesiometer, campimeter, clinometer, craniometer, dynamometer, ergograph, esthesiometer, goniometer, Hipp's chronoscope, olfactometer, the *Schlitteninductorium*, spirometer, tachyanthropometer, thermesthesiometer (Hurley 1996: 100; Horn 2003: 96). The multiplication of instruments devoted to rendering the invisible visible mirrored the multiplication of physical stigmata whose superfecundity had also vexed the criminologists. Instead of alighting on a single reliable indicator of criminal pathology, criminological discourse searched relentlessly for a definitive answer to the question 'What signifies criminality?'

In spite of all the hardware, the turn to instrumentation did not produce the definitive empirical results that the criminologists had hoped for. But in cataloguing criminal anthropology's comprehensive intensity, Gabriel Tarde betrayed a poetic sensibility:

> Every instrument for measuring or which was known to contemporary medical science and to psychophysics, the sphygmograph, dynamometer, aestheseometer, etc., had already been employed by Lombroso for the purpose of characterizing in the language of figures or of graphic curves, singular arabesques, the manner in which thieves or assassins breathe, in which their blood flows, their heart beats, their senses operate, their muscles contract, and their feeling is given expression, and by this means to discover through all the corporal manifestations of their being, considered as so many living hieroglyphics to be translated, even through their handwriting and their signatures submitted to a graphical analysis, the secret of their being and of their life. In this manner he had discovered, especially by means of three sphygmographic tracings, that malefactors are very responsive to the sight of a gold coin or of a good glass of wine, and much less to the sight of a 'donna nuda,' in a photograph to be sure.
>
> (Tarde 1903/1912: 63–4)

With its ready deployment of metaphor and alliteration, and its appropriation of folk tales and myth, criminology's eloquent language often contradicted its prosaic positivist ambitions.

Language

Discourse analysis privileges the role of language in structuring and framing possibilities for action, meaning and interpretation. Criminological texts were a captivating assemblage of words, numbers and images. Lombroso's effusive description of his examination of the brigand Villella's skull, for example, might well have been a post hoc rationalisation of events, but its legacy was a compelling origin myth:

> At the sight of that skull, I seemed to see all of a sudden, lighted up as a vast plain under a flaming sky, the problem of the nature of the criminal – an atavistic being who reproduces in his person the ferocious instincts of primitive humanity and the inferior animals. Thus were explained anatomically the enormous jaws, high cheek bones, prominent superciliary arches, solitary lines in the palms, extreme size of the orbits, handle-shaped ears found in criminals, savages and apes, insensibility to pain, extremely

acute sight, tattooing, excessive idleness, love of orgies, and the irresponsible craving of evil for its own sake, the desire not only to extinguish life in the victim, but to mutilate the corpse, tear its flesh and drink its blood.

(quoted in Jalava 2006: 419)

Although this dramatic passage undoubtedly contains some unusually arresting imagery, its lyricism was far from unique within criminal anthropology, a discourse which was often written for the mass market. In April 1891, Ronald Fletcher delivered his retiring presidential address to the Anthropological Society of Washington (Fletcher 1891). Although his aim was to give his audience an impartial account of the work of the 'New School of Criminal Anthropology', Fletcher's language was distinctly sensationalist. His description of the murderer's 'cold concentrated look' would not have looked out of place in Bram Stoker's *Dracula*, which was still some six years away from publication:

Sometimes the eye appears injected with blood; the nose is often aquiline or hooked, always large; the ears are long; the jaws powerful; the cheek-bones widely separated; the hair is crisp and abundant; the canine teeth well developed, and the lips thin; often a nervous tic or contraction, upon one side of the face only, uncovers the canine teeth, producing the effect of a threatening look or a sardonic laugh.

(Fletcher 1891: 206)

Power

Perhaps the most important aspect of discursive historical work is the analysis of power. Power takes many forms. Some forms prohibit and oppress (*sovereignty*, for example), while others encourage and enable (*empowerment*). Some target the body (*discipline*), others focus on the mind (*interpellation*). Although power is always immanent in discourse, the precise form it takes varies depending on the circumstances (Hook 2007). It should be clear by now that criminological discourse was saturated with a variety of different modes of power (Foucault 1979). In what follows I shall briefly describe four such modes that circulated through the discourse of *Homo criminalis*: discipline, charisma, patriarchy and pastoralism. Other interpretations are doubtless possible. It is clear, for example, that *biopower* remains a feature of criminological discourse (Garland 1997; O'Malley 1999; Rose 2000).

Discipline

Language is the bridge between power and knowledge. How an object is described frames the range of possible ways in which it can be acted upon. The choice of metaphor is not a trivial matter; metaphors have consequences. Take, for example, the metaphor of *disease*, which is occasionally used to describe social phenomena. Once this metaphor acquires a currency and has become socially acceptable, it becomes easy to think of the phenomenon as a *contagious* risk that should be *contained* or *quarantined* and eventually *eradicated*. Eugenicist G. Frank Lydson (author of *Sexual Crimes Among the Southern Negroes*, c.1893 and *That Bogey Man the Jew*, 1921) argued in *Diseases of Society* (1904) that rapists should be castrated and all habitual criminals sterilised: 'The confirmed criminal . . . is simply excrementitious matter that should not only be eliminated, but placed beyond the possibility of its contaminating the social body' (Lydson 1904, quoted in Rafter 1997: 124). W. Duncan McKim's proposal for a 'tremendous reduction in the amount of crime' was even more extreme: 'the *very* weak and the *very* vicious' should be afforded a '*gentle, painless death*' by gassing with carbonic acid (McKim 1900, quoted in Rafter 1997: 124). The conceptualisation of criminality as an inherent biological flaw rendered the disciplinary treatment of criminals more likely. In effect, the people 'most concerned with crime control were receptive to the idea of the criminal as a biologically distinct and inferior being' (Rafter 2006: 166). In 1870, J. Bruce Thomson had claimed that crime was 'incurable ... hereditary in the criminal class' and transmitted 'like other hereditary maladies' (Thomson 1870: 496). He called for transportation to the colonies, the breaking up of criminal communities and lengthy sentences for habitual criminals. He concluded on a pessimistic note: 'The criminal hereditary *caste* and character, if changeable, must be changed slowly, and how to do it must be to sociologists and philanthropists always a *questio vexata*, one of the most difficult state problems' (Thomson 1870: 498).

Patriarchy

As has already been discussed, the male-dominated enterprise of criminology was fascinated by the female offender. In 1890, Gustav Tarde claimed that criminal offences were the 'cutaneous eruptions of the social body; at times indices of a serious illness, they reveal the introduction, through contact with neighbors, of foreign ideas and needs in partial contradiction of national ideas and needs' (Tarde 1890, quoted in Leps 1992: 51). Constructed as a diseased, primitive and childlike entity, the crowd was an emblem of the problems that beset mass society. But crowds were conceptualised as *feminine*; vulgar and unruly – and therefore amenable to patriarchal control (Leps 1992: Ch. 3). The female body did not lose its pathologies when it became conflated with the social body.

'Women's preference for strong scents,' Adalbert Albrecht asserted, 'is to be explained only by the fact that they do not smell as keenly and therefore endure strong odours better' (Albrecht 1910: 79). Criminals were widely believed to have an inferior sensibility compared to law-abiding citizens. Lombroso predictably invoked a hierarchy to explain the problem, claiming that sensibility was highest in con artists but lowest in robbers. Criminals were more likely to be sensitive to the effects of metals and magnets and have acute eyesight. Garofalo pointed to the widespread practice of tattooing among criminals as evidence of their relative insensitivity to pain. Because 'the normal woman is naturally less sensitive to pain', wrote Lombroso and Ferrero, women would possess less compassion – 'the offspring of sensitiveness' – compared to men (Lombroso and Ferrero 1895: 150–1). Women were also assumed to be less sensitive to pain compared to men because of the burdens of childbearing. Women's cruelty was a consequence not only of their weakness, according to Albrecht, but also of their deficient sensibility to pain. Other deleterious consequences followed from this:

> Compared to that of men the morality of women is also inferior. They know only one honour, honour of sex. This inferior morality, too, comes from their lesser sensibility and intelligence, for also in the latter respect women are inferior. The highest plane of intelligence, genius, is completely lacking among women.
>
> (Albrecht 1910: 79)

Charismatic authority

Lombroso's acolytes regarded him as a genius. Ottolenghi called him a 'titanic figure' (Ottolenghi 1908, quoted in Gibson 2002: 135). According to one scholar, 'the father of modern criminology' was 'a scientific Columbus who opened up a new field for exploration, and his insight into human nature was compared to that of Shakespeare and Dostoevsky' (Wolfgang 1972: 287). Albrecht argued that because the science was 'so intimately connected with the name of Lombroso . . . no one can dispute his right to be considered the godfather of criminal anthropology'. He was 'one of the great men of the nineteenth century whose names were familiar to everyone, who were read by many but studied by comparatively few' (Albrecht 1910: 72). The indefatigable Lombroso wrote more than 30 books and published some 1000 articles during his career, becoming one of the most prominent intellectuals in late nineteenth-century Italy (Gibson 2006: 141). He devoted enormous efforts to propagating his theory, disseminating his ideas in a continuous stream of publications (Wetzell 2000: 30). Lombroso clearly possessed a surfeit of what Max Weber called *charismatic authority*, a personological style characteristic of spiritual leaders, warrior heroes and archetypal figures like the 'sorcerer, the rainmaker, the medicine man' (Weber 2006: 60). At times of relative social and political calm, Weber suggested, the normal requirements of everyday life were usually administered by bureaucrats following systems of rational rules in the interests of social harmony. At times of social strife, however – periods of 'psychic, physical, economic, ethical, religious [and] political distress' – leaders were required who possessed a quite different array of 'gifts of the body and spirit'. Charismatic authority came to the fore during such periods of crisis.

Pastoralism

In contrast to disciplinary power which is indifferent to the subject's will, pastoral power works with the approval of those it targets. In spite of the biological determinist character of the discourse surrounding Criminal Man, paradoxically the born criminal was also thought to be capable of reform. Many criminologists voiced enthusiasm over the penal experiments that took place at Elmira, the state reformatory at New York (Winter and Ellis 1891; Williams 1896). The Catholic chaplain Francis Lane spent 12 years working with the young offenders at Elmira (Lane 1934). Here, the inmates were taught trades and provided with a 'good diet, athletic exercises, military training, an elaborate system of baths, massage, and other methods known as belonging to scientific gymnastics' (Fletcher 1891). Of 324 inmates paroled in one year, 148 went directly to employment at the trades they had learned in the reformatory. Power, like all aspects of discourse, can itself operate in contradictory modes (O'Malley 1999).

Chapter summary

In this chapter I have undertaken an historical analysis of a psychological object, Criminal Man, *Homo criminalis*. I have tried to show that an entity that appeared to be solid and unassailable at one moment in history, from another vantage point can be regarded as having been created by an array of contingent circumstances. My aim here, in other words, has been to demonstrate that an entity which ideology ontologised as a *natural kind* is better understood as a *human kind*; that is, as an effect of discourse, produced in and by history. According to Kurt Danziger, whose work informs the historical approach to psychological discourses adopted here, much of contemporary psychology naively believes that the objects of current psychological science 'are the real, natural objects and that past discourse necessarily referred to the same objects in its own quaint and subscientific way'. But what this approach to history overlooks is 'the possibility that the very objects of psychological discourse, and not just opinions about them, have changed radically in the course of history' (Danziger 1990b: 336). I have attempted to show here that because psychological objects are dynamically moving targets, and not stable, elemental, axiomatic, nor universal truths, we can only properly understand them if we employ historical analysis.

References

Albrecht, A. (1910) 'Cesare Lombroso. A glance at his life work'. *Journal of the American Institute of Criminal Law and Criminology*, **1**(2), 71–83.

Billig, M. (1988) *Ideological Dilemmas: A Social Psychology of Everyday Thinking*. London: Sage.

Brinkmann, S. (2005) 'Human kinds and looping effects in psychology: Foucauldian and hermeneutic perspectives'. *Theory and Psychology*, **15**, 769–91.

Brown, S. and Stenner, P. (2009) *Psychology without Foundations: History, Philosophy and Psychosocial Theory*. London: Sage.

Burman, E., Aitken, G., Alldred, P., Allwood, R., Billington, T., Goldberg, B., Gordo López, A. J., Heenan, C., Marks, D. and Warner, S. (1996) *Psychology Discourse Practice: From Regulation to Resistance*. London: Taylor and Francis.

Carson, J. (2007) *The Measure of Merit: Talents, Intelligence, and Inequality in the French and American Republics, 1750–1940*. Princeton, NJ: Princeton University Press.

Cattell, J. McK. (1890) 'Mental tests and measurements'. *Mind*, **15**, 373–81.

Clausson, N. (2005) 'Degeneration, fin-de-siècle gothic, and the science of detection: Arthur Conan Doyle's *The Hound of the Baskervilles* and the emergence of the modern detective story'. *Journal of Narrative Theory*, **35**(1), 60–87.

Clouston, T. S. (1894) 'The developmental aspects of criminal anthropology'. *The Journal of the Anthropological Institute of Great Britain and Ireland*, **23**, 215–25.

Cooter, R. (1984) *The Cultural Meaning of Popular Science: Phrenology and the Organization of Consent in Nineteenth-century Britain*. Cambridge: Cambridge University Press.

Corcos, A. (1997) *The Myth of Human Races*. East Lansing, MI: Michigan State University Press.

Danziger, K. (1990a) *Constructing the Subject: Historical Origins of Psychological Knowledge*. Cambridge: Cambridge University Press.

Danziger, K. (1990b) 'Generative metaphor and the history of psychological discourse', in D. E. Leary (ed.) *Metaphors in the History of Psychology*. Cambridge: Cambridge University Press.

Danziger, K. (1993) 'Psychological objects, practice, and history'. *Annals of Theoretical Psychology*, **8**, 15–47.

Danziger, K. (1994) 'Does the history of psychology have a future?' *Theory and Psychology*, **4**, 467–84.

Danziger, K. (1996) 'The practice of psychological discourse', in C. F. Graumann and K. J. Gergen (eds) *Historical Dimensions of Psychological Discourse*. Cambridge: Cambridge University Press.

Danziger, K. (1997) *Naming the Mind: How Psychology Found its Language*. London: Sage.

Danziger, K. (2008) *Marking the Mind: A History of Memory*. New York: Cambridge University Press.

Davie, N. (2006) *Tracing the Criminal: The Rise of Scientific Criminology in Britain, 1860–1918*. Oxford: Bardwell Press.

Dean, M. (1999) *Governmentality: Power and Rule in Modern Society*. London: Sage.

de Giustino, D. (1975) *Conquest of Mind: Phrenology and Victorian Social Thought*. London: Croom Helm.

Demos, J. (1988) 'Shame and guilt in early New England', in C. Z. Stearns and P. N. Stearns (eds) *Emotion and Social Change: Toward a New Psychohistory*. New York: Holmes and Meier.

Derksen, M. (2005) 'Against integration: why evolution cannot unify the social sciences'. *Theory and Psychology*, **15**, 139–62.

Dixon, T. (2003) *From Passions to Emotions: The Creation of a Secular Psychology*. Cambridge: Cambridge University Press.

Draaisma, D. (2000) *Metaphors of Memory: A History of Ideas about the Mind*. Cambridge: Cambridge University Press.

Fink, A. E. (1938) *Causes of Crime: Biological Theories in the United States*. Philadelphia: University of Philadelphia Press.

Fletcher, R. (1891) 'The new school of criminal anthropology'. *American Anthropologist*, **4**(3), 201–36.

Foucault, M. (1972) *The Archaeology of Knowledge*. (Trans. A. M. Sheridan Smith.) New York: Pantheon Books.

Foucault, M. (1979) *Discipline and Punish: The Birth of the Prison*. (Trans. Alan Sheridan.) New York: Vintage Books.

Foucault, M. (1988) 'The dangerous individual', in L. D. Kritzman (ed.) *Politics, Philosophy, Culture: Interviews and Other Writings 1977–1984*. New York: Routledge.

Garland, D. (1997) '"Governmentality" and the problem of crime: Foucault, criminology, sociology'. *Theoretical Criminology*, **1**(2), 173–214.

Garland, D. (2007) 'Of crimes and criminals: the development of criminology in Britain', in M. Maguire, R. Morgan and R. Reiner (eds) *The Oxford Handbook of Criminology*, 4th edn. Oxford: Oxford University Press.

Gibson, M. (2002) *Born to Crime: Cesare Lombroso and the Origins of Biological Criminology*. Westport, CT: Praeger.

Gibson, M. (2006) 'Cesare Lombroso and Italian criminology: theory and politics', in P. Becker and R. F. Wetzell *Criminals and their Scientists: The History of Criminology in International Perspective.* Cambridge: Cambridge University Press.

Gibson, M. and Rafter, N. H. (2006) *Criminal Man by Cesare Lombroso.* Durham, NC: Duke University Press.

Gould, S. J. (1981) *The Mismeasure of Man.* Harmondsworth: Penguin.

Gregory, R. J. (2004) *Psychological Testing: History, Principles, and Applications*, 4th edn. Boston: Allyn and Bacon.

Hacking, I. (2007) 'Kinds of people: moving targets', *Proceedings of the British Academy*, **151**, 285–318.

Hagner, M. (2003) 'Skulls, brains, and memorial culture: on cerebral biographies of scientists in the nineteenth century'. *Science in Context*, **16**, 195–218.

Hook, D. (2007) *Foucault, Psychology and the Analytics of Power.* London: Palgrave.

Horn, D. G. (2003) *The Criminal Body: Lombroso and the Anatomy of Deviance.* London: Routledge.

Horn, D. G. (2006) 'Making criminologists: tools, techniques, and the production of scientific authority', in P. Becker and R. F. Wetzell *Criminals and their Scientists: The History of Criminology in International Perspective.* Cambridge: Cambridge University Press.

Hull, C. L. (1943) *Principles of Behavior.* New York: D. Appleton-Century.

Hurley, K. (1996) *The Gothic Body: Sexuality, Materialism, and Degeneration at the Fin-de-siècle.* Cambridge: Cambridge University Press.

Jalava, J. (2006) 'The modern degenerate: nineteenth-century degeneration theory and psychopathy research'. *Theory and Psychology*, **16**, 416–32.

Kellor, F. A. (1900) 'Psychological and environmental study of women criminals'. *The American Journal of Sociology*, **5**(4), 527–43.

Lamont, P. (2007) 'Discourse analysis as method in the history of psychology'. *History and Philosophy of Psychology*, **9**(2), 34–44.

Lane, F. J. (1934) *Twelve Years in a Reformatory: A Report of the Activities and Experiences of a Catholic Chaplain during Twelve Years' Service in the Elmira Reformatory.* New York: Elmira Reformatory.

Laqueur, T. (1990) *Making Sex: Body and Gender from the Greeks to Freud.* Cambridge, MA: Harvard University Press.

Leps, M. C. (1992) *Apprehending the Criminal: The Production of Deviance in Nineteenth-century Discourse.* Durham, NC: Duke University Press.

Lombroso, C. (1911) *Criminal Man According to the Classification of Cesare Lombroso, Briefly Summarized by his Daughter Gina Lombroso Ferrero, with an Introduction by Cesare Lombroso.* New York and London: G. P. Putnam's Sons.

Lombroso, C. and Ferrero, G. (1895) *The Female Offender.* New York: D. Appleton.

Lutz, C. (1988) *Unnatural Emotions: Everyday Sentiments on a Micronesian Atoll and their Challenge to Western Theory.* Chicago: University of Chicago Press.

Martin, J. and Sugarman, J. (2001) 'Interpreting human kinds: beginnings of a hermeneutic psychology'. *Theory and Psychology*, **11**, 193–207.

Maruyama, K. (1991) 'The discovery of adenosine triphosphate and the establishment of its structure'. *Journal of the History of Biology*, **24**(1), 145–54.

Michell, J. (1997) 'Quantitative science and the definition of measurement in psychology'. *British Journal of Psychology*, **88**, 355–83.

Mitchell, J. (2000) 'Normal science, pathological science and psychometrics'. *Theory and Psychology*, **10**, 639–67.

Morrison, W. D. (1892) 'The study of crime'. *Mind, N.S.* **1**(4), 489–517.

Norenzayan, A. and Heine, S. J. (2005) 'Psychological universals: what are they and how can we know?' *Psychological Bulletin*, **135**, 763–84.

Nye, R. (1976) 'Heredity or milieu: the foundations of European criminological theory'. *Isis*, **67**, 335–55.

O'Malley, P. (1999) 'Volatile and contradictory punishment'. *Theoretical Criminology*, **3**, 175–96.

Parker, I. (1992) *Discourse Dynamics: Critical Analysis for Social and Individual Psychology*. London: Routledge.

Parker, I. (1994) 'Discourse analysis', in P. Banister, E. Burman, I. Parker, M. Taylor and C. Tindall *Qualitative Methods in Psychology*. Buckingham: Open University Press.

Pick, D. (1989) *Faces of Degeneration: A European Disorder, c. 1848–1918*. Cambridge: Cambridge University Press.

Potter, J. and Wetherell, M. (1987) *Discourse and Social Psychology*. London: Sage.

Rafter, N. H. (1997) *Creating Born Criminals*. Champaign, IL: University of Illinois Press.

Rafter, N. H. (2005) 'The murderous Dutch fiddler: criminology, history and the problem of phrenology'. *Theoretical Criminology*, **9**(1), 65–96.

Rafter, N. H. (2006) 'Criminal anthropology: its reception in the United States and the nature of its appeal', in P. Becker and R. F. Wetzell *Criminals and their Scientists: The History of Criminology in International Perspective*. Cambridge: Cambridge University Press.

Randall, W. L. (2007) 'From computer to compost: rethinking our metaphors for memory'. *Theory and Psychology*, **17**(5), 611–33.

Richards, G. (1987) 'Of what is history of psychology a history?' *British Journal for the History of Science*, **20**(2), 201–12.

Richards, G. (2010) *Putting Psychology in its Place: Critical Historical Perspectives*, 3rd edn. London: Routledge.

Roediger, H. L. (2008) 'Why the laws of memory vanished'. *Annual Review of Psychology*, **59**, 225–54.

Rose, N. (1991) *Governing the Soul: The Shaping of the Private Self*. London/New York: Routledge.

Rose, N. (1996) *Inventing Our Selves: Psychology, Power and Personhood*. London/New York: Routledge.

Rose, N. (2000) 'Government and control'. *British Journal of Criminology*, **40**, 321–39.

Scull, A. (2009) *Hysteria: The Biography*. Oxford: Oxford University Press.

Smith, R. (1998) 'The big picture: writing psychology into the history of the human sciences'. *Journal of the History of the Behavioral Sciences*, **34**, 1–14.

Smith, R. (2005) 'The history of psychological categories'. *Studies in the History and Philosophy of the Biological and Biomedical Sciences*, **36**, 55–94.

Smith, R. (2007) *Being Human: Historical Knowledge and the Creation of Human Nature*. Manchester: Manchester University Press.

Smyth, M. M. (2004) 'Exploring psychology's low epistemological profile in psychology textbooks: are stress and stress disorders made within disciplinary boundaries?' *Theory and Psychology*, **14**, 527–53.

Susman, W. I. (1984) 'Personality and the making of twentieth-century culture', in W. I. Susman *Culture as History: The Transformation of American Society in the Twentieth Century*. New York: Pantheon.

Tarde, G. (1903/1912) *Penal Philosophy* (Trans. Rapelje Howell.) Boston: Little, Brown.

Tate, C. and Audette, D. (2001) 'Theory and research on "race" as a natural kind variable in psychology'. *Theory and Psychology*, **11**, 495–520.

Thomson, J. B. (1870) 'The hereditary nature of crime'. *Journal of Mental Science*, **15**, 487–98.

Thomson, M. (2006) *Psychological Subjects: Identity, Culture, and Health in Twentieth-century Britain*. Oxford: Oxford University Press.

Trendler, G. (2009) 'Measurement theory, psychology and the revolution that cannot happen'. *Theory and Psychology*, **19**, 579–99.

Van Wyhe, J. (2004) *Phrenology and the Origins of Victorian Scientific Naturalism*. Aldershot: Ashgate Publishing.

Weber, M. (2006) 'The sociology of charismatic authority/the nature of charismatic authority and its routinization', in P. D. Marshall (ed.) *The Celebrity Culture Reader*. London: Routledge.

Wetzell, R. F. (2000) *Inventing the Criminal: A History of German Criminology, 1880–1945*. Chapel Hill, NC: University of North Carolina Press.

Wiener, M. J. (1990) *Reconstructing the Criminal: Culture, Law, and Policy in England, 1830–1914*. Cambridge: Cambridge University Press.

Williams, H. S. (1896) 'Can the criminal be reclaimed?' *North American Review*, **163**(2), 207–18.

Willig, C. (2001) *Introducing Qualitative Research in Psychology: Adventures in Theory and Method*. Maidenhead: Open University Press.

Winter, A. and Ellis, H. (1891) *The New York State Reformatory in Elmira (1891)*. Whitefish, MT: Kessinger Publishing.

Wolfgang, M. E. (1972) 'Cesare Lombroso', in H. Mannheim (ed.) *Pioneers in Criminology*, 2nd edn. Montclair, NJ: Patterson Smith.

Žižek, S. (1997) 'Ideology I: No Man is an Island . . .' Accessed April 4, 2011. http://www.lacan.com/zizwhiteriot.html.

PART III

Representations

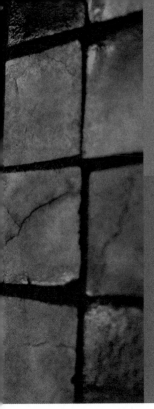

Chapter 11

Future directions for qualitative research

Paul Duckett

Introduction

Back to the past

The growing proliferation of books in psychology on qualitative methods in recent years (e.g. Richardson 1996; Kopala and Suzuki 1999; Willig 2008; Forrester 2009) as well as new journals dedicated to the subject (e.g. *Qualitative Research in Psychology*) are signs that qualitative research methods have become a much more prominent feature of psychological research, certainly since the mid-1990s and certainly in the UK. For example, qualitative methods were recognised in the benchmark guidelines of the Higher Education Council for England in 2002 and then by the British Psychology Society (BPS). This means psychology students in the UK are now expected to be taught qualitative methods in their undergraduate training. The growing popularity of qualitative methods is suggested by the boast made by the BPS Qualitative Methods in Psychology section that they have the largest membership of any BPS section.

So, the future of qualitative methods in psychology is looking bright. However, to say that qualitative methods have become more established in psychology is perhaps not the best way of describing events. Qualitative methods have always played an important role in the development of psychology (psychologists have always used qualitative means of gathering and making sense of their empirical data and still do, albeit not always systematically or transparently). Rather it is more the case that in the past few psychologists wrote about the role which qualitative research played in psychology; those that did write about this were not widely read and when they were read they weren't well remembered. This might have been because of: a strongly held belief in the supremacy of quantitative methods and a scepticism over the value of qualitative methods; fewer opportunities to publish qualitative research in psychology journals; and peer pressure to conform to the image of 'lab-coated scientist' rather than 'baggy trousered philanthropist'. It is likely to be a complex mix of reasons. An example of how qualitative research has been written out of the history of psychology is provided by the way Wilhelm Wundt's (1832–1920) contributions to psychology are remembered. Wundt called for psychology to grow with two branches – a qualitative, exploratory branch in partnership with a quantitative experimental branch. His call for the former has been little noted and he has become more commonly known for calling for the latter (Hamilton 1994; Punch 1994). Indeed, he is now referred to as the founder of experimental psychology. While it is true that he mostly used experimental methods, he did not feel that this was a sufficient method for psychology on its own.

In thinking about the future of qualitative methods in psychology, it is instructive to make use of elements of its history to understand the trajectory that qualitative methods might be on. Others (e.g. Denzin and Lincoln 2000) have offered authoritative accounts of the historical development of qualitative research in general so I will not rehearse that material here. Rather, I wish to concentrate on one particular point in the development of qualitative research in psychology and from that to consider the prudence of the direction qualitative research has subsequently taken. That point in history is what is widely referred to as the 'crisis in social psychology', the point after which qualitative methods came to receive greater recognition in the discipline.

The crisis began during the 1970s as a reaction against a growing body of social psychological work that was deemed socially irrelevant (it was not seen to be producing findings or theory that had a practical application in addressing the major social problems of the time); was viewed to be artificial (research was largely based on experimental work conducted on university students in university laboratories); and was felt to be losing its moral dimension (research was failing to address moral concerns and had adopted morally questionable practices – such as deceiving participants and subjecting them to distress). An example, now infamous, was the Milgram obedience studies which, it was argued, were artificial experiments that subjected research participants to unnecessary harm. Though Milgram's studies provided important and critical insights into human nature and the nature of bureaucracy (see Bauman 1989; Billig 2008), the findings from that research have been largely overshadowed by discussion of the ethics of the research. It became one of a number of studies that were embroiled in vitriolic critiques of the use of experimental, laboratory-based methods in psychology.

The crisis in social psychology was happening during a crisis in science more broadly, referred to as a period of 'epistemological disarray' (Hamilton 1994). It was a time when the basic tenets of positivist and experimental science were challenged by the theories of constructivism, herme-neutics and, epistemologies and methodologies wedded to relativism, deconstructionism and psychoanalysis (described elsewhere in this book). Even the basic tenets of positivism within the physical sciences were being questioned through the re-emergence in physics, mathematics and economics in the 1970s of the challenges posed by theories in quantum physics. It was also a time when feminist theory was making greater incursions into the social sciences, questioning the veracity and legitimacy of the objective, neutral standpoint claimed for by positivist scientists. These cultural shifts were occurring at a time of considerable political upheaval across Europe and the USA (Paris student demonstrations in 1968; economic and political instability caused by the Oil Crisis in 1973; protests against the Vietnam War during the late 1960s and early 1970s; the scandal of Watergate that broke in 1972, and so on). Public faith in the authority of professionals, politicians and other so-called 'experts' (and of the concept of 'big government' more generally) was shaken considerably. For psychology, the notion of psychologists as objective, neutral observers came under scrutiny and a recognition of the subjective, reflexive and politically driven psychologist began to slowly emerge through feminist (e.g. Miller 1976) and radical (e.g. Brown 1973) psychology texts. The canopy of diverse social identities (Klein 2000) that were gaining increased cultural recognition in the industrialised West throughout the 1960s and 1970s (new racial, sexual, cultural and political identities) made it increasingly obvious that the typical psychological researcher was not in fact neutral and faceless, but actually had the face of a white, middle-class, heterosexual male. Moreover, it became apparent that psychology appeared to assume that everyone else had a white, male, middle-class heterosexual face too. The alternative identities and voices that were becoming more visible and louder in society begged the question as to why some people (women, black and Asian people, disabled people, lesbian, gay, bisexual and transgendered people, and so on) were not being represented by psychology. It was becoming increasingly clear that psychological theory was not an objective science but an arbitrary one that produced a particularised view of human nature (one based on one social group's particular interests).

Quantitative methodology mostly (aside from the development of postpositivism) appeared to offer little room to accommodate the challenges posed by new cultural trends and alternative scientific perspectives. Qualitative methodology appeared to offer an alternative way of doing things. It held the promise of delivering work that was: socially relevant (it could be more readily grounded in people's 'real' experiences); authentic (it could more easily be conducted in the 'real' world); moral (it could be more easily made accessible and transparent in terms of its ethics and politics); and could accommodate and represent multiple selves and diverse subjectivities (as the subjectivity of both researchers and participants were viewed as enhancing rather than, as in quantitative methods, polluting the data). So, qualitative methods, by showing how they could meet growing concerns about the ethics of psychological research, gained some ground at this time and saw the beginnings of the break-up of the monopoly of quantitative methods in psychology.

Critiquing ethics

So, the focus on research ethics has become a central concern in qualitative methodology and has created scope for qualitative methods to grow in psychology (with the promise that qualitative methods might temper some of the criticism of the discipline that arose during the crisis in social psychology). So what were these research ethics? Well, there is not any one particular ethical framework for research that all subscribe to. Miles and Huberman (1994), for example, list seven different frameworks. However, a common, generic ethical position has emerged. Murphy and Dingwall (2001) summarise it as containing four principles:

- *non-maleficence* – avoid causing participants harm
- *beneficence* – promote benefits for participants in particular and society in general
- *autonomy/self-determination* – ensure participants have some control over the research
- *justice* – treat all people as equals.

These principles are co-joined in the overall maxims of 'informed consent' and the 'right to withdraw' – the procedure by which the autonomy of the participant is seen as ultimately protected and harm towards the participant is seen as ultimately avoided. It gives the participants the power to ask questions of and to say no to the researcher and, with all being equal, all participants have the right to walk away.

The principles of redressing power inequalities between researchers and participants (justice), and promoting the transparency and accountability of psychological research so that participants occupy active research roles (autonomy and self-determination) was taken up by qualitative research and used as a means of criticising psychological research that relied on passive, ill-informed or misinformed 'subjects'. It was a means of gaining greater recognition for qualitative research in the discipline. Whilst both qualitative and quantitative research could avoid harming participants and could equally aim to promote positive outcomes for both participants and society, it was qualitative methods in particular that came to be seen as the champion for redressing the disempowered research roles occupied by participants – qualitative methods offered the prospect of participants having greater control over the research process and outcome.

However, these ethical principles have been criticised for unnecessarily constraining the type of research that can be done and for carrying unhelpful ideological assumptions that might be maintaining psychology as a culturally and politically blinkered discipline in the social sciences. Once as a researcher you have convinced your peers (usually convened through an ethics committee) that participants in your research will be protected from harm, that your research will do some good, and that participants have some autonomy and control in the research process (even if that is restricted to the use of informed consent and the right to withdraw), a project is largely viewed as satisfying the most pressing ethical demands. Research where any of these ethical principles are not met ordinarily requires additional scrutiny by ethics committees and may be delayed or blocked. So, it seems sensible to ensure that your research methods are selected and used in such a way that satisfies those ethical principles. However, this might result in the design of the research having to be adapted in a way that means the wrong methods end up being used or the methods might be used in a way that renders them unable to deliver meaningful results (Murphy and Dingwall 2001):

Example 1: Research methods need to be fully formalised prior to the research commencing so they can be fully scrutinised by a research ethics committee. This can mean an inductive, organic research methodology that follows an iterative and evolving process (where the methods are co-developed with research participants as part of the research process) being compromised or even abandoned – an ethics committee might judge that a project cannot be given ethical clearance because the research methods to be used are not clearly specified from the outset. (Ramcharan and Cutliffe 2001).

Example 2: Having to ensure that participants are fully briefed or debriefed about the purpose of the research (informed consent) makes it extremely difficult, perhaps impossible, to use non-participant covert observation and the researcher might instead be forced to use participant observation or more overt forms of non-participant observation – where the researcher's purpose and presence in a setting are known to those being observed. This might result in participants behaving differently to how they might have previously have acted.

Example 2 is particularly interesting. We find that covert forms of research are largely viewed as problematic and more stringent tests of beneficence are applied to such research (Calvey 2008). Calvey cites the advice given by the Economic and Social Research Council (ESRC) in the UK, a major funder of research in the social sciences and humanities:

> The broad principle should be that covert research must not be undertaken lightly or routinely. It is only justified if important issues are being addressed and if matters of social significance which cannot be uncovered in other ways are likely to be discovered.
>
> (ESRC 2005: 21)

Here, covert research becomes the method of 'last resort' because participants can neither give their informed consent nor exercise their right to withdraw. It is interesting that this is happening at a time when 'the people' are gaining more access to technologies of surveillance (e.g. miniaturised cameras, recording devices and data storing and sharing technologies) that have historically been used against them by governments and corporations. 'The people' are now using these technologies more and more against those institutions that used to snoop on them. Qualitative methods in psychology appear to be retreating in the opposite direction – the increased regulation of systems of covert surveillance through increasingly bureaucratised systems of research ethics. That is not to suggest that psychology should seek always to be in step with popular opinion or cultural trends, but it is an interesting reflection nonetheless.

The ethical principles of consent and withdrawal largely operate as moral absolutes (they are largely unquestioned). As such, they are protected from critical scrutiny (no one asks who benefits from them) and the question of whether the application of those ethical principals has particular epistemological and methodological effects (prevent us from knowing certain things and from asking certain questions) is not sufficiently attended to. It also deflects attention away from how ethics might work politically, that is: How might an ethical principle prevent researchers from asking certain question of certain participants because of the nature of the power relations they have with them?

Nader notes how the ethics of 'studying down' (researching those who have less power than us) can be very different from 'studying up' (researching those who have more power than us). She quotes her student who is considering the problem of studying up when required to use ethics designed for studying down:

> How can we gain access to the same kinds of information as when we 'study down' without being dishonest (i.e. fake secretary or other role)? If we did get information without letting informants know we were social scientists, how could we publish it? It seems that the only 'open' way of doing a study would end up being fairly superficial – questionnaires and formal interviews as versus what we learn by participant observation.
>
> (Nader 1972: 304)

Nader further draws out the distinction between 'public' and 'private'. Ethics that have been largely developed to protect the private matters of participants do not necessarily transfer well to the study of the public matters of participants (such as studying the activities of governments, corporations and public realm social institutions) and upon phenomena that have a direct public impact (such as the public administration of social and corporate policymaking). Our ethical principles largely prevent us from studying, in any meaningful way, how the powerful work in the public domain. Ethics have developed to protect and empower the individual foremost and with an understanding primarily geared to ethically responding to the scenario of the researcher working with *power over* rather than *power under* those they research. This compromises the opportunity for researchers to study the powerful as the researcher is obliged to give such participants the right to control the research process (in terms of the right to informed consent, the right to withdrawal, and the right to exercise autonomy and self-determination during the research process – having a say in how data is collected, analysed and disseminated). This permits the powerful to close the door to you as a researcher or to open the door to you on the understanding that it is their agenda which will dominate and their version of reality which will be disseminated, or to block your research entirely (the powerful unlike the powerless have the resources to stop you publishing and potential to stop your research, see Monbiot 2000). A researcher seeking to question a multinational pharmaceutical corporation, for example, on issues of corporate corruption could be turned away or told what to say or threatened with a legal action.

Psychology has not always operated with the type of ethical principles that it does now. Indeed, today's requirements over obtaining informed consent and ensuring participants have a right to withdraw might have stymied some of the most important psychological research that was conducted in the past such as the work of Erving Goffman (1961) and David Rosenhan (1972) into the appalling conditions in psychiatric institutions. It is likely that the managers of those institutions, along with senior psychiatrists and local government officials, would have stopped that research happening on the basis of it being covert. There is a strong history of covert observational work conducted in the social sciences, that pre-dated the most recent, focused, some might say frenzied, attention on research ethics. Ethical rules that arguably served as a key to fully open the door of psychological issues to qualitative inquiry might mean that much of the important work that remains to be done might suffer delay and obstruction in the face of the scrutiny of research ethics committees that view deception and coercion as anathemas to the research enterprise.

Research ethics committees have become increasingly bureaucratised in the past two decades or more and researchers are becoming increasingly conditioned to develop their research proposals in a way that will proceed smoothly through ethical scrutiny (Richardson and McMullan 2007). Some have argued that the process of seeking ethical approval for a project has become little more than a routine (Sin 2005) or form of ritualistic practice. It has, for some, become little more than a form-ticking exercise where the thought of questioning or problematising ethical codes is rarely considered and, if it is considered, is viewed as foolhardy.

So, informed consent along with meeting the requirements of particular articulations of the concepts of justice, autonomy and self-determination can result in some methods being viewed as unacceptable, can render other methods as ineffective and can keep us researching down (studying the powerless) and away from researching up (studying the powerful). The way qualitative work, but not such work alone, deals with ethics might be constraining the ability of qualitative work to deliver all that is expected of it in terms of addressing contemporary social problems. The ethical principles are applied in ways that might render them insensitive both to methodological considerations and sociopolitical context.

The way qualitative methods have developed along with a set of ethical principles that are designed to protect the powerless perhaps reveals an inherent class bias – the fascination of the rich with the lives of the poor. As such, qualitative methods may have developed in a way that subtly colluded with the interests of those who have power by protecting them from our inquiring gaze. A response to this could be to call for the generalised application of ethical principles to be rejected and a 'situated ethics' to be used in their place (Murphy and Dingwall 2001) – an ethics that is not guided by an abstract code but developed and determined in fidelity with the particular cultural, social and political context in which those ethics are to be applied. Thus, rather than deceit being proscribed, it might be used only for certain methods in certain situations (i.e. when observering powerful individuals, groups and organisations). This would not be a case of disassociating qualitative research from research ethics, but about questioning how ethics are used and why they are there.

The history of psychology's engagement in ethics in research in particular might have looked very different had psychology spent more time researching the powerful rather than the powerless and the course of qualitative methods in psychology might have taken a distinctively different turn. There is a further critique of the application of ethics in qualitative research that they are blind to cultural context. Specifically, the argument is that the ethical principles that have been adopted by qualitative research in psychology are predicated on the assumption that individual autonomy is a fundamental human right and as such they carry particular cultural assumptions tied to how the industrialised West's political and economic systems now largely operate (described below). Here, a future turn for qualitative research in psychology might be to strip it of its Western bias and class bias – a call for qualitative methods in psychology to undergo a thorough process of decolonisation.

Decolonising methods

Linda Tuhiwai Smith (1999) has developed a critical and authoritative case for decolonising research methodologies. She describes the risk of researchers using methods that only permit them to see the world through the eyes of a particular cultural group (typically, the group which has most cultural power). As such, research methods might deliver data that is little more than a confirmation of the preconceptions held by those who have power over those they study. In general, research might deliver to us little more than a oblique insight into the views of academics dressed up as the views of their research participants or, as Spivak puts it more acerbically: 'the banality of leftist intellectuals' lists of self-knowing' (Spivak 1988: 70).

The problem of colonisation is usually characterised as the way the cultural systems of beliefs, behaviour norms and social rituals of countries that have the greatest economic, political and military power are imposed on those countries that have the least amount of such power. The culture of the powerful becomes hegemonic as it is ingrained and sustained in the colonised country through processes of socialisation, informal and formal systems of education and the norms that govern civil and political society (Gramsci 1971). In its most recent manifestation and of most relevance to the argument here is the colonisation of Western psychological knowledge over non-Western indigenous psychologies. The USA and UK are major exporters of psychological knowledge to the rest of the world. Scholars from these countries have more opportunities to publish and present their work (coming from relatively resource rich universities) while the global use of English privileges them still further.

The need to decolonise psychology has been voiced by new and fast-growing areas of the discipline such as: indigenous psychology (Allwood and Berry 2006); feminist psychology and psychology of women (Kidder and Fine 1997; Wilkinson 1996); and a psychology of disabled people (e.g. Goodley and Lawthom 2006). Much of the progress made has been through qualitative methods employed in these new areas. So far largely absent is a psychology of the working class and underclass. As discussed above, qualitative psychology may need to be decolonised through attending to the problem of psychology being primarily about the study of the poor for the advancement of the rich. We may need to attend to the cultural assumptions that are carried by qualitative research, particularly in relation to the ethical principles that have largely guided or at the very least accompanied it. These ethics are based on a respect for the individual's right to self-determination and autonomy – values carried by Western capitalist consumer economic systems that extol the virtues of heightened competitive individualism and promote individual choice and autonomy as the stalwart values of a healthy economy. So, the project of decolonisation might ask us to look at the use of qualitative methods in psychology and consider whether those methods might have become a vehicle of colonisation for class interests and interests of particular economic systems. This is something I am subjecting my own work to:

> Our methodology was also grounded in a consumerist culture where the heightened influence of individualism and growing spread of consumerism [have] led to the increasing power and influence of the consumer's voice and choice.
>
> (Duckett *et al.* 2010: 171)

Individualism and an emphasis on participant/citizen autonomy and self-determination contrast with alternative economic, political and cultural systems that emphasise the import-ance of the collective over the individual, of interdependence over independence and of duty over personal freedom. Under such systems the duty of participants to take part in research might carry as much or more weight than the participants right not to. The present ethical arrangements that dominate qualitative research would make such a stance mostly unpalatable and be labelled 'coercion'.

The need for a heightened cultural awareness (being aware of the cultural norms which might be carried by the methodologies we employ and how those norms might impact both the knowledge we acquire from particular cultural and political contexts, and also how our investi-gations might impact those contexts in terms of a colonising trend) and heightened reflexivity (in terms or recognising where we are in the world and our social, cultural and political positioning towards others) are key here.

This is not to suggest that any of the present ethical principles that dominate qualitative work should be abandoned, but might suggest the need for a reflexive account of how qualita-tive methods are used in psychology and how some methods might be used more often and be more commonly accepted because of the weight of the political and economic systems that sit behind them. This forms part of a more general critique of psychology in the UK – that it acts as though it is engaged in a European colonial project – seeking to spread European values wider (Howitt and Owusu-Bempah 1994); and that when it seeks to help those who have been marginalised by the dominant social, economic and political systems of the West, it does so by getting those individuals to change so as to adopt to those systems rather than challenging their legitimacy. Coupled with the criticism of a class bias in studying the poor rather than the powerful, qualitative methods might need to attend to Nader's (1972) plea that we should not study the poor and the powerless because everything we find out about them will be used against them.

Overcoming the qualitative vs. quantitative divide

There is another historical feature of qualitative work in psychology that needs discussion. As qualitative methods have become established they have largely rested on a dichotomous relationship with quantitative methods. Research methods have largely undergone a process of bifurcation with qualitative and quantitative methodologies becoming set up as binary oppositions involving epistemological and methodological choices that take you down one route or the other. Methodological decisions have mostly been grounded in the logic of the excluded middle (the purported incompatibility between two systems and the lack of availability of an alternative to them – e.g. 'you are either with us or against us'). Qualitative and quantitative methods are described as based on wholly different epistemological and methodological principles (e.g. Becker 1996) and their relationship with each other is often characterised as a war between paradigms (e.g. Lincoln and Guba 1985). However, recent methodological developments are beginning to ask whether this is a false logic.

Polemics such as that of Potter and Wetherell (1987) on the incompatibility of qualitative with quantitative methods have been less evident in recent years and there appears to be a greater level of pragmatism that has taken the arguments away from methodological purity and towards methodological pluralism. The new position has also come from a more direct challenge of the logic of binaries (such as the challenge of queer theory in the social sciences that has sought to transgress conventional binary categories and traverse and break social boundaries). Mixed methods are increasingly being explored, not as a clumsy stitching together of two incompatible systems but as a genesis of a 'third paradigm'. Increasingly, the paradigm war between qualitative and quantitative methods is being overwritten by a narrative of a peaceful co-existence (e.g. Datta 1994).

Some use the term 'hybridisation' to describe a methodology driven by pragmatic need such that a researcher can use both qualitative and quantitative methods without being tied to a specific methodological paradigm. However, the dichotomous relationship between qualitative and quantitative is proving difficult to overcome and the difficulty is not only grounded in epistemological and methodological concerns but is also about ideology – the threat of a redistribution of resources (both material and symbolic) away from one group of psychologists and towards another. Both camps, over many decades, have accrued sufficient rhetoric resources to argue that their method is superior to the other and to justify ring-fencing areas of social science funding off as protected territory. For example, qualitative methods have been described as the preferred, perhaps only, method to be used in studying macro sociological phenomena (Cicourel 1981), public health issues (McKinlay 1995) and critical forms of inquiry, even though quantitative data has been important in these areas (such as epidemiological evidence that offers a critical perspective on public health issues, see Wilkinson and Pickett 2010) and even though quantitative data can be a powerful source of evidence used in work that promotes social justice (Parker and Burman 1993).

The bifurcation of qualitative and quantitative methods has been particularly pronounced in psychology where these paradigm wars are often times pronounced. This is to such an extent that the term 'positivism' has become a pejorative term for those working in some areas of psychology that are associated with qualitative methods (such as critical psychology). The future relationship between qualitative methods and quantitative methods in psychology is likely to be weighed down by these historical acrimonies and the 'third paradigm' remains under-theorised with mixed methods research either viewed as adventuresome or naïve depending on how well disposed one is to the notion that qualitative and quantitative methods are compatible (e.g. Jick 1983). Also, attempts to establish this third paradigm are finding that some areas of qualitative method are perhaps more amenable to being reconciled with quantitative approaches. Methodological approaches based on theories of symbolic interactionism (such as content analysis) might work alongside quantitative methods relatively untroubled – indeed, the methods might blur together at times (such as when content analysis is used to deliver frequency counts on themes that occur in transcripts). However, other approaches based on phenomenology, social constructivism, psychoanalysis and hermeneutics might be much harder to reconcile with quantitative methods. Indeed, phenomenological and hermeneutic research in particular have developed in a way that views linking the results of this research to quantitative research as largely, if not wholly, unnecessary (Flick 2009). Here perhaps is one of the greatest challenges ahead and returns us back to the future.

Back to the future

Social media as text

The types of social text available to qualitative researchers have been changing dramatically in recent years, most notably through the proliferation of social media in many Western countries as a result of an exponential growth in information communication technologies. Social networking internet sites, web blogs, and so on have dramatically increased the volume and diversity of social media outputs. This is creating a greater array of texts available to social scientists that are relatively easily captured (through digital recording) and an increasing number of representations of lived experience. These new media outputs are becoming important sources of data for qualitative research and are starting to reduce qualitative researchers' reliance on more traditional sources of data (face-to-face interviewing, surveying and in-situ observing). More and more researchers are not only using these new forms of social text as data but also creating new social texts as data through adopting existing methods to these new media (such as conducting email interviews and chat room focus groups). This is creating new methodological questions for qualitative researchers in terms of how to use these new forms of data (including questions around sampling, editing, analysis and ethics). In relation to ethics, researchers are already being warned of the temptation of engaging in non-participant, covert methods (such as snooping on emails, online discussion and personal web pages):

> Critical psychologists need also to be cautious about the ethical issues raised by the various forms of virtual (but potentially invasive) voyeurism that technological advances make possible. As researchers more interested in data interpretation than its source, we must resist being so beguiled by the ease of snooping that we undermine the very social justice agenda we are so proud to claim.
>
> (Stainton-Rogers 2009: 347)

This might be a sign that qualitative methods in psychology still have some way to go before it can claim to be class-aware and decolonised. For example, it is not clear whether Stainton-Rogers' warning would also apply to researchers using documents released on such websites as 'wiki leaks' – i.e. snooping on powerful governments and corporations. Perhaps a more immediate concern is that the class bias might be present in only a mute acknowledgement so far of the class-created digital divide between those who can access the new forms of communication and those who cannot, based on their access to the material resources required to take part in this new world of social media text production.

We may find that new social media become a new method of colonisation – whereby the resource rich are primarily the producers and the poor are primarily the consumers. Alongside the more practical risk that the sheer number of social texts available might soon overwhelm researchers, social media might suggest another turn of direction open to qualitative methods in psychology.

It may be time for qualitative research in psychology to more fully embrace the alternative perspective offered by psychoanalysis and genetic structuralism – a hermeneutic analysis of what lies beneath the text. This might not only be a sensible response to how social media are saturating the world with more and more texts, but also as a response to how those texts might become a new voicepiece of the powerful. Structuralist or psychoanalytic perspectives highlight the role of unconscious psychological structures and subterranean cultural, economic and political systems in determining the nature of social arrangements and experiences. Qualitative methods might use the opportunity offered by these perspectives to move further beyond the text – to look at what sits beneath the text and at how human behaviours are culturally, politically and socially produced (e.g. Foucault 1978, 'technologies of the self'). This might be difficult to accomplish as qualitative methods may not only have suffered a history of being sidelined following a bifurcation of methodology from the outside (the split between quantitative and qualitative methods described above) but also from the inside. So far, qualitative work has become dominated by two interpretative frameworks: one that focuses on participants' subjective experiences (symbolic interactionism and phenomenology) and one that focuses on the social conditions whereby those experiences have come about (ethnomethodology and social constructivism). There is a danger that qualitative researchers can sometimes find themselves trapped between these two dominant approaches in an undertheorised, underpopulated middle ground and that psychology might find comfort from psychoanalysis as a means of escape from this particular binary.

Chapter summary

When looking to the future of qualitative research in psychology we might be mindful of how the focus on ethics that opened up greater opportunities for qualitative methods in the discipline might have also worked, increasingly so recently, as an essentially conservative force. Qualitative research might need to force a rethink on ethics if it is to avoid becoming more regressive than progressive. It might also be the case that psychology has been slow to respond to the need for decolonisation and slow to recognise the need to acknowledge class bias. It might be time (as qualitative researchers in psychology scrutinise ethics, scrutinise the quantitative-qualitative paradigm wars and their traditional data sources are being replaced by social texts) to consider slipping beneath the dominant modes of delivering ethics, discussing paradigms and deciphering texts.

References

Allwood, C. M. and Berry, J. (eds) (2006) 'Indigenous psychologies'. *International Journal of Psychology*, **41**, 4.

Bauman, Z. (1989) *Modernity and the Holocaust*. New York: Cornell University Press.

Becker, H. S. (1996) 'The epistemology of qualitative research', in R. Jessor, A. Colby and R. A. Shweder (eds) *Ethnography and Human Development*. Chicago: University of Chicago Press.

Billig, M. (2008) *The Hidden Roots of Critical Psychology*. London: Sage.

Brown, P. (ed.) (1973) *Radical Psychology*. New York: Harper.

Calvey, D. (2008) 'The art and politics of covert research: doing "situated ethics" in the field'. *Sociology*, **42**(5), 905–18.

Cicourel, A. V. (1981) 'Notes on the integration of micro- and macrolevels of analysis', in K. Knorr-Cetina and A. V. Cicourel (eds) *Advances in Social Theory and Methodology: Towards an Integration of Micro- and Macro-Sociologies*. London: Routledge and Kegan Paul.

Datta, L. (1994) 'Paradigm wars: a basis for peaceful coexistence and beyond'. *New Directions for Programme Evaluation*, **61**, 53–70.

Denzin, N. and Lincoln, Y. S. (eds) (2000) *Handbook of Qualitative Research*. London: Sage.

Duckett, P., Kagan, C. and Sixsmith, J. (2010) 'Consultation with children on healthy schools: choice, conflict and context'. *American Journal of Community Psychology*, **46**(1/2), 167–78.

ESRC (2005) *Research Ethics Framework*. Accessed May 15, 2011. http://www.esrcsocietytoday.ac.uk/ESRCInfoCentre/opportunities/research_ethics_framework/index.aspx?ComponentId.

Flick, U. (2009) *An Introduction to Qualitative Research*, 4th edn. London: Sage.

Forrester, M. (ed.) (2009) *Doing Qualitative Research in Psychology: A Practical Guide*. London: Sage.

Foucault, M. (1978) *The History of Sexuality*. New York: Pantheon.

Goffman, E. (1961) *Asylums: Essays on the Social Situation of Mental Patients and Other Inmates*. New York: Doubleday.

Goodley, D. and Lawthom, R. (eds) (2006) *Disability and Psychology: Critical Introductions and Reflections*. Basingstoke: Palgrave Macmillan.

Gramsci, A. (1971) *Selections from the Prison Notebooks*, in Q. Hoare and G. Nowell Smith (eds). London: Lawrence and Wishart.

Hamilton, D. (1994) 'Traditions, preference, and postures in applied qualitative research', in N. Denzin and Y. Lincoln (eds) *Handbook of Qualitative Research*, Thousand Oaks, CA: Sage.

Howitt, D. and Owusu-Bempah, J. (1994) *The Racism of Psychology*. Hemel Hempstead: Harvester Wheatsheaf.

Jick, T. (1983) 'Mixing qualitative and quantitative methods: triangulation in action', in J. v. M. Maanen (ed.) *Qualitative Methodology*. London: Sage.

Kidder, L. H. and Fine, M. (1997) 'Qualitative inquiry in psychology: a radical tradition', in D. Fox and I. Prilleltensky (eds) *Critical Psychology: An Introduction*. London: Sage.

Klein, N. (2000) *No Logo*. Toronto: Knopf Canada.

Kopala, M. and Suzuki, L. A. (eds) (1999) *Using Qualitative Methods in Psychology*. London: Sage.

Lincoln, Y. S. and Guba, E. G. (1985) *Naturalistic Inquiry*. London: Sage.

McKinlay, J. B. (1995) 'Towards appropriate levels: research methods and healthy public policies', in I. Guggenmoos-Holzmann, K. Bloomfield, H. Brenner, and U. Flick (eds) *Quality of Life and Health: Concepts, Methods and Applications*. Berlin: Blackwell.

Miles, M. B. and Huberman, A. M. (1994) *Qualitative Data Analysis: An Expanded Sourcebook*. Thousand Oaks, CA: Sage.

Miller, J. B. (1976) *Toward a New Psychology of Women*. Boston: Beacon.

Monbiot, G. (2000) *Captive State: The Corporate Takeover of Britain*. London: Macmillan.

Murphy, E. and Dingwall, R. (2001) 'The ethics of ethnography', in P. Atkinson, A. Coffey, S. Delamont, J. Lofland and L. Lofland (eds) *Handbook of Ethnography*. London: Sage.

Nader, L. (1972) 'Up the anthropologist: perspectives gained from studying up', in D. Hymes (ed.) *Reinventing Anthropology*. New York: Random House.

Parker, I. and Burman, E. (1993) 'Against discursive imperialism, empiricism and constructivism: thirty-two problems with discourse analysis', in E. Burman and I. Parker (eds) *Discourse Analytic Research: Repertoires and Readings of Texts in Action*. London: Routledge.

Potter, J. and Wetherell, M. (1987) *Discourse and Social Psychology: Beyond Attitudes and Behaviour*. London: Sage.

Punch, M. (1994) 'Politics and ethics in qualitative research', in N. Denzin and Y. Lincoln (eds) *Handbook of Qualitative Research*. Thousand Oaks, CA: Sage.

Ramcharan, P. and Cutliffe, J. R. (2001) 'Judging the ethics of qualitative research: considering the "ethics as process" model'. *Health and Social Care in the Community*, **9**(6), 358–66.

Richardson, J. T. E. (ed.) (1996) *Handbook of Qualitative Research Methods for Psychology and the Social Sciences*. Oxford: BPS and Blackwell Books.

Richardson, S. and McMullan, M. (2007) 'Research ethics in the UK: what can sociology learn from health?' *Sociology*, **41**(6), 1115–32.

Rosenhan, D. (1972) 'On being sane in insane places'. *Science*, **179**, 250–8.

Sin, C. H. (2005) 'Seeking informed consent'. *Sociology* **39**(2), 277–95.

Smith, L. T. (1999) *Decolonising Methodologies: Research and Indigenous Peoples*. Auckland: Zed Books.

Spivak, G. C. (1988) 'Can the subaltern speak?', in N. Cary and L. Grossberg (eds) *Marxism and the Interpretation of Culture*. Urbana, IL: University of Illinois Press.

Stainton-Rogers, W. (2009) 'Research methodology', in D. Fox, I. Prilleltensky, and S. Austin (eds) *Critical Psychology: An Introduction*. London: Sage.

Wilkinson, R. and Pickett, K. (2010) *The Spirit Level: Why Inequality is Better for Everyone*. London: Penguin.

Wilkinson, S. (ed.) (1996) *Feminist Social Psychologies: International Perspectives*. Bristol, PA: Open University Press.

Willig, C. (2008) *Introducing Qualitative Research in Psychology*. Maidenhead: Open University Press.

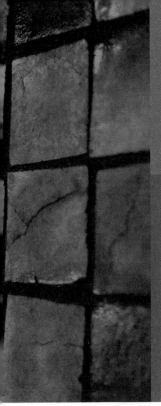

12

New and emerging forms of representation

Rebecca Lawthom

Introduction

In this chapter I explore emerging directions for qualitative research. The preceding chapters have covered orientations of qualitative research and particular methods in detail. It would be impossible to map the total landscape of qualitative research, although Denzin and Lincoln regularly report, reflect and update the map (see Denzin and Lincoln 2003, 2005). This task of orienteering is also made richer and more difficult as methodological inquiry is common to many disciplines, and psychology is but one discipline which is connected and related to a host of others.

The task here then is to map some of the possibilities and representations for current/future qualitative research in psychology. First, I provide a wider context (of discipline, culture and time) in which to position these emerging approaches. Second, I outline particular trends which are reflected in the literature. Third, I utilise some examples of this kind of work that myself and other colleagues have engaged in. Fourth, drawing on this and other work, I also present some advantages of disadvantages around these emergent methods and representations.

The context for emergent representations

We are currently entering a critical time in qualitative research as radical voices fight for scientific credibility in a time of austerity. In the current climate 'science' and what counts as science are being contested. In UK higher education institutions and elsewhere funding cuts for undergraduate programmes are prioritising STEM subjects – science, technology, engineering and mathematics. This privileging of traditional dominant views of science serves to undermine and downplay the potential influence of 'non-scientific' or hermeneutic social sciences. A further issue becomes evident as dominant experimental ways of positivist knowing are becoming enshrined as evidence. This weakens the potential for qualitative and more creative approaches to science. In the UK, the higher education funding cuts may well have wider ramifications around issues of what gets taught and hence what is considered important culturally. There is, however, a ray of light in that research funding councils are urging academics to be interdisciplinary or transdisciplinary in terms of engaging with knowledge, methods and approaches from other disciplines. This does present us with a possibility for being creative and looking for new possibilities of data collection, representation and forms of analysis. In this chapter as I map emerging forms of representation, you will note how we gain insight from such diverse disciplines as social and cultural anthropology, human geography and sociology, tourism studies and performance studies.

The wider context in terms of the scientific and academic community impacts upon the landscape of qualitative work generally. Within this diverse movement, it has been argued that qualitative work can be seen in terms of moments. The eighth moment upholds a concern for social justice issues and an ethic of communitarian, egalitarian and critical caring that underpins this research project. Denzin and Lincoln (2005: 1118) argue that 'the new participatory, feminist, and democratic values of interpretive qualitative research mandate a stance that is democratic, reciprocal, and reciprocating rather than objective and objectifying'. However, whilst inclusion and democratic practice in research are desired – can these emergent methods provide possibilities here? I shall return to this issue later in the chapter.

Pathway towards emerging representations in the social sciences

Creative methodological approaches see data as more than word-based – data can be gained from multisensory engagement and represented in different forms. The old adage of ethnography where researchers rendered the strange familiar assumes that 'going native' involves much more data than written renderings of culture. When we visit somewhere different from our own familiar setting – even if we have been there before, we are struck by the different look of the buildings and landscape, the feel/temperature of the environment, the smells offered and the different accent/language being spoken – indeed, what Crouch and Desforges (2003) term the sensuous nature of the 'tourist encounter'. If we want to learn, understand and represent other people's lives then we need to engage in multisensoriality. Many of the preceding chapters engage explicitly with rich constructions of subjectivity but most of these implicitly rely on the visual – observation, reading text, generating stories, analysing written transcripts. Whilst as researchers, we utilise a range of senses to extract and collect data – listening, seeing, touching – when representing this data we often present word-based text. In terms of a sensorium here (the way in which senses experience and interpret environments) vision is often privileged – the dominance of occularcentrism. Indeed, Titchkosky (2010) argues that even within the sensorium – the way in which senses are organised, that vision is very much prioritised. Carothers (1959) compared the impact of literacy on African native sensory life. He was arguing that people who live in an oral-aural world know none of the personal or detached attitudes of a visual–literate people. Moreover, the latter assume that ways of seeing and organising the world are natural to them and senses are organised so that vision is very much prioritised.

Howes (2005) notes the 'linguistic turn', which was prominent in the 1960s, has been privileged by the social sciences and humanities. This is reflected in an approach where human thought is understood 'as structured by, and analogous to language, so one may best look to linguistics for models of philosophical and social interpretation' (p. 1) Academia is of course hyperliterate and hence reading, writing 'discourse' has held much sway in interrogating social systems. The over-reliance on word-based text requires a sensory turn. Indeed, Howes (2005) claims it (the social sciences and humanities) has taken a sensual revolution: 'Once the encompassing grip of "the science of signs" (modelled on linguistics) is broken, we are brought – perhaps with a gasp of surprise or a recoil of disgust – into the realm of the body and the senses' (p. 1).

Serres (1985, cited in Howes 2005) and others have critiqued the sensorial poverty of contemporary theory. The lack of theory around sensorial understandings can be linked to Western or Global North ideas which associate senses with nature, 'innocent' or savage'. Senses historically have symbolised that which is antithetical to culture and civilisation. This seeming split of the civilisation versus untutored sensation cannot be supported. However, the human sensorium is of course not a natural state – it is, like humans, always social. Classen (2005) notes that supposedly primitive people living in intimate contact with nature have sensory experiences which are permeated with social values. Sounds, touches and tastes are immersed in meaning and ordered within hierarchies to enforce and express the social and cosmic order. Serres argues that the domination of language needs a revolt from the senses, but the empire of signs here will need to be replaced by the empire of the senses (many empires).

What might an approach that involves more than 'reading' subjectivity and cultures look like? Sensing itself is not a topic for study – rather, as social scientists, we use senses as media through which we can interpret and experience aspects of culture such as gender, colonialism and material culture. Of course there is an inherent paradox here as this richness is subsequently written and communicated through language. An aim of this sensorial revolution then is to recover perception from the laboratory. Science and traditional forms of psychology situate perception as private, internal, apolitical and ahistorical ignoring the role of culture. Sensation, however, like meaning, is socially constructed and senses are cultural systems. Howes and other theorists argue that scientists generally fail to consider cultural factors in their study of perception and usually fail to recognise sciences as a product of culture. To sense culture we need some new language; for example, the term 'emplacement' suggests the interrelationships between body, mind and environment.

This kind of argument is interesting because when trying to make sense of our own experience we implicitly use emplacement. If I am trying to learn Iyengar yoga for the first time – whilst I may read a text about it, or watch a DVD or social media site to see yoga positions – there is no substitute for doing or trying the positions. Here I am using emplacement to learn and do – reading manuals is insufficient. In this section I have argued for a richer sense of understanding which involves less reliance on word-based text and moves towards using other senses and hence other representations.

This brief introduction communicates the full range of sensory knowing and alternative representations available to us – even though most of what is commonly represented as psychological data is written and visual. How might a psychology researcher undertake a sensorially rich ethnography where visual data is supplemented by other forms? To convey some of the richness of the field I have mapped and provide tasters (note the language of the senses) of some approaches. I start with those which may seem more familiar (engaging with words) and then present some visual approaches, ending with what may be seen as radically different forms of sensory-based data.

Engaging with words rather differently

Earlier chapters, and indeed this one, encourage readers to immerse themselves into a vat of words. Different approaches use different words (lifeworld, psyche, feminism) to understand and construct subjectivity and experience. There is a plethora of frameworks to understand what is 'real', how to interpret words and what the informant and the researcher mean. In most of these forms, data is presented back through narratives, themes or discourses – portions of texts are actual replicas of speech or interviews. In these cases, the reproduction of words (as evidence) presents us with something tangible with which to judge the interpretation or the absence of words (in certain accounts) and also allows theorising. The sheer variability of qualitative approaches (some of which are covered in this text) allows the reader to explore the interpretation of text alongside the actual text.

The apparent dualism between fact/truth and fiction is worthy of exploration. For certain theorists, to produce writing which is creative and interesting we should question the 'truth' of data (Banks and Banks 1998). The role of fiction and non-fiction in communicating research findings is interesting and other researchers have creatively narrated life histories which may be composite forms of experience (see Goodley *et al.* 2004). Bochner and Ellis (2002) and Ellis (2004) address ways in which autoethnography can be innovatively represented in alternative writing forms. Experimental writing formats can be utilised to incorporate data and fiction into pieces as diverse as Japanese haiku to other forms of poetry (such as ethnographic poetics, Denzin 1997). These forms of writing around poetic representation can offer the researcher a way of merging participant 'voice' with researcher 'voice'. Both Richardson (1997) and Denzin (2003) have written about the potential of artistic expression to bring new theoretical insights. Whilst Richardson's work uses interview-based data which is turned into a story, this poetic represen-tation of interview data allows 'pleated texts' to emerge, richly conceptualising the possible layers of meaning. An alternative approach, investigative poetry used by Hartnett (2003), combines autobiography, critical ethnography and political underpinnings to explores issues of social justice. Whilst poetry is not for every researcher or project, this method offers a rather different communicative device. The example below presents a case study.

Case study

A doctoral student (Dawson 2007) wanted to explore the human–companion animal bond particularly in the context of companion animal euthanasia. The sensitivity of the topic warranted an approach which used a more relational ontology and engaged with feelings. She engaged with organic inquiry (OI), rooted in transpersonal psychology as a way of connecting companion animal owners with animals and the environment. Creative approaches were utilised and rich participant narratives or euthanographies (Couser 2004) were obtained around the decision to euthanase companion animals. The OI methodology embraces spirituality and encourages the researcher to 'live the methodology' (Curry and Wells 2003). Utilising personal experience of euthanasia, professional experience (as a veterinary nurse) and rich narratives, the researcher developed a sequence of research poems (Langer and Furman 2004). The processing of data involved an iterative process of research conversations, reflexivity, developing poems and sharing them with participants, and then further development of the poems. Dawson utilised a poetic approach to sharing the narrative collected called stanza narrative (McLeod and Balamoutsou 2000) where participants had their own words read to them and meanings clarified. Following this experiences, Dawson developed research poems with each participant (Langer and Furman 2004) as a way of representing core aspects of the euthanasia experience. This approach allowed lived experience to be honoured through verbatim word usage. In this beautifully crafted study, the researcher also utilised a poem of self-dialogue – a soliloquy in order to reflect upon professional and personal identities.

In this section, I have briefly sketched potentially different approaches to working with words. However, in these approaches covered, words are still king although poetic approaches can offer a rather different lens on the world. In the next section, I turn to a visual lens.

Visual representations

The axiom that we are living in an increasingly visual age seems a truism. Gombrich (1996) not only argues that we are living in a visual age but that 'we are entering a historical epoch in which the image will take over from the written word' (1996: 41). Thinking about the visual as data often leads to a reductionist approach of dealing with 2D data (pictures, advertisements, photographs). However, the bombardment of pictures we are experiencing through the visual is also about the experience of 3D. Objects and buildings carry meanings, as do clothing and body language. Whilst psychologists have historically been interested in eye contact and personal space as ways of regulating communication and contact, the interpretation of this provides rich visual data. The increasing surveillance of life (through CCTV) and personal technologies poses questions about visibility, privacy and the use of space. As I argued earlier, the visual medium (looking, observing) is routinely utilised in many (if not all) of the methodological approaches from hard to soft science. What is rather different is the way in which the visual gets 'read' or translated. Parker (1999) coming from a discourse analytic position uses a broad approach to discourse in critical text work. Here, methodological issues of reading and representation are explored in critical descriptions of how we might read such things as advertising, bodies, comics, film, letters, organisations, sign languages and other language systems. Engaging with the visual this text shows that discourse may be studied wherever there is meaning, and extends the principles of discourse research beyond conversations, interviews, newspaper articles and fiction to gardens and sign language. Whilst Parker (1999) argues for wider consideration of what is a text, the analysis is of course represented through word. There is a body of work which engages directly with the visual: 'Visual inquiry is no longer just the study of the image, but rather the study of the seen and observable' (Emmison and Smith 2000: ix).

Emmison and Smith (2000) argue that in broadening the concept of visual research, it can offer possibilities for linking the visual to social science and cultural theory. For example, ideas around display and status can link to Goffman's work on interaction whilst the issues of visibility, surveillance and privacy can be linked to Foucault and Elias. Postmodern theorists have long argued for deeper analysis of the visual spectacle (Baudrillard 1998; Lash 1988). In contrast, it has also been argued that humans have always lived in visual cultures. Hull (1990) and Michalko (2002) write from positions of blindness to argue that sight is king in quotidian practices and of course this dominance of sight (as primary in the sensorium) extends to research. Whilst there is broad agreement that the visual is important, the question of how to research it is rather more difficult. The primacy of the word and the premium placed on it need little rehearsal. Chaplin (1994) shows how the development of social science has privileged verbal forms of communication:

> In social sciences, therefore, a photograph depends on caption and textualisation to give it authentic and precise social scientific meaning. In this way it loses its autonomy as a photograph, and thus any claim to make a contribution 'in its own right'. In social science, as in most other discipline areas images needs words, while words do not necessarily need images.
>
> (Chaplin 1994: 207)

Certain theorists have argued that the absence of the visual (predominantly photography) is very much linked to the political nature of the 'relations of viewing' which is around the generation and consumption of images. Tagg (1988) has linked the development of photography to a broader concern for the surveillance, regulation and control of populations. There is a pattern of 'studying down' as particular groups of people became visual studies – street kids, the underclass, etc. Particular social sciences such as anthropology have embraced imagery of far-distant cultures where readers have little knowledge. Here the implicit colonial discourses and power relations, plus the quality of 'primitive as other', historically allowed photographs to be taken without fear or moral contagion.

Whilst there is a tradition of visual engagement in psychology, historically this pivots around clinical observation (children, families) and visual perception-style tasks. A new text (Reavey 2011) paints a rich picture, showcasing the potential for visual methods in psychology. The theoretical, methodological, ethical and analytical issues which shape the way in which visual qualitative work is undertaken span diverse visual forms of data. These include photography, documentary film-making, drawing, internet media, model making, walking and map drawing, video recording and collages.

There is much potential within visual research to work participatively. The increasing use of the camera (and mobile phone technology) presents opportunities for greater inclusion in the research process (Rose 1997; Reavey and Johnson 2008). For example, the photo elicitation process allows the researcher to actively involve participants. The researcher takes photos as part of the study and then uses these as prompts within subsequent in-depth studies. Here the image is used to generate more information – predominantly verbal. Another form is 'autophotography' where the researcher enables the participant to take photos and then the researcher analyses the material.

Within research, the use of photography as a method is becoming more popular, and whilst there are variants on a theme, photovoice seems to be the most popular (Wang et al. 1998). The advantages of this particular approach, which allows photographs to be read in context, is that participants can feel empowered, articulate and with a sense of community (Newbury 1997).

The context of photographs is particularly important in allowing meaning to emerge. Whilst certain theorists take a realist stance in relation to the image, as the camera captures a moment as an observation (Price and Well 1997), other theorists see images as more complex (Pink 2001). A scientific realist approach positions the content of images as reflecting realistic representation of visual evidence. In comparison, the reflexive approach takes into account the broader context of the image, allowing richer interpretations to emerge. Banks (2001) and Kuhn (1995) suggest that when looking at an image questions are asked such as: What is it of? What is the content? Who took it? Why? How do others read it?

Banks (2001) defines 'good' visual research as that which engages with both internal (local) and external (wider) narratives and is therefore multivocal. Whilst the use of visual data raises question of validity and interpretation, the democratising nature of photography can allow participants to 'speak' in particular ways and settings. Kellock (2009) explored children's well-being utilising an array of visual methods in school settings. Her approach engaged with small groups of children using experiential walks to map well-being and feelings dictionaries using photos taken by children and ascribed labels. Children also made visually annotated diaries of daily activity around well-being. Using an immediate form of child-produced photography (here Polaroid) allowed children to make methodological and analytical decisions within the research process. Whilst visual methodologies can enrich understanding of human experience and provide a window on aspects of lives rarely considered (Holliday 2004), it adds complexity to the research process (as the case study below demonstrates).

Case study

The project outlined here utilises a method developed by Haworth (2010) and is richly reported elsewhere (Kellock *et al.* 2011; Mountian *et al.* 2011). As a group of researchers, we had began using visual methods in participative ways across a range of projects. Mindful of the critiques of visual research but committed to working in settings with people, we pondered the applicability of the visual to community psychological ways of working (Kagan *et al.* 2011). To address issues and as development we engaged in a visual creative project. The research into activity and well-being in daily life uses the experience sampling method (ESM). Traditionally, the method uses questionnaire diaries and electronic pagers which are pre-programmed to bleep at randomly selected times during the day to indicate response times. The research here uses a mobile phone to indicate response time eight times a day for seven consecutive days, extended to include images taken at each signal with the mobile phone/camera. The data is gathered by each individual and so the photo represents the choice of the participant (within an ethical framework). The data provides a picture at each signal, an approach which was first used by Haworth (2010) as a part of his research into creativity and well-being.

This approach offers many possibilities of interpretation of this visual methodology considered to be an artistic object for contemplation; as individual visual profiles for comparative research; or as analysis of themes across a group of individuals, and between groups. As the rich data is provided across a week, each day yields eight photographs and other data. Focusing on the visual data can then be done individually, in a group and comparing immediate and retrospective responses to the photographs. Aside from yielding rich data (which allowed exhibition opportunity) the process and analysis gave much insight into the possibilities and problems of this approach. Participants reported: feeling surveilled (although all photos were autonomously taken), changing behaviour to present a picture of self; how the documented nature of the week enhanced memory; how well the week represented a 'normal' week. Space precludes richer discussion of many of the themes which emerged but the experience of participating and then analysing the visual offered insight into ways in which the visual can work.

Using creative approaches explicitly as ways of engaging in participative research presents interesting challenges. Work (spanning academic and practitioner circles) that links creative engagement in art practices with enhanced health and well-being uses creative approaches (e.g. Sixsmith and Kagan 2005; Kilroy *et al.* 2007). Art practices here are loosely defined as activities ranging from singing, making art products, photography, creative writing or utilising creative methods which are transformed into dissemination products (for example, films, magazines). Here, methods are not utilised therapeutically but as a means to engage people as collaborators in, and agents of, promotion of their own health and well-being. The process of engagement in creative work enables participants, art practitioners and researchers to reflect rather differently on the process (Lawthom *et al.* 2007). Indeed, the question of when and how to use creative methods (predominantly visual) is one which needs careful consideration (Lawthom *et al.* 2011).

Space precludes extensive coverage of the wider field but projects that colleagues have been involved with include: collaborative film making (Woolrych and Sixsmith 2008; Kagan and Michallef 2009); participatory photo-taking (Kellock 2009); talking heads; storyboards; and experience sampling methods (Haworth 2010; Kellock *et al.* 2011; Mountian *et al.* 2011). These projects focused on health-related issues such as flow, well-being, intergenerational understanding and urban regeneration, deriving from a community psychology approach. The creative practices here are employed collaboratively where accessibility and accountability become real issues. Diverse stakeholders in these projects represent members of the public (such as community residents and migrants), interested researchers and professional artists. Whilst collaboration and participation are often guiding principles of community psychology work, tensions can arise around outputs and interpretation of meanings (see Mountian *et al.* 2011). The project outputs arising from this kind of research include traditional academic outputs as well as artistic products such as exhibitions, films, magazines, etc. Not only do visual creative approaches demand radically different ways of working with people, but the outputs, the 'texts', can have multiple meanings. Whilst these creative methods and outputs appear to be more accessible to participants in research enterprises, they are not without challenge.

In this section I have presented emerging representations of visual work – alongside possibilities and tensions afforded by this way of working. In the next section, I present a radically different engagement of senses in research which may tantalise your tastebuds for doing research differently.

The radically different

Sensory ethnography (Pink 2009) engages seriously with the multisensoriality of experience, perception, knowing and practice. In Chapter 5 on ethnography, you were presented with the assumptions and practices of ethnographic work. Whilst this work engages with encounters through the senses, it tends to report back using the written word:

By a sensory ethnography, I mean a process of doing ethnography that accounts for how this multi-sensoriality is integral both to the lives of people who participate in our research and to how we, ethnographers, practice our craft.

(Pink 2009: 1)

Pink's (2004) research on housework demonstrates that the 'sensory home' which participants experienced through sound, vision, touch and smell is indeed multisensorial. Here, decisions about what and when to clean are made through visual cues (looking dirty), olfactory cues (smelling unhygienic) and touch (dusting). In another sensorially informed research project, Roseman (2005) discusses the importance of song among the Temiar people of Kelantan, Malaysia. These are indigenous forest-dwelling people whose existence is being impacted upon by rainforest deforestation, land alienation and Islamic evangelism. However, to understand their world there is a need to engage in culturally meaningful ways (here, song) in order to see how song enables sense making.

Critics of the sensory approach may problematise the arts-based nature of the work. However, the applied potential for more sensory approaches is interesting. Lammer (2007) uses video in a radiography unit to understand how sociality and multisensoriality affect interactions in clinical contexts. She argues that multisensuality may encourage empathy and heightened sensibilities amongst health professionals.

Lisa Law (2005) explores how displaced Filipino domestic workers try to emplace themselves by reproducing the sensory comforts of home in the city core of Hong Kong. Sensescapes (the rich interplay of the senses) require that we attune to sensation in a cultural context. Cultural geographer Lisa Law accounts for the diaspora in Hong Kong who evoke a 'sense' of home through sights, sounds, tastes and aromas for which there is no affordance within the city. The Filipino takeover of the business district is denounced on aesthetic and hygienic grounds by dominant members of society. This sensuous reconstruction of space by migrant workers during leisure hours provides a testimony to the politics of differing sensory strategies for making sense of the city. Law posts senses as 'situated practices' – a move from visual consumption of Hong Kong to aural recognition of Little Manila. Here, women create new ways of engaging with the city and recover from domestic-based sensory reculturation. It is difficult to find a method that engages explicitly with sensory landscapes. Sensory landscapes of cities suggest less conventional forms of ethnic politics and reveal how diasporic populations find original ways of engaging with urban life. Little Manila is a hybrid site (Hong Kong and Philippines, domestic worker and Filipino). The alternative sensorium here is constructed through cooking, photos and letters.

Whilst there are some innovative examples of sensory-based ethnography, there are no conventions or techniques for how to evoke the visual-textual in ethnographic texts (Pink 2009). The doing of this kind of work invoked careful consideration of ethics around process and then extending into outputs. The sensory ethnography of domestic spaces (Pink 2004) could potentially identify homes through the visual so photography was not included in outputs. The question of how to represent the sensorium is clearly ethical but also practical. Reports, journal articles and books provide limited and costly options for visual and other sensory evocation. For example, sound ethnography and the making of soundscapes can provide rich data, but how to represent this practice? Wrightson (2000) and Adams and Bruce (2008) used recorded soundwalks to represent acoustic environments. Feld (2001) developed a rainforest soundwalk which not only represents what places sound like but invites us to hear the 'sonic everyday' of others. This kind of soundscape practice not only extends beyond the academic audience but can increase awareness using other senses. Moore (2003) researched Protestant and Catholic soundscapes within Northern Ireland. He compares sounds, services, drumming and violence, linking current hearing (and seeing) to the past. Biella (2009) suggests that producing a sense of intimacy in ethnographic representation can enable a more moral project of increasing awareness (here intercultural). As noise and sound are increasingly familiar soundscapes for Global North citizens, the tuning in to sound becomes increasingly important.

The approaches discussed above pose interesting questions about creative production and whether this can constitute intellectual inquiry. In the modern arts and humanities, theorists have always structured a gap between practice and analysis. Performance practices have always contributed to knowledge but the idea that performance (e.g. a soundscape) can be more than creative production, and in itself can constitute intellectual inquiry and contribute new understanding and insight, challenges our notions of what gets valued as knowledge (Riley and Hunter 2009).

I hope the immersion within the sensory has tempted you with some inspiring models of possibility. Whilst the sensory may appear to be a radical departure from the everyday notion of 'science', it seems more analogous to human experience which is involved in the sensorium every day.

Chapter summary

Bruner (1986) argues that there are two ways of knowing: the paradigmatic and the narrative. The paradigmatic is based on positivism and a science which involves classification, and categorisation, whilst narrative knowing is located in meaning making and storytelling. In this chapter I have been arguing for and presenting the case for the latter. This approach, however, is not without critics.

Critics of qualitative research generally have well-rehearsed 'problems' with the interpretation and unscientific nature of messy qualitative data . These issues are legacies of a traditional scientific rationalist model which wrongly assumes that science is and can be objective. For these newer methods, however, subjectivity is privileged which brings issues of evaluation of quality to the fore. Words or text-based data have spawned a plethora of diverse analytical frameworks that range from discourse and the psychoanalytic through to experience. Whilst we must be careful not to become entranced with methodolatry, there is a need to embrace and be playful. Silverman (2007), in a chapter subtitled 'On Bullshit and Tonsils', argues that qualitative research in using these art-based approaches is defined less as 'science' and more as 'artistic' performance. He states that these approaches can be gripping but factually inaccurate. Silverman locates this kind of research as 'postmodern' advocating that 'anything goes' in a paradigm which prefers 'ethnodrama, story and poetry' to clear refutable statements about research findings. The preceding chapters of this book have engaged with research findings which are anything but clear and refutable – hence a need for qualitative methods and analysis. In Silverman's agenda for qualitative research he argues that talk, interaction, documents and other artefacts can offer revealing data:

> Good research, perhaps like good art, in some senses needs to stand outside the taken for granted assumptions that inform our everyday life. The aim need not be to criticise the world around is (although it may be) but to allow us a fresh gaze at the way we live.
>
> (Silverman 2007: 147)

I would argue that engagement in alternative representations of data forces us to step out of a hyperliterate culture. These emergent methods, however, can require skill development. To enact participatory approaches may well involve collaboration around photo/film, sound production, song writing, cooking, art production or other such tasks. These ways of working require rather different research engagement styles and researcher skills. Radically departing from the traditional interview or text-based engagement will require researchers to critically examine their own skill set and also their ability to collaborate. The call from research councils to be transdisciplinary requires that research training engages not only with methods per se but also research assumptions (epistemology and ontology). Collaboration across disciplines needs appreciation of the situatedness of knowledge if it is to be successful (Hesse-Biber and Leavy 2008).

The potential to include participants more democratically in data gathering and analysis is an advantage of some of the approaches covered here. Indeed, for analysis and dissemination, a movement away from text-based immersion seems to hold promise. However, the offer to participate in research (whilst originating from a socially just agenda) may not be seen as important to informants. Cooke and Kothari (2001) talk about the tyranny of participation in the lives of individuals who are being exhorted to increasingly take part in areas of civil life. Many of these emergent approaches assume that the researched will want to participate, to embrace the experience of doing research and to gain useful knowledge. Is research participation in the form of data collection and at times analysis yet another form of tyrannical participation? If analysis is done without participants, then we need to know whose interpretation is present.

These emergent forms of representation will not appeal to all, as researcher reflexivity is forefronted. Pelias notes that these kinds of texts are '[a]methodological call, writings that mark a different space. They collect in the body: an ache, a fist, a soup' (2004: 11). In texts which do engage with arts-based work, the term practices is often used rather than methods (Sinner *et al.* 2006). This perhaps reflects the hybrid nature of the work which can be a research tool and a practice for change. Janesick (2001) and others have noted that qualitative researchers do more than gather and write; they compose, orchestrate, weave and choreograph. They are instrumental in research and in practice – 'artist-scientists'. As Hesse-Biber and Leavy (2006) note, it is often the development of new theories and corresponding insights about the social world which provoke the development of new research tools. In increasingly uneasy times, where doubt and uncertainty are essential elements of the scientific process (Jha 2011), these alternative forms of qualitative representation offer something new to the mix. I hope that the senses are tapped and the chapter has tantalised you to explore something a little more.

References

Adams, M. and Bruce, N. (2008) 'Soundwalking as a methodology for understanding soundscapes'. *Proceedings of the Institute of Acoustics*, **30**(2), 552–8.

Banks, A. and Banks, S. P. (eds) (1998) *Fiction and Social Research: By Fire or Ice*. Lanham, MD: AltaMira Press.

Banks, M. (2001) *Visual Methods in Social Research*. London: Sage.

Baudrillard, J. (1998) 'Simulcra and simulations', in M. Poster (ed.) *Jean Baudrillard, Selected Writings*. Palo Alto, CA: Stanford University Press.

Biella, P. (2009) 'Visual anthropology in a time of war', in M. Strong and L. Wilder (eds) *Viewpoints: Visual Anthropologists at Work*. Austin, TX: University of Texas Press.

Bochner, A. and Ellis, C. (eds) (2002) *Ethnographically Speaking: Autoethnography, Literature and Aesthetics*. Lanham, MD: AltaMira Press.

Bruner, J. S. (1986) *Actual Minds, Possible Worlds*. Cambridge, MA: Harvard University Press.

Carothers, J. C. (1959) 'Culture, psychiatry and the written word'. *Psychiatry*, **22**, 307–20.

Chaplin, E. (1994) *Sociology and Visual Representations*. London: Routledge.

Classen, C. (2005) 'McLuhan in the rainforest: the sensory worlds of oral cultures', in D. Howes (ed.) *Empire of the Senses: The Sensual Culture Reader*. Oxford: Berg.

Cooke, B. and Kothari, U. (eds) (2001) *Participation: The New Tyranny?* London: Zed Books.

Couser, G. T. (2004) *Vulnerable Subjects: Ethics and Life Writing*. Ithaca, NY: Cornell University Press.

Crouch, D. and Desforges, L. (2003) 'The sensuous in the tourist encounter: introduction: the power of the body in tourist studies'. *Tourist Studies*, **3**, 5–22.

Curry, D. and Wells, S. J. (2003) *An Organic Inquiry Primer for the Novice Researcher*. Seattle, WA: Liminal Realities.

Dawson, S. E. (2007) 'Companion animal euthanasia: the lived paradox of the human–companion animal bond'. Unpublished PhD thesis, Manchester Metropolitan University.

Denzin, N. K. (1997) *Interpretive Ethnography: Ethnographic Practices for the 21st Century*. Thousand Oaks, CA: Sage.

Denzin, N. K. (2003) *Performance Ethnography: Critical Pedagogy and the Politics of Culture*. Thousand Oaks, CA: Sage.

Denzin, N. K. and Lincoln, Y. S. (2003) 'Introduction: the discipline and practice of qualitative research', in N. K. Denzin and Y. S. Lincoln (eds) *Collecting and Interpreting Qualitative Materials*. London: Sage.

Denzin, N. K. and Lincoln, Y. S. (2005) *The Sage Handbook of Qualitative Research*, 3rd edn, London: Sage.

Ellis, C. (2004) *The Ethnographic I: The Methodological Novel about Autoethnography*. Lanham, MD: AltaMira Press.

Emmison, M. and Smith, P. (2000) *Researching the Visual*. London: Sage.

Feld, S. (2001) *Rainforest Soundwalks* (CD). Santa Fe, NM: Earthear.

Gombrich, E. (1996) 'The visual image: its place in communication', in R. Woodfield (ed.) *The Essential Gombrich: Selected Writings on Art and Culture*. London: Phaidon.

Goodley, D. A., Lawthom, R., Clough, P. and Moore, M. (2004) *Researching Life Stories: Method, Theory and Analyses in a Biographical Age*. London: Routledge Falmer.

Guba, E. G. and Lincoln, Y. S. (2005) 'Paradigmatic controversies, contradictions, and emerging influences', in N. K. Denzin and Y. S. Lincoln (eds) *The Sage Handbook of Qualitative Research*, 3rd edn. London: Sage.

Hartnett, S. J. (2003) *Incarceration Nation: Investigative Prison Poems of Hope and Terror*. Lanham, MD: AltaMira Press.

Haworth, J. (2010) 'The way we are now'. *Leisure Studies*, **29**(1), 101–10.

Hesse-Biber, S. N. and Leavy, P. (2006) *Emergent Methods in Social Research*. Thousand Oaks, CA: Sage.

Hesse-Biber, S. N. and Leavy, P. (2008) 'Pushing on the methodological boundaries: the growing need for emergent methods within and across the disciplines', in S. N. Hesse-Biber and P. Leavy (eds) *Handbook of Emergent Methods*. New York: Guilford Press.

Holliday, R. (2004) 'Reflecting the self', in C. Knowles and J. Sweetman (eds) *Picturing the Social Landscape: Visual Methods and the Sociological Imagination*. London: Routledge.

Howes, D. (ed.) (2005) *Empire of the Senses*. New York: Berg.

Hull, J. M. (1990) *Touching the Rock*: *An Experience of Blindness*. London: SPCK.

Janesick, V. J. (2001) 'Intuition and creativity: a pas de deux for qualitative researchers'. *Qualitative Inquiry*, **7**(5), 531–40.

Jha, A. (2011) 'We must learn to love uncertainty and failure says leading thinkers'. Accessed January 15, 2011. www.guardian.co.uk.

Kagan, C., Burton, M., Duckett, P., Lawthom, R. and Siddiquee, A. (2011) *Critical Community Psychology: Critical Action and Social Change*. Chichester: Wiley.

Kagan, C. and Micaleff, A. M. (2008) *Active and Positive Parenting: Composite Evaluation Report*. Manchester: RIHSC.

Kellock, A. (2009) 'Children's perceptions of well-being through photography'. Unpublished PhD thesis, Manchester Metropolitan University.

Kellock, A., Lawthom, R., Sixsmith, J., Duggan, K., Mountian, I., Haworth, J. T., Kagan, C., Brown, D. P., Griffiths, J. E., Hawkins, J. E., Worley, C., Purcell, C. and Siddiquee, A. (2011) 'Using technology and the experience sampling method to understand real life', in S. N. Hesse-Biber (ed.) *The Handbook of Emergent Technologies in Social Research*. Oxford: Oxford University Press.

Kilroy, A., Garner, C., Parkinson, C., Kagan, C. M. and Senior, P. D. (2007) 'Towards transformation: exploring the impact of culture, creativity and the arts on health and wellbeing'. Paper presented at The Critical Friends Event, Manchester, Arts for Health.

Kuhn, A. (1995) *Family Secrets*. London: Verso.

Lammer, C. (2007) 'Bodywork: social somatic interventions in the operating theatres of invasive radiology', in S. Pink (ed.) *Visual Interventions: Applied Visual Anthropology*. Oxford: Berg.

Langer, C. L. and Furman, R. (2004) 'Exploring identity and assimilation: research and interpretive poems'. *Forum Qualitative Social Research* (online journal), **5**(2). www.qualitativeresearch.net.

Lash, S. (1988) 'Discourse or figure? Postmodernism as "regime of signification"'. *Theory, Culture and Society*, **5**, 311–36.

Law, L. (2005) 'Home cooking: Filipino women and geographies of the senses in Hong Kong', in D. Howes (ed.) *Empire of the Senses: The Sensual Culture Reader*. Oxford: Berg.

Lawthom, R., Kagan, C., Richards, M., Sixsmith, J. and Woolrych, R. (2011) 'Being creative around health: participative methodologies in critical community psychology', in C. Horrocks and S. Johnson (eds) *Advances in Health Psychology: Critical Approaches*. Basingstoke: Palgrave Macmillan.

Lawthom, R., Sixsmith, J. and Kagan, C. (2007) 'Interrogating power: the case of arts and mental health in community projects'. *Journal of Community and Applied Social Psychology*, **17**(4), 268–79.

McLeod, J. and Balamoutsou, S. (2000) 'A method for qualitative analysis of psychotherapy transcripts'. Accessed November 30, 2004. http://shs.tay.ac.uk.shtjm/Articles.htm.

McLuhan, M. (2005) 'Inside the five sense sensorium', in D. Howes (ed.) *Empire of the Senses: The Sensual Culture Reader*. Oxford: Berg.

Michalko, R. (2002) *The Difference that Disability Makes*. Philadelphia, PA: Temple University Press.

Moore, P. (2003) 'Sectarian sounds and cultural identity in Northern Ireland', in M. Bull and L. Bank (eds) *The Auditory Culture Reader*. Oxford: Berg.

Mountian, I., Lawthorn, R., Kellock, A., Duggan, K., Sixsmith, J., Kagan, C., Hawkins, J., Haworth, J., Siddiquee, A., Worley, C., Brown, D., Griffiths, J. and Purcell, C. (2011) 'On utilising a visual methodology: shared reflections and tensions', in P. Reavey (ed.) *Visual Methods in Psychology: Using and Interpreting Images in Qualitative Research*. London: Routledge.

Newbury, D. (1997) 'Talking about practice: photography students, photographic culture and professional identities'. *British Journal of Sociology of Education*, **18**(3), 421–34.

Parker, I. and Bolton Discourse Network (1999) *Critical Textwork: An Introduction to Varieties of Discourse and Analysis*. Buckingham: Open University Press.

Pelias, R. J. (2004) *A Methodology of the Heart: Evoking Academic and Daily Life*. Lanham, MD: AltaMira Press.

Pink, S. (2001) *Doing Visual Ethnography*. London: Sage.

Pink, S. (2004) *Home Truths: Gender, Domestic Objects and Everyday Life*. Oxford: Berg.

Pink, S. (2009) *Doing Sensory Ethnography*. London: Sage.

Price, D. and Well, L. (1997) 'Thinking about photography: debates, historically and now', in L. Wells (ed.) *Photography: A Critical Introduction*. London: Routledge.

Reavey, P. (ed.) (2011) *Visual Methods in Psychology: Using and Interpreting Images in Qualitative Research*. London: Routledge.

Reavey, P. and Johnson, K. (2008) 'Visual approaches: using and interpreting images', in C. Willig and W. Stainton-Rogers (eds) *The Sage Handbook of Qualitative Research in Psychology*. London: Sage.

Richardson, L. (1997) 'Skirting a pleated text: de-disciplining an academic life'. *Qualitative Inquiry*, **3**, 295–304.

Riley, S. R. and Hunter, L. (eds) (2009) *Mapping Landscapes for Performance as Research*. New York: Palgrave Macmillan.

Rose, G. (1997) 'Situating knowledge: positionality, reflexivities and other tactics'. *Progress in Human Geography*, **21**(3), 305–20.

Roseman, M. (2005) 'Engaging the spirits of modernity: Teimar songs of a changing world', in D. Howes (ed.) *Empire of the Senses: The Sensual Culture Reader*. Oxford: Berg.

Serres, M. (1985) *Les cinq sens: philosophie des corps mêlés*. Paris: Grasset.

Sixsmith, J. and Kagan, C. (2005) *Arts for Mental Health: Final Report*. Manchester: Manchester Metropolitan University.

Silverman, D. (2007) *A Very Short, Fairly Interesting and Reasonably Cheap Book about Qualitative Research*. London: Sage.

Sinner, A., Leggo, C., Irwin, R., Gouzouasis, P. and Graer, K. (2006) 'Arts based education research dissertations: reviewing the practices of new scholars'. *Canadian Journal of Education*, **29**(4), 1223–70.

Tagg, J. (1988) *The Burden of Representation*. Amherst, MA: University of Massachusetts Press.

Titchkosky, T. (2010) 'Access and the sensorium'. Paper presented to Theorising Normalcy Conference, Manchester, May.

Wang, C. C., Wu Kun Yi, Zhan Wen Tao and Carovano, K. (1998) 'Photovoice as a participatory health promotion strategy'. *Health Promotion International*, **13**(1), 75–86.

Wrightson, K. (2000) 'An introduction to acoustic ecology'. *Soundscape: The Journal of Acoustic Ecology*, **1**(1), 10–13.

Woolrych, R. and Sixsmith, S. (2008) *Understanding Health and Well-being in the Context of Urban Regeneration: Manchester Case Study. Final Report*. Manchester: Manchester Metropolitan University.

Chapter 13

Writing up

Peter Banister

Introduction

This chapter covers a number of important intertwined areas. It starts by looking at ways in which one should present findings, and emphasises that qualitative methods should place emphasis on reflexivity. Consideration of ethical issues is vital in any psychological research, and should especially permeate qualitative methods. Personal and cultural values are also an important area to consider. The chapter concludes by making some points about the role of psychology in social change.

The first point to remember is that there is no one 'right' way to write up; what you are trying to do is produce something which accurately reflects your work and communicates your findings, so that the reader can follow them and understand your conclusions. Some of the points covered below are common to all report writing, whilst some are more specific to qualitative research. A lot may depend upon who the intended audience is. There will be differences between writing up a report for a government department, for journal publication, for a professional publication, or for a student practical or dissertation. You are aiming to share your understandings with others. The precise way in which this can be best done will obviously be partly dependent on the actual methods which you have used. What this chapter does is to provide a number of suggestions that should be of use. The general model advocated is producing a report suitable for journal publication.

General considerations

Although it sounds a very trivial point, language is important. Thus, remember that you are not writing up an 'experimental report'. Use appropriate discourses: avoid using 'experiment', 'experimenter', 'subject', etc.; instead, talk about the 'researcher', 'co-researchers' (or 'participants'), etc.

What is perhaps initially difficult to do (as this goes against traditionally accepted methods of writing up scientific reports), it is generally desirable in writing up qualitative reports to use the first person (e.g. 'I'), rather than reporting the research in the more traditional stylised impersonal fashion. This is not essential, but it may help to emphasise the somewhat different philosophy underlying qualitative research, as it helps to acknowledge the position of the researcher as owning the research. However, conventions do vary here as to the acceptability of such a position. Do remember that there is a danger in doing this; forgetting that you as an individual will have information that only you are privy to, and assuming similar knowledge in the reader. Thus, if you are writing in the first person, be careful to ensure that you do not lapse into unsubstantiated assertion, that you make it very clear as to who you are, that your assumptions and position are clearly stated, and that pre-existing relationships with participants are clarified.

Often, it is useful to write with a mixture of the active voice (e.g. I joined the fans at an away match) and the passive voice (e.g. football programmes were examined). In particular, do use the active voice if you want to stress that the agent of the activity is important.

There is a need to be aware of sexism in the use of language and steps should be taken to avoid it; thus, for example, never use 'he' to refer to people in general. Use 'he or she', or (preferably) try to write in such a way that it is not necessary to make general statements in the third person singular. By using 'they', all such problems are avoided, but it must be noted that this may create the further problem of producing the fiction of a genderless participant.

Be careful to make sure that your use of verb tenses is systematic. In general, the accepted method in research is to use the past tense in the introduction and methods sections (e.g. football matches were attended), and the present tense when it comes to looking at the results and subsequently discussing them (e.g. findings may indicate that . . .).

Always keep in mind that the main point of a write-up (at which many published articles are poor) is to communicate clearly your findings to others, to share your understandings of your results, to tell others what has been learnt from your particular piece of research.

A key point to aim for is replicability (but not in the quantitative sense). Ideally, the model here should be to present sufficient detail about what you actually did to enable the reader to pick up your report, and to repeat your study from the information provided. Even if the readers do not wish to replicate your study, they should be provided with sufficient material to allow them clearly to understand what it was that you did. This means that they should be able to clearly visualise the setting, the participants, etc. from what has been written. Aim for conciseness wherever possible.

As has already been stressed above, reflexivity is a very important aspect of writing up reports (both qualitative and quantitative), and must be included.

It is often useful to make a plan for your report, before you begin to write it up. This needs to be flexible, but it will help you to produce a better structured report. The area of interest that you are researching into needs to be kept in mind, possibly written down on a card to keep in front of you, aiding relevance and focus. Bem (1991) makes the interesting point that there are often two possible reports which can be written: the report you thought you were going to write when you started; and the report that makes the best possible sense of your findings. The natural scientific method suggests that one follows an inexorable process, starting from a literature review and proceeding in a linear fashion, step by step, while real-life research practicalities may be somewhat different to this. Bem rightly concludes that usually it is the second report which one should write, and this is the one which you will need your plan for. Often the most interesting findings are the serendipitous ones. Willig (2008) similarly contrasts a 'recipe' approach (the 'right' way to do things) with 'adventure' (research as exploration).

The report writing up and the bibliographic reference list will always take a long time. Using a tool such as *EndNote* may be worth considering here. Give yourself some leeway, as reports can usually be improved by reviewing them, and extra time is inevitably needed for such a process (and spellchecking and proofreading). There are a number of ways in which a review can be carried out. The simplest is to write a draft report, and then to put it on one side for a few days, turning to something else in the meantime; then return to it and re-read it. The extra few days will allow you to become more detached from it, and the extra distance will allow it to be looked at more as an outsider. A more difficult but preferable alternative is to show the report to a colleague or friend who is unfamiliar with your research to see if they can follow the write-up. This view from a different perspective will check for clarity, replicability, etc., but will also provide an alternative slant on your work, and can help to point out things which you have missed, including offering alternative explanations.

Structure of a report

What follows here is a general outline of a typical write-up, following standard journal practice. Some of what follows may thus repeat what is covered elsewhere, but despite this many researchers still have a lot of trouble with this activity. It is felt that any repetition here may help to lead to improved report writing.

A general guideline to bear in mind is that the shape of a report is ideally like that of an hourglass, starting off in the introduction with very general considerations, and continuing to gradually focus in on the specific area of interest. The methods and the results narrowly attend to the research itself, while the discussion gradually widens out again to broader issues. As Bem (1991: 456–7) says:

> If your study is carefully executed and conservatively interpreted, you deserve to indulge yourself a bit at the two broad ends of the hourglass. Being dull only appears to be a prerequisite for publishing in the professional journals.

It is suggested that the report is easier to follow if it is subsectioned. In a lengthy report it is often useful to subsection further, both to enable the reader to appreciate the structure of your report and to help you, as the writer, to produce a more carefully thought out and developed argument.

Title

The title should clearly and succinctly indicate the area of study, and should inform precisely what the study is about. Remember that a number of databases concentrate on article titles. Thus someone searching a database (such as *PsycLit*) may only discover the relevance of your article for their research if your title clearly indicated the precise nature of your study. The title, as well as being as informative and specific as possible, should endeavour to be concise; as a broad rule of thumb, it should never go beyond 12 words. Snappy or punning titles may attract the reader's attention, but should generally be avoided.

Contents

Although this is not generally necessary in articles, in other contexts it is often useful, to enable the reader to find the relevant parts quickly; pagination also helps here.

Abstract

Practice concerning abstracts varies, some journals preferring a 'conclusion' or a 'summary' at the end of an article, but the usual practice is to provide an 'abstract' at the beginning of the report. This should give a succinct summary of what the research was designed to investigate, what precisely was done, what was found and how the results were interpreted. As with the title, remember that databases (e.g. *Psychological Abstracts*) often rely on this section, so ensure that appropriate keywords are included. Given that qualitative methods are fairly distinctive, it might be useful to give some indication here as to the type of analysis that was used (e.g. naturalistic observation, feminist interview, discourse analysis, etc.). Thus, by the end of this section, the reader has a very clear general picture of your study. As a general rule of thumb, 150 words might be a suitable upper target to aim for.

Introduction

It is often useful to subsection this part of the report, especially if it is a long one. If this is done, provide a brief outline of the section's structure. This will aid both the reader and the writer to follow better the thesis of this portion of your write-up. With qualitative reports sometimes it is worth explaining at the outset why the study was undertaken.

Remembering the hourglass suggestion earlier, start off with a general introduction to the area. Commence at the macro level (e.g. 'social behaviour', 'gender expectations') before gradually concentrating on the precise area of interest (e.g. 'queuing behaviour'; 'mothers' gender expectations of their children'). Briefly review relevant and up-to-date literature in the area before going on to more detailed critical discussion of studies which are of direct relevance to your research. Do realise that often you may come across absences and gaps in published research, which your study will attempt to remedy. This literature review should end with a clear statement of what the study is going to investigate, possibly indicating any expectations about what the findings are likely to be. Often, you will have read far more than you are likely to need, and there is a temptation, which should be avoided, to put in as many as possible, in order to demonstrate how wide your reading has been.

Most importantly, in a study that relies on qualitative methodology, this section should also include a brief justification for the precise methods adopted in the research, indicating clearly why they were chosen. What should be argued here is why it is considered that qualitative methodology in general and the chosen method in particular may be the most appropriate to answer the particular research question under investigation. Alternatives should be briefly considered, and the reasons for their rejection should be made clear to the reader. It is critical to include this, and it might raise issues that need to be returned to in later parts of the report.

The reader should, by the end of this section, have a very clear idea of what you are intending to do, why you are doing it, how you are doing it and why you have chosen this particular way to investigate it. To some extent, the introduction is an exercise in 'selling': it needs to convince the reader that this will be an interesting and worthwhile study, and that it is going to use the most suitable research methods possible.

Method

This section should provide sufficient detail to allow the reader to replicate the study on the basis of the material presented. 'Methods' often take too much for granted, or simply leave out vital information. Some justification for the method chosen may occur here, particularly detailing why the specific variety of method which is to be used has been chosen. The precise structure of this section will obviously differ depending on the particular methodological approach being used, but in general needs to include the following points:

1 *Give a general outline of the design of the study*, making it clear to the reader what the general methodology is (for instance, 'this is a participant observation study, where the people being observed were not aware of the researcher's identity', or 'this is a feminist interview').

2 *Give an outline of any pilot studies that were carried out.* Such studies are often vital to attempt to iron out potential pitfalls. Practice interviews, for instance, may indicate that important questions have been left out, or may need to be rephrased. Trial observations will indicate what is possible and what is impossible to observe in a given social situation. Clear indications should be given as to what procedural and other changes were made as a result of pilot work. Reliability checks can also be carried out at this stage.

3 *Give details as to your participants were*, and how precisely they were selected (indicating any prior links between them and yourself). Provide as much detail as possible of the participants (demographic and other), bearing in mind principles of anonymity. If it was felt necessary to carry out any selection or control procedures, then the reasoning behind such preliminaries needs to be spelt out, with reference to the appropriate literature. If (for instance) discourse analysis is being carried out, the reasons for the choice of the precise texts used need to be stated.

4 *Some indication is needed as to who the researcher is*, including demographic and other social characteristics (these might affect the research).

5 *A clear description should be given of the location of the study.* If it is outside, then do not forget variables such as the weather. If it is inside, then include variables such as extraneous noise, lighting and interruptions.

6 *Stipulate clearly when the study took place*, including both the date and the time. You may also want to include some chronology of the development of your interpretations.

7 *Give precise details of the procedure followed*, from (if appropriate) the initial approach made to the participant to any 'debriefing' or feedback. The way in which a study is introduced to the co-researcher, for instance, may influence what is subsequently found; an example of

this might be calling oneself a 'psychologist', which may well conjure up images such as the 'psychoanalyst' for many members of the public. If this does occur, then the participant may be more concerned with presenting themselves as being mentally healthy, rather than indicating what they really think. This has occurred to the author of this chapter. When I was carrying out work on vibration-induced white fingers (see Banister and Smith 1972), forestry workers initially refused to take part in the study until they were reassured that psychologists were interested in other things than Freudian theory and their sex lives. To avoid problems of this nature, it is often better to describe oneself as a 'researcher', perhaps from a specific institution, interested in a particular area (i.e. you should take into account co-researchers' perceptions of the nature of the investigation).

8 *An outline needs to be provided as to what precisely was recorded and how.* If (for instance) interview transcripts were subsequently produced, these need to be put in the appendices, preferably with each line separately numbered, to aid subsequent easy reference to them. How and when these transcripts were produced needs to be stated, along with a key as to what form of notation is being used (to indicate pauses, inflections, paralinguistic aspects, etc.). An example of this is given in Jefferson (1987).

9 *If any permission was needed for the study to be carried out*, this should be included here. If a contract was made between the researcher and the participant, this also should be referred to here, including commitments made and adhered to.

10 *Ethical issues* (as stressed in detail below) need to be very carefully considered in any study, and must be included here. Even if it is felt that the method involves no ethical concerns (which is probably impossible), this nonetheless needs to be thought through and clearly stated.

Analysis

Once again, the exact format to be followed here will depend on the precise methodology used, so the following is intended more as general points to bear in mind. Sometimes, it may be more appropriate to combine the analysis and discussion sections. If you are doing a thematic analysis of interview material, for instance, it would be best to do this as one section, and then go on to discuss wider issues.

Overall, what should be aimed for is a clear and unambiguous statement as to what was found, to enable the reader to understand it from the material presented. Remember that some readers will only look at some sections of the report, and it is much more 'user friendly' to try to ensure that each section can be clearly understood if read alone. It is often useful to start by reminding the reader what precisely the study was looking at, to go on to give an overall general picture of the results, and finally to examine them in detail. Some of the more specific aspects might be placed in the appendices.

If any attempt has been made to validate the data (e.g. through triangulation, through repetition over time or with different people, etc.), then this should be included in this section. Make it clear which points seem to be well established from your work and which are more speculative.

As has been mentioned above, often unsolicited and unexpected comments from the participants prove as interesting as answering the research question. It is thus often worth including such remarks in this section, as they not only help to give some idea of the 'flavour' of the research, but also may provide explanations of the results gained as well as useful pointers for future research. If this is done, however, do remember your commitments to the co-researcher and related ethical issues.

Discussion

As has been mentioned above, it may be more appropriate to combine the analysis and discussion sections. In many ways, the discussion is the most important part of your whole write-up. Again, it should start with a brief reminder to the reader as to what the focus of interest is, and should then go on to present an overall summary of the findings. These should be discussed in detail with reference to the purposes of the study (as argued in the introduction) and relevant literature. Do remember that there may be a whole variety of reasons why your findings differ from previous findings. These include: differences in methodology (does discourse analysis tap material at a less conscious level, for instance?); in sampling (who co-researchers are may well lead to different results); in the researcher's impact on the situation (your demographic characteristics, your skill in utilising qualitative methods, your expectations); in the environment (extraneous noise, interruptions), as well as differences related to time and space. (Studies carried out in another culture and/or at another time may not be universally generalisable.)

What this section should provide is an interpretation of the findings and their meaning. Are they in line with expectations, what generalisations can one make from them, what unexpected results are there and how might they be interpreted? Bem (1991) makes the somewhat heretical suggestion that if your results are startlingly new, and lead to a new theory, it might be worth going back and rewriting the whole report so that it begins with the new theory.

Reflexivity

What is extremely important here is the provision of a reflexive analysis, which could be in a separate subsection. Reflexivity is vital in qualitative analysis. There is a need to include a section that stands back from your study and looks at it, analysing how appropriate the methods were in retrospect, what it felt like to be the researcher doing the study, what it might have felt like to be a participant (including any reports from the participants themselves), what flaws in the design came to light in the experience of completing the study, how it might be improved if it were to be replicated in the future, what other ways it could have been done and what further research needs to be done. The emphasis here should thus be on constructive criticality; the realisation of the relative nature of social reality, that there are multiple realities, the questioning of whatever it is that one does, the refusal to be satisfied with outcomes, the seeking of alternatives and other possibilities. Qualitative methods may avoid many of the problems faced by other methods of doing research, but nonetheless aspects of research still need to be carefully considered. In particular, such methods may involve features which are potentially exploitative.

Reflexivity should involve both thinking about oneself and thinking about one's research. Wilkinson (1988) defines these two aspects as 'personal' and 'functional' reflexivity respectively, but points out that the two are very closely intertwined. It needs to be realised that inevitably any researcher will have biases, interests, predilections, values, experiences and characteristics that will affect the research and your interpretations of it.

Discussion with participants and colleagues will help to gain a broader picture, but reflexive writers must be aware of their limitations. Thus you should always be questioning in a disciplined manner what it is that you have done, asking yourself whether your choice of methods was appropriate, what alternatives could have been utilised, what your impact on the setting, situation, participants, results, etc. was, what alternative interpretations might be put forward.

Sometimes keeping a diary as your research progresses is very useful here. Thus, as well as thinking carefully about your own particular study (and yourself), you also need to think about more macro issues, which include research methodology and questioning psychology itself (what Wilkinson 1988 calls 'disciplinary reflexivity'). Power relationships are likely to be particularly important, and must always be given due consideration.

References

References must be given of all cited literature, systematically using the standard procedure, as in journal articles. If some material has been gathered from a secondary source, this should be made plain to the reader; if you are quoting from such material, then do remember that secondary sources can be misleading. Idiosyncratic interpretations can be given of the work of others (sometimes to fit an argument), and at times inaccuracies will creep in (like the debate over whether Watson's Little Albert study initially involved a white rabbit or a white rat).

Appendices

These are often useful to help the reader understand precisely what it was you discovered in your research, and how you set about doing it. It also allows space to put material which is too bulky or detailed for the report itself. Such material will allow the reader to follow better the arguments put forward, and may even permit reinterpretation of the material. Appendices should be clearly labelled and paginated; they can include raw material, transcripts, details of pilot studies, etc.

Ethics

Quite rightly, and as has been emphasised above, psychologists have become increasingly worried about ethical issues concerned with research. Indeed, this has been part of the impetus behind the turn towards more qualitative methods. In this context, the argument between Zimbardo (1973) and Savin (1973) concerning the famous Stanford mock prison work is particularly interesting as an illustration of debates on the ethics of experimentation (see also McDermott 1993 for a commentary by Zimbardo on this controversy). Many feel that qualitative methods have the potential to avoid a number of the usual ethical pitfalls of more conventional psychological methods.

There are now published ethical guidelines for conducting research and the reader is urged to consult those of the American Psychological Association (2010) and the British Psychological Society (2011); the full text of these guidelines should be essential reading for any researcher. All psychologists who are engaged in research are expected to abide by the principles espoused in these documents.

Ethical concerns must be part of the fundamental design of any research project, and ideally any proposed research (including undergraduate, A level and GCSE practical work) should be talked through with an ethics committee and/or colleagues, to ensure that the research does not, as a minimum, contravene the published ethical principles. The proposal should also be talked through with members of the population with whom the research is going to be carried out. The broader perspective so gained will help to reduce the possibility that the proposal is too one-sided, and may assist it to take on board such issues as (for example) living in a multicultural society. It must be emphasised that many think the current guidelines do not go far enough, and need to be further discussed and developed; the guidelines themselves are constantly reviewed and modified, rather than being fixed. Guidelines do not tell us much directly concerning what to do if one observes somebody committing a criminal act, or doing something which is harmful to another. There are also current debates as to whether it is ethical to take photographs of people in public social situations without their permission; something that the paparazzi may frequently do, and contemporary worries regarding paedophilia are suggesting that it is no longer appropriate to take photographs of children in public social situations without due permission being attained.

It is important to stress that the guidelines are not a set of rules that must be abided by, and if you do so then this absolves you of any ethical responsibility; rather they are things that need to be thought about and carefully and responsibly considered, and that ethical dilemmas and problems are never simply resolved, but need to be carefully considered. As the American Psychological Association (2010) stress in their ethics code: 'the development of a dynamic set of ethical standards for psychologists . . . requires a personal commitment and lifelong effort to act ethically' (p. 2). It also points out that 'the Ethical Standards are not exhaustive. The fact that a given conduct is not specifically addressed by an Ethical Standard does not mean that it is necessarily either ethical or unethical' (p. 1).

The guidelines are rightly very clear on a number of points. These will be outlined first in general terms and then their impact on qualitative research will be considered. An overall principle is that of the welfare and protection of participants in research. It must be emphasised that studies should, among other things, be concerned with establishing mutual respect and confidence. We should respect participants as individuals; we must treat them as having fundamental rights, dignity and worth. Moreover, we should be appreciative and grateful for their helping us. Participants should leave the research situation with their self-esteem intact, feeling glad to have made a valued contribution to a worthwhile piece of research and happy to take part in further studies in the future.

The following paragraphs take as their general framework the British Psychological Society (2011) guidelines. A vital point that the guidelines rightly emphasise is the necessity of avoiding anything that has any possibility of harming the individual taking part in the study. The definition of 'harm' here includes discomfort and embarrassment. Any potential threats to psychological well-being, mental or physical health, values, attitudes, self-worth or dignity must be fully thought through. Thus, all possible psychological consequences for the participants need to be carefully considered and discussed with colleagues, including *inter alia* the study from the standpoint of the participant.

There is a paramount underlying precept of informed consent; participants in a study should be very clear as to what the research entails, and should have agreed to take part. Why we are carrying out our particular research should be made clear to them, along with full details as to what is proposed. Any aspect that might conceivably affect willingness to take part in the study needs to be brought to the attention of the other. Often, it is useful to draw up a full written contract with the other, explaining the procedures, what you intend to do with the results and how confidential or anonymous they are going to be, giving the other the right to terminate the study at any point, to withdraw or modify their contribution (for instance, it is desirable common practice for co-researchers in interviews to be given a copy of the interview transcript, with the invitation to modify or delete anything), to refuse to answer any question, etc. The guidelines recognise that some potential participants may not be able to give consent; research studies involving children or those with various impairments are obvious examples here. In such cases, those *in loco parentis* or similar positions must give their consent. People should never feel pressurised into taking part. (This is often difficult to ensure, especially in situations involving explicit power relationships between participants, such as in prisons or in universities.)

If for some reason withholding of information, misinformation, misleading or even deception is deemed to be essential to ensure that a more accurate picture is gained, this should only be exceptionally done, and only after detailed discussions with colleagues and disinterested independent advisers have produced no suggested feasible alternatives (and it is agreed that it is necessary for the research to be carried out). If this does take place, it is essential that participants are fully debriefed, the reasons for the misinformation being fully spelt out, and again guaranteed the right to withdraw their contribution to the research. This session should also include a discussion with participants concerning their experience of the research, in particular checking for misconceptions and any negative effects.

As a general principle, report write-ups should guarantee confidentiality or anonymity, unless explicit identification of participants is discussed and agreed in advance. Publication of results should ideally be of such a form as to guarantee anonymity for individual participants, and should not have the potential to cause harm to persons who might identify themselves from such a report. However, it must be realised that in many cases when examples are being used of, for instance, a participant's interview comments, although these can be readily anonymised they will inevitably not be confidential as they will be reported in full in the write-up. Thus, these limitations to confidentiality need to be made very clear to your participants.

Researchers utilising qualitative methods are usually aware of possible harmful consequences, and indeed prefer to use methods that treat and respect the other in the research situation as an equal; thus, full and open discussion is usually encouraged, which it is hoped will minimise any problems in this area. By their nature, qualitative methods tend to be less intrusive, but there is still the need to guard against potential harm to the psychological well-being (e.g. self-esteem) of participants. The method is generally far less reactive (i.e. the actual act of carrying out research has less of an effect on what is found) than more quantitative methods, which again is an advantage.

Similarly, this very openness generally means that research often fulfils the desirable general principle of 'informed consent', avoiding problems of deception which beset a lot of psychological work. The very use of terms such as 'participants' (or 'co-researchers', depending on the precise methodology adopted) rather than 'subjects' emphasises the realisation of the imbalanced power relationships inherent in much research, and attempts to address and remedy such problems.

On the other hand, deliberate attempts are made in some circumstances to study people in real-life contexts when they are unaware that they are being used as part of a study; examples here include some kinds of both participant and non-participant observation. Here, the principle of 'informed consent' is usually impossible to maintain. The British Psychological Society guidelines explicitly point out that in such circumstances we must respect the privacy and psychological well-being of the people being studied. Unless we have obtained informed consent, we should really only observe in situations where observation by strangers is normally expected. Thus, we should restrict ourselves to settings such as public social situations, but even then we need to be aware that variables such as local cultural values need to be taken into account, and as has been stressed above there may be limitations in such situations.

Qualitative methods also have specific problems when it comes to the writing of research reports. The general aim of confidentiality and anonymity is much harder to guarantee, especially in using people from a limited population. A guarantee of anonymity is no assurance that a participant will not be recognised; interviews within my institution with staff, for instance, mean that who the participants are is obvious to colleagues. Therefore special care needs to be taken in writing up such research, which should be done sensitively and with the realisation that at least it is likely that participants will be able to recognise themselves. These potential limitations need to be made clear to the participants.

It should be realised that one's responsibility as a researcher does not end at the end of the research. As is mentioned in Chapter 4, observation has been called an 'act of betrayal' by some, as it is making public something which previously is private, often to the benefit of the researcher and to the detriment of the observed.

This leads on to an important ethical debate that is related to the whole issue of the relationship between psychology and social change (which is briefly considered below): namely, in whose interests is the researcher being carried out? One of Savin's (1973) criticisms of the Stanford Prison Experiment is that it was not carried out primarily to reform prisons, but to aid the careers of the researchers. One position that could be adopted here (which goes beyond the standard ethical guidelines) is that one should not carry out research purely for the benefit of the researcher. Ideally, there should be possible benefits to the participant, possibly in general terms (e.g. contributing to the debate on improving prison conditions for prisoners), if not in specific terms. Sometimes these benefits may be incidental to the participant, but nonetheless valuable; for instance, there may be value in talking to somebody else about one's experiences since being diagnosed as suffering from a serious illness which may prove to be beneficial to the co-researcher.

The role of values

Again, this is intertwined with many of the points above, but it is worthy of its own heading to signify its importance, even if only briefly mentioned here. 'Values' have already been touched upon above. In this context, one is admitting that a researcher and research cannot be value-free, and that the general 'objectivist' notion that science can be value-free is impossible, given that we are all rooted in a social world that is socially constructed. Psychology (at least in the West) has general values (even if these are often left implicit) of communicating broadening knowledge and understanding about people, with a commitment to both freedom of inquiry and freedom of expression.

Inevitably, researchers themselves will have their own notions as to what the 'right', the 'correct', way of doing things is, and this needs to be clearly recognised in carrying out and writing up research. One also needs to admit one's values, and to stipulate them clearly. This is not to say that such revelations will minimise their impact, but it is a step in the right direction at least to admit their existence.

In this context, an important point to remember is that one's choice of research methods will inevitably influence the outcome of the research; different research techniques generate different kinds of material, ask different questions and produce different answers. As a very minimum, one should at least acknowledge that this occurs.

Psychology and social change

Inevitably, the question needs to be asked as to what use research is. Here, we could get tied up in interminable arguments about 'pure' versus 'applied' research. This distinction, however, is rather an artificial one, as all research will have some implications (even if one is not aware of it at the time). In terms of our own values, we would prefer to see research as having outcomes that directly relate to the 'real world', but this is not to decry other forms of research. The insights gained by some qualitative studies, for instance, may be sufficiently interesting to persuade psychologists who prefer more traditional ways of doing research to re-examine their principles (which in itself would be a laudatory outcome). Overall, though, I would concur with Shepherd (1993: 42):

> Most people working at the sharp end, however, would of course take a different line again. What matters to them, indeed what should matter to all of us, is not philosophical arguments about the superiority of one research methodology over another, rather the utility of research results.

The implications and implementation of findings are of importance and need to be carefully addressed in writing up research; as has been stressed above, research inevitably involves both values and moral dilemmas.

Another question that needs to be touched upon here is the thorny one of who pays for the research, and what the real motivation is for doing it. At the very least this needs to be made overt in any write-up and there is a need to try to establish the limits of the independence of the researcher from whoever is paying for the research. Who the gatekeepers are (which may also include journal editors and reviewers) is important, and this needs to be acknowledged.

It must also be realised that there are ethical issues involved in the utilisation of research results. Such results can be misused in other settings and cultures and can be used to further political and social ends. It is thus important to attempt to state clearly the limits of what it is that one has found, and to try to anticipate and forestall possible misinterpretations. Responsibility does not end with publication and we need always to be aware of who is using our results and for what ends.

When it comes to assessing this utility of qualitative research results, however, it might be worth bearing in mind that there are very different criteria which can be used here. Reason and Rowan (1981) raise questions as to what appropriate validity criteria might be for looking at research, emphasising that we need to go beyond asking 'Is it right?' to ask 'Is it useful?' and 'Is it

LIVERPOOL JOHN MOORES UNIVERSITY
LEARNING SERVICES

illuminating?' Sapsford (1984) picks this up, suggesting that we can assess research by the three criteria of agreement (do participants agree with the accounts of life which we, as researchers, provide them with?); consensus (is there general agreement?); and plausibility (does the research make sense of all the evidence?). Thus an appropriate criterion when considering qualitative research is to adopt that of examining the illumination provided by the research, rather than just asking about the validity of the results. What qualitative methods may be about is attempting to enhance understanding of the social world by helping to reveal the multifaceted nature of social reality. The change is one for psychology as well as one for our conceptualisation of that world; moreover, it may be a change for the researcher.

Chapter summary

This chapter has provided a detailed guide on how to write up a qualitative research project, with due emphasis on the differences to writing up a quantitatively based project. In particular, emphasis has been laid on the importance that the writing up should include reflexivity, ethical considerations and acknowledgement of the researcher's personal and cultural values.

Useful reading

Forrester, M. A. (2010) *Doing Qualitative Research in Psychology: A Practical Guide*. London: Sage.

Miles, M. B. and Huberman, A. M. (1994) *Qualitative Data Analysis*, 2nd edn. London: Sage.

Robson, C. (2011) *Real World Research*, 3rd edn. Oxford: Blackwell.

Willig, C. (2008) *Introducing Qualitative Research in Psychology*, 2nd edn. Maidenhead: McGraw-Hill.

References

American Psychological Association (2010) 'Ethical Principles of Psychologists and Code of Conduct'. Accessed December 12, 2010. http://www.apa.org/ethics/code/index.aspx.

Banister, P. and Smith, F. V. (1972) 'Vibration-induced white fingers and manipulative dexterity'. *British Journal of Industrial Medicine*, **29**, 264–7.

Bem, D. J. (1991) 'Writing the research report', in C. M. Judd, E. R. Smith and L. H. Kidder (eds) *Research Methods in Social Relations*, 6th edn. Fort Worth, TX: Holt, Rinehart and Winston.

British Psychological Society (2011) *Code of Human Research Ethics*. Leicester: British Psychological Society.

Jefferson, G. (1987) 'Appendix: transcription notation', in J. Potter and M. Wetherell (eds) *Discourse and Social Psychology*. London: Sage.

McDermott, M. (1993) 'On cruelty, ethics and experimentation: a profile of Philip G. Zimbardo'. *The Psychologist*, **6**, 456–9.

Psychological Abstracts. Washington, DC: American Psychological Association.

PsycLit. Washington, DC: American Psychological Association.

Reason, P. and Rowan, J. (eds) (1981) *Human Inquiry: A Sourcebook of New Paradigm Research*. Chichester: Wiley.

Sapsford, R. (1984) 'Paper 10 – a note on the nature of social psychology', in R. Stevens (ed.) *D307 Metablock*. Milton Keynes: Open University Press.

Savin, H. B. (1973) 'Professors and psychological researchers: conflicting values in conflicting roles'. *Cognition*, **2**, 147–9.

Shepherd, S. (1993) 'Review of "Suicides in Prison" by Liebling, A'. *Inside Psychology*, **1**(2), 42.

Wilkinson, S. (1988) 'The role of reflexivity in feminist psychology'. *Women's Studies International Forum*, **11**, 493–502.

Willig, C. (2008) *Introducing Qualitative Research in Psychology*, 2nd edn. Maidenhead: McGraw-Hill.

Zimbardo, P. G. (1973) 'On the ethics of intervention in human psychological research with special reference to the "Stanford Prison Experiment"'. *Cognition*, **2**, 243–55.

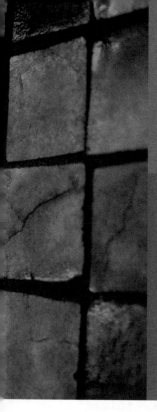

Chapter **14**

Problems in/of qualitative research

Erica Burman and Pauline Whelan

Introduction

The discourse of problems

Focusing on problems in qualitative research might seem an odd way to end a textbook promoting qualitative research in psychology. Clearly each of the qualitative approaches discussed in this book have their own specific domains of inquiry with associated strengths and weaknesses, which each chapter has discussed. In this chapter we take up some of the more general, supposed limitations of qualitative research that are commonly encountered across a range of health, education, policy and practice arenas to which psychological research contributes. But rather than accepting this discourse of 'problems', which would already be to concede too much to the discursive terrain of quantitative research by which – as we will argue – qualitative research is too often evaluated, our approach instead is to explore these 'problems' as problems: that is, as topics and resources for further investigation. Hence in this chapter we explore why and how these problems arise, rather than seeking to 'solve' them, and in so doing to arrive at a better understanding of the contexts of and for our work, and the nature of our interventions. This invites a more considered response instead of becoming absorbed in a defensive posturing that occludes the vibrant debates taking place between and amongst qualitative researchers. In line with their various philosophies of reflection and inquiry, we prefer to engage with these 'problems' as incitements to further conceptual elaboration that will strengthen understanding of what research is and does, the claims that can be made for specific approaches, and indeed the terms on which such claims could be warranted.

To arrive at the structure of this chapter we have drawn on the debates circulating within the qualitative research community and attempted also to address the kinds of concerns that qualitative researchers are faced with in convincing wider audiences of the value of their work. Hence we deal with not only questions of conceptual frameworks but also questions of epistemology, legitimacy, ethics, power relations and justification. While we are mindful of how helpful specific examples can be, we have decided not to single out particular studies as illustrative of the problems we describe. In part this choice arises out of ethical-political concerns, since it would seem invidious to target specific culpable authors or studies, especially as these are commonly encountered issues. Moreover, to identify specific examples would be to imply that these problems are individual matters, whereas the key point we want to make is that these questions of theoretical and political framing and rhetorical address – which structure the problems of justification, credibility, interpretation and application qualitative researchers deal with – are in fact general, relational and institutional matters faced by all researchers in communicating their work. (This issue does also face quantitative researchers, although they are less frequently obliged to account for themselves in this way.) For significant reasons (and with significant consequences) that we address below, too much energy is being devoted to defending the legitimacy of qualitative research at the expense of promoting discussion about precisely what it is about such work that is inspiring, distinctive or valuable in other ways. There is a further problem posed by the focus on 'problems', which is the danger of getting lost in a spiral of navel-gazing and legitimacy claims and so forgetting the ethical and political commitments that motivated us to engage with qualitative research in the first place. The point is not (or not just) that all these problems exist but rather how we acknowledge and navigate them in our research practice.

Problems of epistemology

The title of this book, *Qualitative Methods in Psychology*, draws our attention to the 'how' of psychological research. However, a focus on methods or methodology in qualitative research can sometimes work to obscure epistemological positions so that how we conduct our research begins to seem more important to us than the consequences of what we do. Psychology has a long disciplinary history of ignoring epistemological issues and this 'epistemophobia' (Chamberlain 2000) has resulted in a discipline where epistemological assumptions are often furtively embedded in research projects without any serious consideration of their appropriateness or function. There should be an alarm bell ringing here because we know that implicit assumptions in psychology have been among the most dangerous problems of the discipline. It is similarly hazardous to believe that we can avoid adopting some kind of epistemological position altogether. Epistemological inquiry involves the philosophy of the nature of knowledge (involving such questions as: Who is a knower? What counts as knowledge?), while all research adopts a position on politics, power, values and truth, even if that adoption sneaks into the research unannounced. Put simply, no research operates in an epistemological vacuum and we do have a problem if we think we can conduct our research without addressing epistemological questions.

The obscuring of epistemological commitments is a ~~problem~~ in academic research in many fields, but there are also specific reasons why we should be particularly attuned to this ~~problem~~ within the discipline of psychology. The perpetual agonising over methodological issues that has occurred in psychology almost since its inception (Danziger 1985) has often given rise to a prioritisation of methodological concerns over more basic questions of epistemology. This preoccupation with methodology has also frequently descended into 'methodolatry' where researchers have come to worship a method so completely that they have lost sight of the purpose and politics behind their research (Chamberlain 2000). The research then becomes one where the 'tail of methodology wags the dog of inquiry' (Lather 2006: 47). Qualitative psychologists are not exempt from falling into this little trap and it is frequently the case that qualitative psychologists begin their research by choosing a method of inquiry rather than engaging in a thorough consideration of the underlying epistemological framework (Salmon 2003).

Splitting methodology off from epistemological assumptions is a dangerous move because it supports the fiction that psychological research can operate outside politics (St. Pierre 2004). Explicitly engaging with epistemological issues allows us to clarify our position on the key questions of values, politics, power and truth and the implications of the positions we adopt. This forces us to realise that we cannot have any meaningful debate about methodology without understanding the philosophy behind it (St. Pierre 2000). We must consider what can be known (epistemology) before thinking about how we can come to know it (methodology). Avoiding epistemological questions yields even further confusion when incommensurable concepts are muddled together and where we find, in research reports, for example, positivist notions of bias and replicability interspersed with interpretivist rejections of objectivity and universal truths.

Despite the modest resurgence of qualitative methods within Anglo-US psychology, qualitative methods often operate in politically hostile conditions, where the 'gold standards' of research remain firmly weighted with evidence-based practice and randomised controlled trials. There is then some cause for celebration when qualitative methods are adopted and recognised, but we need to be careful not to fall into the essentialist trap of believing that all qualitative methods are necessarily a good thing. The celebration should be about what we can achieve using qualitative methods – by developing strategies to tackle oppressive psychological practice, for example – rather than simply paying homage to the fact that we are 'using' qualitative methods or because of their increasing popularity.

There is a free bonus in attending to epistemology in qualitative psychology and this takes the form of discovering the epistemological legacy of inspiring radical research within psychology that operated from marginal positions (e.g. feminist and queer research). Addressing epistemological questions reminds us that qualitative research 'carries on its strong, supple back the epistemologies of the Other' (St. Pierre and Roulston 2006: 678). This radical legacy foregrounds the political potential of qualitative research and the ethical commitments that should underpin our qualitative work. We need to avoid becoming deterministic about the relation between methods and politics and recognise that the separation of epistemology from methodology threatens to undermine our ethical-political commitments. To prevent drowning in methodological nuances, we have to leave breathing space for crucial epistemological questions around power, values, truth and politics.

~~Problems~~ of legitimacy

Another key ~~problem~~ that qualitative researchers often encounter is how to justify their methodological orientation. This ~~problem~~ is particularly pertinent because of the temporarily favoured position of conducting qualitative research in applications for state research funds. In part this development is a reflection of the increasing acceptability and even mainstreaming of (some varieties of) qualitative research – a shift that is perhaps a matter for some celebration – as indicated by the fact that the British Psychological Society Qualitative Methods in Psychology Section established in 2006 is now the biggest section in the organisation; while within the American Psychological Association the proposal to create a new division on Qualitative Inquiry gave rise in August 2010 to a 'Qualitative Inquiry' section being established within APA's Division 5. Quite what this section – which was formerly named 'Evaluation, Measurement and Statistics' – will be called remains a matter of debate, but the fact of this incorporation seems important. A related development has been that the British Psychological Society demands a qualitative research component for accredited degrees, giving rise to the need for detailed texts addressing the forms of qualitative research undertaken within specific areas of psychology (see e.g. Willig and Stainton-Rogers 2008). The ~~problems~~ of legitimacy take particular form within the discipline of psychology and we now turn to explore the ~~problem~~ of 'mixing methods'.

One strategy to further the legitimacy of qualitative research has been to use it alongside quantitative approaches. Yet the current popularity of 'mixed methods' is in our view something of a mixed blessing for qualitative researchers. This is because any such 'mixture' tends to revert to dominant (quantitative) models for its criteria for legitimation. While also a reflection of wider political pressures – the rise and rise of demands for evidence-based practice and the definition of randomised control trials as the 'gold standard' of ('scientific') research has never been stronger – this reversion arises because mixed methods derive from classical experimentalism (Denzin *et al.* 2006) which enforces a simple, orderly view of the world and marginalises particular forms of qualitative work (e.g. feminist, critical race, queer theory) while merrily ignoring key epistemological differences (see previous section above). Moreover, the combination of quantitative and qualitative research leads to a watering down of the rationale for and claims of qualitative research, where qualitative research gets thrust into a purely technocratic role of 'what works' (St Pierre 2000, 2004; Maclure 2005). The rationale for qualitative research becomes one of exploration that quantitative work then 'confirms'. Significantly, this contrived separation typically works to exclude the participants from any meaningful role in the research, rendering the work, contrary to the aspirations of much qualitative research, neither democratic nor dialogical (Denzin *et al.* 2006).

In Chamberlain's (2000) typology of methodolatry in qualitative research, 'mixed method' researchers fall into the category of 'agnostics' – that is, people who 'do not really understand what qualitative research is, and have little or no interest in finding out' (p. 288). They are recognisable by claims of having 'also' conducted qualitative research, supplementing questionnaires with open-ended questions or with interviews conducted with a small number of participants. Typically the analysis of this qualitative material is rather descriptive and atheoretical, accompanied by claims of adding depth, richness or context. As Chamberlain notes: 'Qualitative research is more than this, but the term is used so broadly that it is possible to include also anything under this heading that does not involve the statistical analysis of numbers' (2000: 288).

One problem with mixing quantitative and qualitative work concerns evaluations of size in relation to quality, or the scope of the claims that can be made from the research. Qualitative researchers often focus on seemingly localised topics and frequently work with small numbers of research participants (at least relative to much quantitative research), which cannot be reconciled with the positivism and quantitative preoccupations of much of psychology. This 'small' work is sometimes motivated by the need to attend to issues that would otherwise fall off the political agenda (the so-called 'statistical outliers') and we might be reminded here that part of the motivation behind the resurgence of qualitative research in psychology was to meaningfully engage with marginalised voices. Beyond the ethical impetus to attend to these 'small issues', it often emerges during the course of our research that these initially marginal-seeming concerns resonate with much larger issues and the insights gained from our 'small, localised' projects have far greater implications and applications than we could have predicted before we embarked on our research journey. In contexts where we are called upon to justify our recourse to qualitative methods, we need to beware methodological objections to 'small sample sizes' or 'small issues' because these typically either code for political objections, or represent fundamental misunderstandings of the epistemological basis of the work that we do (St. Pierre 2004). Size-related quality assessments are inherently problematic because they belong to a quantitative evaluative framework that is incommensurable with qualitative research.

A related problem arising from the mixing of methodological approaches concerns the model mobilised of how these approaches relate to each other. A realist model of 'triangulation' predominates that takes different methodological approaches as generating perspectives on the 'same' phenomenon, without appreciating how these frameworks in fact constitute their problem in radically divergent ways. Failure to do this not only strips qualitative research of its constructionist commitment to viewing its phenomenon or topic from its specific analytical framework, but actually juxtaposes different representations as if they could all be set alongside each other on the same topological plane. If such a plane exists, it is only within a quantitative paradigm. As Mason (1996: 149) notes:

> It implies a view of the social world which says there is one, objective, and knowable reality, and all that social researchers have to do is work out which are the appropriate triangulation points to measure it by.

We need to move away from this model to treat all approaches as generating distinct perspectives or representations that cannot be combined, since they are incommensurable. This point also goes for combinations of qualitative approaches, which cannot be compared and contrasted except from a particular perspective, whose assumptions and implications would need to be declared and open to evaluation. Hence while researching a topic from a variety of methodological frameworks may well enrich the understanding of the phenomenon at issue, there is no easy way to move across the different representations generated. There are implications for the kinds of truth claims that can be made from such inquiries – as multiple and diverse rather than unitary and consensual. As Mason continues:

> You are highly unlikely, therefore, to be able to straightforwardly use the 'products' of different research methods or sources to corroborate (or otherwise) each other. If you are expecting to use triangulation

in this sense, you are likely to become very confused about matters of validity, because you will have more than one data set which will seem to inexplicably point in different directions.

(Mason 1996: 149)

The point in combining different methodological approaches should be to open up interpretations rather than to close them off, as is the case in realist models of mixing methods.

Before we move on, we might note that just because qualitative research is now regarded in some contexts as acceptable, this does not mean that it should be valued as somehow intrinsically a good thing or (morally) superior to quantitative research. To do this would be to commit another kind of methodolatry, one of mistaking the methodological approach for the politics. Indeed, qualitative research is still subject to many of the same (as well as different) ethical-political problems that characterise research in general – of colonising people's experiences (Morgan 1981), still worse rendering their survival or resistance strategies visible and so legible and surveillable by the dominant where these may have arisen precisely because of their hidden or ambiguous character (Scott 2008). Indeed, we might note that qualitative research can all too easily be co-opted to perpetuate precisely the kind of exclusions that it was introduced to overcome. One way this can happen is when the reification or fetishising of particular methods displaces the social justice motivations of qualitative research and results in the stigmatising of particular groups of people (e.g. in the deployment of qualitative methods to further oppressive corporate marketing campaigns).

A further danger of the popularity of qualitative research in service policy-related research is that it might be preferred because it is seen as a cheap option (Craig 1996); doing a small-scale study is usually less resource-intensive than a larger one (and this is of course a good reason too!). Yet concerns have been noted by qualitative health researchers that such economic priorities underestimate the time and analytical resources required to complete a coherent, viable and valuable study, with the result that a qualitative study is designed as merely a small-scale version of or for a quantitative investigation – not only subordinating the qualitative to the quantitative but overlooking the key differences of claims and strengths of each (Yardley and Bishop 2008).

There are two possible strategies open to qualitative researchers in dealing with legitimacy problems. The first is one of refusing the discourse of 'science' that renders qualitative research deficient or inferior. On this point we might note that those working in the natural sciences typically dismiss the idea that any kind of psychology is scientific anyway (Derksen 1997), while quantitative psychologists have rarely engaged with philosophical questions of science (Michell 1997; Trendler 2009). Instead qualitative researchers have embraced new discursive registers, for example, emphasising distinctive features of qualitative inquiry such as 'fidelity' or 'authenticity', 'meaning-in-context' that extend to 'a prophetic, feminist postpragmatism that embraces an ethics of truth grounded in love, care, hope and forgiveness' (Denzin *et al.* 2006). Other strategies have included reclaiming or redefining what 'science' is (mobilising examples from the history of science, especially of psychology, which of course started from a qualitative tradition of introspection with Willhem Wundt); whilst also highlighting specific cultural assumptions structured into particular discourses of science, so that, for example, the French word for 'experiment' is 'experience' – highlighting specifically Anglophone binaries/agendas at work (Chalmers 1999).

On the other hand, in relation to the charge of being 'unscientific', we might note that there are also claims that there is nothing intrinsically unscientific about the use of qualitative methods in psychology, as far as the traditional realist understanding of science is concerned (Michell 2004), so rejecting the 'narrow scientism' that prioritises evidence-based practice and randomised control trials (RCTs), rather than science per se. Criticisms can also be levelled at the spurious claims to science fostered by new methodologies of neoliberal governance such as 'systematic review' which disguise what may be a very unsystematic process by couching it in pseudoscientific terms (Maclure 2005).

There are also disciplinary, rather than specifically, political confusions that are played out via methodological disputes, as where there are ~~problems~~ of 'scaling up'. Qualitative research deals in specificities and particularities, while the demands of policy agendas for large-scale applications and interventions can make the research topics taken as the focus for qualitative researchers appear 'too small' or not relevant for wider populations. 'Why should we design our services around the needs of this (numerically small) group?' is a refrain often heard in relation to designing provision for people from minority ethnic backgrounds or people with disabilities. Yet the point here is not that all groups share all these features (as the quantitative discourse of 'scale' would presume), but that in taking up the recommendations arising from the research to make services accessible to these groups, they become accessible to many more. Hence, while qualitative research may address some unique or exceptional topics or arenas, this does not mean that its analyses have no application to others (while equally there is a key political point of principle that lack of wider relevance or applicability should not become a criterion to reject or criticise qualitative research). Rather what is important is to recognise that a key strength of qualitative research is its specificity and corresponding depth of focus, which allows for the documentation of particular constellations of contexts and relationships that might not become apparent using other approaches. The art of designing a good piece of qualitative research is to elaborate a form of investigation that is small enough to be explored in depth, that somehow exemplifies wider issues, so (as the poet William Blake put it) 'seeing the world in a grain of sand'. Tiny as the grain of sand may be to the naked eye, it nevertheless exquisitely encapsulates a host of wider structures and relationships. Maintaining the analogy, dismissing analysis of that sand grain as not having relevance to beaches, mineral stocks, water levels, land masses and associated practices of agriculture, tourism or disaster management is to miss a key opportunity to build a picture of delicate but important systemic links.

~~Problems~~ of selection, interpretation and reflexivity

Conducting qualitative research always involves demarcating our field of inquiry and selecting research material to include in the representation of our research. In the social sciences, 'representation' combines political and pictorial senses of the term so that how we speak or act on behalf of particular groups and how we register our academic opinions are intimately bound up with how we describe and present our research. Alongside negotiating ~~problems~~ of selection, we need to address ~~problems~~ of interpretation and ensure that we neither indulge in convoluted over-analysis nor, conversely, that we merely summarise our research material. We stumble into a related ~~problem~~ if, ruminating on whether we should accept our participants' stories as irrefutably authoritative or disregard them as cases of 'false consciousness', we forget to situate our analysis (and our participants' material) within prevailing structures and ideologies (Kitzinger and Wilkinson 1997). ~~Problems~~ of selection and interpretation are unavoidable in any qualitative analysis and as we make our way through these issues, ~~problems~~ of reflexivity necessarily emerge.

In qualitative research, ~~problems~~ of selection include the decisions we make about how to circumscribe our field of research as well as how we choose particular material to include in the representation of our analysis. We might also note how the term 'selection' has particularly unfortunate historical connotations (with Nazi genocide) that should at least invite reflection on the relationships between psychological research, racism and war (see Wexler 1983; Terre Blanche *et al.* 2006). A 'selection' ~~problem~~ we often encounter involves debunking the idea that qualitative analysis is really only a case of researchers 'cherry-picking' material to support their own favourite arguments or positions (Hollway and Jefferson 2000). Responding to this ~~problem~~ typically involves pointing out that all researchers (qualitative and quantitative) are implicated in the selection of their material and to pretend that this is not the case is to fall prey to an untenable case of the neutral observer. Rather than submit to this kind of positivist delusion that vanishes the producer from the research product, qualitative researchers justify the production and selection of material via recourse to the rigour of their respective methodological frameworks as well as committing to processes of reflexivity and ethical accountability. Charges of 'cherry-picking' material can generally be read as political distractions from the more important issue of what it is we do with the material that we have selected, but we also need to ensure that we explicitly account for the 'selections' we have made along the way. Staying with ~~problems~~ of selection, we also need to beware the issue of 'relevance', or more specifically, who defines what is relevant and how we accept or challenge these definitions. While we may aspire to make our research socially relevant, we need to avoid fawning on dominant social policy agendas or simply shaping our research to comply with external pressures to be 'socially useful' (pressures which too often merely translate into calls to be lucrative).

The presentation of research is central to our response to ~~problems~~ of selection, with this assuming a particular shape within the discipline of psychology. Professional psychologists are often considered to be mere regurgitators of common sense, while academic psychologists are sometimes thought to spend their time converting everyday banalities into obscure theories. As qualitative researchers in psychology operating across these two arenas, one of the ~~problems~~ we face is how to present our work in such a way that we convince our audiences of its value. Writing about our research is, in this sense, a craft activity and we aspire to keep our readers convinced and interested. Navigating this ~~problem~~ of choosing material that represents our analysis as well as keeping our research narrative alive should not lead us to a position where we are using our interview transcripts in ways that will individualise or trivialise issues nor simply feed a prevailing popular appetite for personal misery or heroic survival stories. Our task is rather to enliven, as well as enlighten, our research to keep our readers awake, while simultaneously curbing our enthusiasm for delivering the kind of sensational material so beloved of policymakers, who despite claims to validate only quantitative material, are eager for lurid case exemplars.

Of course, presenting our research is bound up with how we interpret and analyse our research material. ~~Problems~~ of interpretation usually fall into one of two categories: either we are accused of making too much of our research material (over-interpreting) or conversely we are accused of not making enough (under-interpreting). Under-interpreting happens when instead of analysing our material, we merely redescribe it. On the other hand, and although it is a strength of qualitative research to develop rich analyses from 'small sample sizes' (relative to much quantitative work), over-interpreting can happen if our line of argument becomes obscured in the weaving of intricate analytical tales. A related ~~problem~~ involves justifying our corpus of material – whether our analysis has drawn on indicative material or on our most diverse or atypical examples. Decisions about how we begin and end our process of analysis are tied not only to the methodological framework we espouse, as you will have read about in the other chapters, but also to our research purposes and aims. Alongside these decisions, we will encounter ~~problems~~ of interpretation if we neglect to contextualise, historicise and connect to material realities and this is one of the reasons why Foucault's work has been so useful for qualitative researchers (e.g. Parker 1992, 2007). It is to the closely related process of reflexivity, which deals with connecting our analysis to structural and ideological issues, that we now turn.

Reflexivity has a pivotal role to play in accounting for the production of our qualitative analysis, as you will have read about in the preceding chapters. However, there are ~~problems~~ associated with reflexivity too and we need to be aware of these so that we can successfully orient our way around them. The first ~~problem~~ occurs when the concept of reflexivity collapses into a self-involved kind of confession so that a catharsis of self-disclosures becomes the end point of our reflexive account. This is a ~~problem~~ nurtured by the co-option of reflexivity to further neoliberal political agendas where – in a familiar de-reradicalising move – quasi-feminist rhetoric is deployed to further old-style individualism (Burman 2006, 2009). In extending cautions about how to employ reflexive analyses, we need to be careful that our approaches to reflexivity do not slip into a narcissistic recentring of the subjectivity of the researcher – the kind of project so endorsed by the neoliberal exhortation to work on ourselves and an incitement notably encouraged at the expense of wider social-political considerations (Rose 1985; Burman 2006). We often deploy reflexive strategies to explore 'what went wrong' with our research and this can usefully expose the limitations of our research practices, but reflexivity is also about exploring why things worked (in contrast to why they did not), as well as questioning why things worked in the ways that they did. Another ~~problem~~ with reflexivity which you may have noticed as you read through the previous chapters is that different modes of qualitative inquiry can espouse different models of reflexivity. Of course this is not really a ~~problem~~ at all (unless we have been duped into believing that all qualitative methods are aspiring to achieve the 'same results' – in which case, see the ~~problem~~ of 'mixing methods' above). Indeed, multiple perspectives can offer fruitful opportunities for engaging with the strengths and weaknesses of respective qualitative approaches to reflexivity (Parker 2005; Burman 2006). On a final reflexive point, we should note that almost all qualitative research practice has derived from the social sciences of Europe and North America (Preissle 2006) and this should encourage us to be on our critical toes by reflecting on the colonial tendencies that such a geographical emergence might entail.

~~Problems~~ of ethics

All research involves ethical ~~problems~~ – the question is how these are engaged with and addressed. The ethics committee checklist bureaucracy ushers in the fantasy that ethical issues can be administered away, but this is only at the cost of sanitising and dehumanising what must always be in some sense a risky encounter, if it is an encounter at all. The responsibilities for and of the researcher are onerous, including to themselves. The current balance of practice towards risk aversion simply works to deny ethical engagement. Questions of informed consent cannot be determined absolutely, or in advance, even with the most robust participant groups (i.e. not those considered 'vulnerable'), but have to be understood as constantly in process as part of the ongoing negotiation of research relationships. Similarly the researcher cannot be entirely responsible for the meanings and associations generated by their questions or interventions – though they can certainly do their best to alert participants so that areas of sensitivity can be managed together in a co-operative and consultative manner. Submissions for ethical approval often require us to work with predefined categories (e.g. 'vulnerable groups', 'sensitive issues'), thus perpetuating the illusion that these are clear-cut, static, easily identifiable and manageable things. In much the same way that the discipline of psychology sometimes reduces people to diagnostic labels, the process of ethical clearance can create a further problem if we are tricked into believing that our participants are nothing more than the descriptive categories we are obliged to box them into for our ethics committee submissions.

Ethical responsibilities are not only generated in contexts where a seemingly 'direct' encounter is taking place, for example, between an interviewer and interviewee. Equivalent considerations arise in the responsibilities incurred by analysing text – including the selection of text, and the meanings subscribed to or reproduced in analysing it and reporting on this analysis (e.g. analysing racist text and so running the risk of legitimising it by reproducing it). There are strategies we can engage with for limiting such consequences, including clearly situating the analysis within a narrative that clarifies the ethical-political rationale and explicitly challenging unwanted readings. Obviously undesirable readings cannot absolutely be prevented, for as researchers we cannot legislate the readings made of our material – we can only indicate why and how particular readings are preferred.

Different research contexts can also give rise to different, as well as the same, ethical problems. We might encounter ethical issues around the disclosure of sensitive material in face-to-face contexts, for example, but these might evolve differently or be differently textured in online environments. We need also to be aware of the dangers of romanticising about the subversive potential of particular contexts, taking into account, for example, how feminist scientists have shown that the much lauded possibilities of cyberspace for transcending traditional embodied hierarchies have been greatly overblown (Wajcman 2007). Analysis of online material also raises particular ethical issues around the identification of participants, who although writing in a public forum might not wish their material to be used for research purposes. Issues of participant anonymity with respect to complex questions around identification and tracing are particularly pertinent here.

Redressing the long history of abhorrent manipulation and control of participants in psychology was part of the moral-political impetus behind the resurgence of qualitative research in psychology. However, we encounter another qualitative research problem if we think that we are engaging in good ethical research merely by 'being nice to people' (Parker 2005: 13) and then come to accept or support morally reprehensible ideas simply to avoid offending our participants. Our ethical commitments in qualitative research involve adopting an explicit political stance and assuming the responsibility of our research positions and actions, which, for the purposes of our research, may mean that it is unethical to accept our participants' views. If our participants are prominent agents of oppressive practices, for example, the ethical impetus of our research would be to challenge their accounts (Burman 2003). Our research always involves determining our ethical accountability, which inevitably extends beyond our immediate academic community, just as our ethical commitments frequently extend beyond the official academic timelines of our research activities.

~~Problems~~ of power

Although we have not explicitly engaged with issues of power so far, implicit throughout all qualitative research is the importance of the researcher assuming their authority and authorial responsibilities. There is a double sense here that draws attention to the question of writing and representation. The model of power in qualitative research is not like weightlifting or a pendulum. Power is not a possession or a unilinear force, but a set of multiple, complex (and contested) relationships that modulate and shift during the research process. Power relations are inevitable and not all determined by the micropolitics of the research encounter. While improving our interview techniques or creating cosier physical research settings might assist us in our research practice and increase the comfort of our participants, the micropolitics of research cannot be magically disappeared away with these kinds of manoeuvres or strategies. Indeed, promoting research encounters as democratic spaces often disguises pernicious forms of covert regulation and control (Burman 2003).

Power considerations should always go beyond the micro level and recognise that power operates at multiple levels. A significant feature of feminist research has been to consistently draw attention to the institutional power dynamics that structure research, including publishing gatekeepers, research council agendas, government policies and so on, and this provides a wealth of material to draw on for exploring power in qualitative research (e.g. Stanley and Wise 1980; Ribbens and Edwards 1998). What is important is to acknowledge and be aware (or as aware as we can be and make this explicit in our accounts) of the varieties and vicissitudes of power relations as they have entered into the formulation, generation, conduct, analysis and reporting of our research. We also need to attend to the difficult questions of who benefits materially and symbolically from the research.

The main ~~problems~~ of power in qualitative research occur when power is ignored. We might expect that 'where there is power, there is resistance' (as Foucault claims) so if we render power invisible it makes it more difficult for strategies of resistance to be seen. While it might not always be ethical for these strategies of resistance to be made too visible (and so render them subject to further policing), we do have a ~~problem~~ if we neglect to attend to the role of power or ignore its constraining and enabling effects on our research practices.

Not a ~~conclusion~~

As we have seen in previous chapters, different research methods adhere to different evaluative criteria and their respective languages of justification may be incommensurable. As qualitative inquirers we recognise the impossibility of static, predefined, universally applicable quality criteria and we reject the rigid definitions of generalisability, validity, reliability and rigour that psychologists have historically held so dear. Being flexible and open in developing new modes to evaluate our qualitative research, however, does not mean that we cast aside the concept of academic scholarship (Parker 2004). As researchers, we need to determine and clearly articulate which principles and priorities we are aiming for and to present plausible, theoretically congruent and grounded arguments to support and situate our qualitative work.

Qualitative research is hardly renowned for resulting in internationally acclaimed artistic masterpieces but Leonardo da Vinci's well-known declaration that 'art is never finished, only abandoned' seems to resonate with the inexhaustibility of the analytic task. There is no such thing as a 'complete' analysis and we need to focus instead on the fruitfulness of our research – we are more concerned with 'where our research goes and what it does there' (St Pierre 2000: 27) than judging our research on a myopic kind of methodological merit. Unlike quantitative psychology, we do not work with fixed quality criteria or rigid definitions of validity, rigour, generalisability, reliability, and so on, and at the very least these concepts require redefinition within a qualitative framework. Rigour and validity can no longer be achieved simply by methodical allegiance to a list of technical procedures because in qualitative research these criteria cease to exist purely as epistemic concepts and instead become bound to the ethics of relational research practice (Lincoln 2001; Lather 2007). The traditional psychological concept of reliability – the idea that we can consistently reproduce the same results – becomes antiquated in qualitative research that specifically aims to drive positive change (Parker 2004). The robotic regularity of human beings assumed in the crudest forms of positivist generalisability is at odds with most kinds of qualitative research, as is the idea that individual life trajectories can be straightforwardly scripted by statistical projections developed from so-called 'random' samples. The qualitative challenge is to develop our own composition and definition of evaluative criteria and to elaborate these criteria with and through the generation of our material, starting with the initial stages of formulating our research questions.

The renunciation of quantitative evaluative concepts, such as generalisability, and the abandonment of the positivist preoccupation with objectivity in research should not, however, lead us to a position where we feel we can say nothing about our research that might be relevant to other contexts (Fine and Torre 2004), or that – after a bout of peculiarly self-absorbed 'reflexivity' perhaps – we come to think that our analysis is nothing more than our own subjective opinion. We do have a problem if we are deploying quantitative quality criteria to evaluate our qualitative research, but the qualitative redescription of these terms can also serve us well in contexts where our research comes under attack and where we need to justify the systematicity, ethics, relevance and importance of what we do (e.g. for qualitative debates on generalisability, see Smaling 2003; Sandelowski 2004; Goodman 2008; for validity, see Fine and Torre 2004; Lather 2007; for reliability, see Parker 2005; for rigour, see Guba and Lincoln 2005).

All this is alongside long-standing political priorities favouring research that makes claims to generalisability and replicability. Here we see how wider political agendas inform research design in the form of the resurgence of positivism (Lather 2006). This, however, institutes a related problem whereby a dispute that is apparently over method (technique) or methodology (research approach) actually codes for a political difference (over what the research is about, or who it is for). While a positivist framework encourages lack of acknowledgement of the ethical-political stance inevitably structured into any investigation, which is (or should be) made explicit in qualitative research, in some contexts making this more visible may render the research less politically acceptable. On the other hand, at least it is clear that the reasons why the research may be deemed inadequate are not to do with the rigour, creativity or commitment with which it was conducted but rather the political 'lack of fit' with prevailing priorities of the funders. Hence we raise this issue out of concern for the ways important political differences in agenda can be masked by methodological debates, with qualitative research sometimes spuriously rejected for reasons that are other than methodological.

This political manipulation of research practices, whether in the form of systematic review mechanisms (Maclure 2005) or other such forms of governmentality and technocracy, raises a final related issue that we would like to address here. The recurrent ~~problems~~ of qualitative research can tell us something about the legacy of regulation and control that characterises the discipline of psychology (Burman 1998), particularly around challenges to legitimacy, credibility and justification. The best work in qualitative research has broken the rules and one of the keys to becoming a good researcher is learning to develop innovative approaches that can overthrow disciplinary norms (Parker 2004). Our discussion of ~~problems~~ here is necessarily incomplete and inconclusive because the temporal specificities and contextual particularities of qualitative research mean that ~~problems~~ are always emergent and in flux. Instead we have attempted to sketch the controversial parameters of our qualitative research activities.

Chapter summary

In this chapter we have explored ~~problems~~ in/of qualitative research as resources and topics that can help us understand the nature of qualitative research practice and the contexts within which this work takes place. Rather than positioning these ~~problems~~ as errors to be eliminated or whitewashed away, we explored how and why they arise out of specific political, disciplinary, relational, historical and institutional contexts. In exploring the conditions of legitimacy and justification within which qualitative research is held to account, we have specifically addressed ~~problems~~ of epistemology, selection, interpretation, reflexivity, ethics and power. Throughout the chapter, our aims were to identify strategies to convince others of the value of qualitative research, as well as to signpost ways of navigating these ~~problems~~.

Common to all the ~~problems~~ we discussed in this chapter is the key issue of political framing, which not only structures quality criteria that force qualitative research into a quantitative evaluative framework, but also permeates the more subtle micro-practices of research relations. By exploring how and why such ~~problems~~ occur in qualitative work, we elaborated the contexts within which our work takes place, as well as the kinds of institutional, disciplinary and relational dynamics that facilitate and constrain all kinds of psychological research. If your qualitative research seems threatened by political incursion, or mired in the conventional or the banal, then the cautionary tales outlined here might help you craft more creative research stories.

References

Burman, E. (1998) 'Disciplinary apprentices: "qualitative methods" in student psychological research'. *International Journal of Social Research Methodology*, **1**(1), 25–45.

Burman, E. (2003) 'Narratives of challenging research: stirring tales of politics and practice'. *International Journal of Social Research Methodology*, **6**(2), 101–19.

Burman, E. (2006) 'Emotions and reflexivity in feminised education action research'. *Educational Action Research*, **14**(3), 315–32.

Burman, E. (2009) 'Beyond "emotional literacy" in feminist and educational research'. *British Educational Research Journal*, **13**(1), 137–55.

Chalmers, A. (1999) *What Is This Thing Called Science?*, 3rd edn. Buckingham: Open University Press.

Chamberlain, K. (2000) 'Methodolatry and qualitative health research'. *Journal of Health Psychology*, **5**(3), 285–96.

Craig, G. (1996) 'Qualitative research in an NHS setting: uses and dilemmas'. *Changes: An International Journal of Psychology and Psychotherapy*, **14**(3), 180–6.

Danziger, K. (1985) 'The methodological imperative in psychology'. *Philosophy of the Social Sciences*, **15**(1), 1–13.

Denzin, N. K., Lincoln, Y. S. and Giardina, M. (2006) 'Disciplining qualitative research'. *International Journal of Qualitative Studies in Education*, **19**(6), 769–82.

Derksen, M. (1997) 'Are we not experimenting then? The rhetorical demarcation of psychology and common sense'. *Theory and Psychology*, **7**(4), 435–56.

Fine, M. and Torre, M. E. (2004) 'Re-membering exclusions: participatory action research in public institutions'. *Qualitative Research in Psychology*, **1**(1), 15–37.

Goodman, S. (2008) 'The generalizability of discursive research'. *Qualitative Research in Psychology*, **5**(4), 265–75.

Guba, E. G., and Lincoln, Y. S. (2005) 'Paradigmatic controversies, contradictions, and emerging influences', in N. K. Denzin and Y. S. Lincoln (eds) *The Sage Handbook of Qualitative Research*, 3rd edn. London: Sage.

Hollway, W. and Jefferson, T. (2000) *Doing Qualitative Research Differently: Free Association, Narrative and the Interview Method*. London: Sage.

Kitzinger, C. and Wilkinson, S. (1997) 'Validating women's experience? Dilemmas in feminist research'. *Feminism in Psychology*, **7**(4), 566–74.

Lather, P. (2006) 'Paradigm proliferation as a good thing to think with: teaching research in education as wild profusion'. *International Journal of Qualitative Studies in Education*, **19**(1), 35–57.

Lather, P. (2007) 'Validity, qualitative', in G. Ritzer (ed.) *The Blackwell Encyclopedia of Sociology*. Oxford: Blackwell.

Lincoln, Y. (2001) 'Emerging criteria for quality in qualitative and interpretive research', in N. K. Denzin and Y. S. Lincoln (eds) *The Qualitative Inquiry Reader*. London: Sage.

Maclure, M. (2005) 'Clarity bordering on stupidity: where's the quality in systematic review?' *Journal of Educational Policy*, **20**(4), 393–416.

Mason, J. (1996) *Qualitative Researching*. London: Sage.

Michell, J. (1997) 'Quantitative science and the definition of measurement in psychology'. *British Journal of Psychology*, **88**(3), 355–83.

Michell, J. (2004) 'The place of qualitative research in psychology'. *Qualitative Research in Psychology*, **1**(4), 307–19.

Morgan, D. (1981) 'Men, masculinity and the process of sociological inquiry', in H. Roberts (ed.) *Doing Feminist Research*. London: Routledge and Kegan Paul.

Parker, I. (1992) *Discourse Dynamics: Critical Analysis for Social and Individual Psychology*. London: Routledge.

Parker, I. (2004) 'Criteria for qualitative research in psychology'. *Qualitative Research in Psychology*, **1**, 95–106.

Parker, I. (2005) *Qualitative Psychology: Introducing Radical Research*. Maidenhead: Open University Press.

Parker, I. (2007) *Revolution in Psychology: Alienation to Emancipation*. London: Pluto Press.

Preissle, J. (2006) 'Envisioning qualitative inquiry: a view across four decades'. *International Journal of Qualitative Studies in Education*, **19**(6), 685–95.

Ribbens, J. and Edwards, R. (eds) (1998) *Feminist Dilemmas in Qualitative Research*. London: Sage.

Rose, N. (1985) *The Psychological Complex: Psychology, Politics and Society in England 1869–1939*. London: Routledge and Kegan Paul.

Salmon, P. (2003) 'How do we recognise good research?' *The Psychologist*, **16**(1), 24–7.

Sandelowski, M. (2004) 'Using qualitative research'. *Qualitative Health Research*, **14**(10), 1366–86.

Scott, J. (2008) 'Everyday forms of resistance'. *Copenhagen Journal of Asian Studies*, **4**, 32–62.

Smaling, A. (2003) 'Inductive, analogical and communicative generalization'. *International Journal of Qualitative Methods*, **2**(1), 52–67.

Stanley, L. and Wise, S. (1980) *Feminist Consciousness and Feminist Research*. London: Routledge and Kegan Paul.

St. Pierre, E. A. (2000) 'The call for intelligibility in postmodern educational research'. *Educational Researcher*, **29**, 25–8.

St. Pierre, E. A. (2004) 'Refusing alternatives: a science of contestation'. *Qualitative Inquiry*, **10**(1), 130–39.

St. Pierre, E. A. and Roulston, K. (2006) 'The state of qualitative inquiry: a contested science'. *International Journal of Qualitative Studies in Education*, **19**(6), 673–84.

Terre Blanche, M., Durrheim, K. and Painter, D. (eds) (2006) *Research in Practice: Applied Methods in the Social Sciences*, 2nd edn. Cape Town: University of Cape Town Press.

Trendler, G. (2009) 'Measurement theory, psychology and the revolution that cannot happen'. *Theory and Psychology*, **19**(5), 579–99.

Wacjman, J. (2007) 'From women and technology to gendered technoscience'. *Information, Communication and Society*, **10**(3), 287–98.

Wexler, P. (1983) *Critical Social Psychology*. London: Routledge and Kegan Paul.

Willig, C. and Stainton-Rogers, W. (eds) (2008) *Handbook of Qualitative Research in Psychology*. London: Sage.

Yardley, L. and Bishop, F. (2008) 'Mixing qualitative and quantitative methods: a pragmatic approach', in C. Willig and W. Stainton-Rogers (eds) *Handbook of Qualitative Research in Psychology*. London: Sage.

Glossary

Please note that terms in this glossary may be interpreted and defined differently by different writers. The glossary has been developed by the co-authors of this book, and should be used in this light.

action research (AR): research that is attempting to improve social practice by changing it and evaluating the impact of change.

axiology: the value of the research.

colonisation: realisation that the cultural systems of beliefs, behaviour norms and social rituals of Western psychological knowledge are given precedence over non-Western indigenous psychologies.

community of practice (CoP): a group of people who share an interest, hobby, and/or profession and who engage in collective learning.

constructivism: the notion that individuals construct an understanding of the world around them through reflection on their own experiences.

conversation analysis: the detailed study of actual talking in natural interactions.

critical disability studies: theory and research that aim to expose the conditions of disabilsm as they work at all levels.

critical hermeneutics: part of phenomenology, which explores how the understandings of participants (often from marginalised groups) are structured by dominant ideologies.

critical narrative analysis (CNA): recognises that narratives can

be critically interrogated in terms of power.

decolonisation: attempt to draw attention to and to avoid the problems of colonisation.

deconstructionism: to identify, question and take apart assumptions and cultural norms.

descriptive phenomenology: emphasises the essential features of lived experience. Such essences are taken as objective and true descriptions of the phenomenon, which stems from the realist ontology of this school of phenomenology.

discourse analysis: a number of different methods that analyse written, spoken or other language which are taken to reflect and reproduce the culture and society in which they have occurred.

discursive psychology: sees discourse as structuring and creating the social world and uses ideas from discourse analysis and conversation analysis to explore how psychological phenomena are constructed and negotiated in language.

emancipatory disability research: research 'with' rather than 'on' disabled people which is aiming to emancipate.

embodiment: the notion that it is through our bodies, our felt sense, or the subjective meanings of our lived

experience that we communicate with and come to know and understand our world.

enlightenment: the recognition that oppressive events and practices are recognised or exposed for what they are and this recognition is used to mobilise oppressed people to work together to fight against them.

epistemology: the study of knowledge.

epoche: where the researcher sets aside assumptions, judgements and prior interpretations before immersing themselves fully in the data.

ethics: part of philosophy that is concerned with what is acceptable.

ethnography: a method that attempts to grasp another's point of view, their relation to life, and to realise their vision of their world through first-hand observation and participation in natural settings.

ethnomethodology: the study of the everyday methods people employ to make sense of their social worlds.

evaluation research: research involving the measurement of programme effectiveness in terms of reaching its desired goals.

existentialism: sees people as having free will, individuality and subjectivity.

feminist research: research carried out by feminists that draws on women's experience of living in a world in which women are seen as being subordinate to men. Such research has the aim to bring about social change and improvement in relation to gender and all the other related forms of inequality and oppression in which gender subordination is implicated.

focus group: interview research carried out with a group of people at the same time.

Foucauldian discourse analysis (FDA): a deeper form of discourse analysis that explicitly and critically takes account of power, objects, techniques and language.

grounded theory: the researcher derives categories for analysis directly from the observations in the field, not from preconceived theories or hypotheses.

hegemonic: the power exerted by a dominant group over others.

hermeneutics: the study of interpretation and understanding.

hybridisation: a methodology driven by pragmatic need such that a researcher can use both qualitative and quantitative methods without being tied to a specific methodological paradigm.

interpretative phenomenological analysis (IPA): the examination of how people make sense of their own life experiences, but with an emphasis also on the researcher, who is seen as influencing the data and the subsequent interpretation of the account.

intersubjectivity: recognised as being between subjectivity and

objectivity, where something is personally experienced by more than one person through an ongoing process of exchange and interaction with others.

Kleinian approach to psychoanalytical research: emphasis on identification, projection and transference within the research setting, which can be interpreted by the researcher. There is an emphasis on social constructionism.

Lacanian approach to psychoanalytical research: emphasises discourse and language, and the unconscious is understood to be the discourse of the other.

lifeworld: how things seem to the perceiver.

methodolatry: researchers have come to worship a method so completely that they have lost sight of the purpose and politics behind their research.

methodology: a particular approach to searching for and generating knowledge.

narrative inquiry: a research method which examines the storied character of psychological and cultural life.

observation: research which relies on techniques of watching and noting naturally occurring phenomena.

ontology: the philosophical study of knowledge and of being.

paradigm: the commonality of perspective that binds theoretical work together.

participatory action research (PAR): emphasises the experiential knowledge of stakeholders such as community members or organisational staff (i.e. the people who are experiencing the problem).

participatory ethnography: ethnographic investigation which directly involves the people on whom the study is being carried out with.

personal construct theory (PCT): arising from the work of Kelly, which emphasises how we personally construe others, the social world and ourselves. It is phenomenological with an individual ontology, resulting from our experiences.

phenomenology: uses participants' accounts of their lived experience, mediated by the research process with the aim of achieving a deep and useful understanding of another's lifeworld.

positionality: the researcher makes clear their own position and how this might affect the research results.

positivism: knowledge is seen as existing as an independent, value-free and objective phenomenon, which is observable and can be measured and verified as existing.

postmodernism: moves away from a world of certainty towards notions that reality is more socially constructed, and is subject to change over time and location.

postpositivism: knowledge is seen as being changeable, and subject to modification in the light of further research.

power: power relations are seen as being central to the production of knowledge and are seen as being inevitable, but need to be acknowledged.

prefigurative action research (PreAR): examines the motivations and practices of those in power such that their positions are understood and power relations intrinsic to those positions are scrutinised.

problems: the scoring through in this context indicates that problems may not necessarily be problems, but they can help to aid understanding.

qualitative: research where the emphasis is on understanding, generally in natural contexts, rather than on measurement and quantification.

realist: assumes that there is some direct access to reality, which exists independently.

reflexivity: as part of the research process, involves both thinking about oneself and thinking about one's research, and one's impact on the research and its results and interpretation.

relativism: assumes that all knowledge is constructed.

scientist: generally refers to those who concentrate on using natural science methods.

social constructionist: individuals are seen as being constructed by their cultural and historical context.

spatiality: refers to our lifespace, which includes others, a variety of natural and cultural objects and cultural institutions.

standpoints: the acknowledgement that inevitably the researcher will be considering the social world from a particular position.

subjectivity: emphasis on individual interpretation, rather than attempting objectivity; an acknowledgement that both researchers and participants will bring to the research encounter their subjectivities.

temporality: an awareness of finiteness of life, of lived time and time left to live.

Index

Locators shown in *italics* refer to figures and boxes.

abstracts
  salience as element of report writing, 197
access, participant
  as consideration for ethnographic research, 81
action research (AR)
  definition, history and characteristics, 22–30
  relationship with evaluation, 30–31
  salience of emancipation, 32–3
  salience of utility, 31–2
action research, participatory (PAR), 24–5
Adams, M., 187–8
adenosine triphosphate (ATP), 144
Ahmed, S., 17
Albert, S., 65
Albrecht, A., 155
Ali (case study)
  use of repertory grid analysis, 109–11, *110*
Allport, G., 138
American Psychological Association (APA), 201, 202, 211
analysis, critical narrative (CNA), 17
analysis, discourse
  role of history in, 149–50
  see also influences e.g. antagonisms; contexts; language; objects, psychological; power; techniques, criminology; themes
  see also subject e.g. 'Criminal Man'
analysis, historical
  salience in the field of psychology, 143–7

analysis, interpretive phenomenological (IPA), 15–16
analysis, interview
  types, characteristics and uses, 90
analysis, psychosocial
  advantages and disadvantages, 122–5
  case study of, 120–22
  recent history of interest in, 116–18
  role in psychosocial research, 118–20
analysis, repertory grid
  case study of use, 109–11, *110*
  role and features, 108, *108*
  see also elements e.g. exploration, conversational
analysis, research
  salience as element of report writing, 199–200
analytical narratives, 130–31
Andrew, M., 112
Angelina (case study)
  narrative interviews, 133–6
Angrosino, M., 138
anonymity, participant
  salience as element of report writing, 203, 204
  salience as practicality of interview process, 96
antagonisms
  salience in psycho-historical discourse analysis, 151–2
Anthropological Society of Washington, 154
APA (American Psychological Association), 201, 202, 211
appendices
  salience as element of report writing, 201

appraisal, participatory rural (PRA), 80
AR *see* action research
Argyle, M., 65
Arthur, S., 53
Atkinson, D., 131
Atkinson, P., 77–8, 84, 95
ATP (*adenosine triphosphate*), 144
authority, charismatic
  salience as element of analysis of power, 156

Bales, R., 65
Banks, M., 185
Bargdill, R., 14
Barnes, C., 23, 95
Bauman, L., 79
Behar, R., 18, 76
Bem, D., 195, 196, 200
Bentall, R., 16
Beresford, P., 133
Beukema, L., 29–30
Biella, P., 188
Billig, M., 102
Blumenfeld-Jones, D., 90
Bogdan, R., 7, 51–2
Boies, H., 148
'born criminal' *see* 'Criminal Man'
Brinkman, S., 91, 95, 96
British Psychological Society (BPS), 73, 165, 201, 202, 204, 211
Brown, L., 28
Brown, S., 146, 147
Bruce, M., 187–8
Bruner, J., 188
Brydon-Miller, M., 33
Burke, L., 131, 137
Burns, D., 38, 44, 45, 52
Burrell, G., 6, 47–8
Burton, M., 23–4
Butt, T., 12, 16, 103

Caelli, K., 5
Calvey, D., 169
Capps, L., 134
Carothers, J., 180–81
Cary, M., 66
case studies
    approaches to visual
        representations in social
        research, 185–6
    ethnographic research on
        disabled children, 82–4
    narrative interviews, 133–6
    process of observation, 69–71
    role of psychoanalysis in
        psychosocial research,
        120–22
    use of repertory grid analysis,
        109–11, *110*
    ways of engaging with social
        research wording, 182–3
Cattall, J. McK., 143
CDS *see* studies, critical
    disability
Chamberlain, K., 211
Champagne, F., 31
change
    salience of centrality in AR,
        25–6
Chaplin, E., 184
Chicago School of sociology, 89
children, disabled
    case study of ethnographic
        research on, 82–4
Chris (case study)
    role of psychoanalysis in
        psychosocial research,
        120–22
Claire, H., 105
Clark, A., 80
Classen, C., 181
Clough, P., 47–8
Clouston, T., 150
Cocks, A., 81, 82
codes, ethical
    as consideration for
        ethnographic research, 81
Colaizzi, P., 7
Colajann, N., 151
collaboration
    role of stakeholder in action
        and evaluation research, 33
    salience as feature of AR, 27–8

confidentiality
    salience as element of report
        writing, 203, 204
    salience as practicality of
        interview process, 96
consent, informed
    as consideration for
        ethnographic research, 81
    salience as element of report
        writing, 202–3
    salience as feature of AR, 29
contents
    salience as element of report
        structures, 197
contexts
    salience in psycho-historical
        discourse analysis, 150–51
conversations
    exploration of as element of
        repertory grid analysis,
        108–9
Cook, M., 79
Cooke, B., 189
Crang, I., 79
'Criminal Man'
    historical discourse analysis of,
        148–57
    history of idea of, 147
Criminal Sociology (Colajann), 151
critical disability studies *see*
    studies, critical disability
critical narrative analysis (CNA),
    17
Crouch, D., 180
culture
    narrative interviews as artefact
        of, 137
Cutliffe, J., 168
cycles (cyclical action research)
    as characteristic of AR, 25

Danny (case study)
    role of psychoanalysis in
        psychosocial research,
        120–22
Da Vinci, L., 219
Darley, J., 63
Darwin, C., 150–51
Dawson, S., 182–3
deconstruction
    narrative interviews as tool of,
        137–8

de Laine, M., 50
Degeneration and Criminality
    (Féré), 151
Denzin, N., 81, 179, 180, 182
Department for Health, 30
Department of Culture Media
    and Sport, 30
description
    as element of
        phenomenological
        analysis, 5
Desfoges, L., 180
Dick, B., 24
Dingwall, R., 167–8
disability
    and inequality, 43–4
    case study of ethnographic
        research on, 82–4
    contribution to understanding
        epistemology, ontology and
        methodology, 48–9, *48*
    definition, 47–8
    feminism and CDS as reactions
        to theories of, 45–6
    see also studies, critical
        disability
discussion
    salience as element of report
        writing, 200
discipline
    salience as element of analysis
        of power, 154–5
Diseases of Society (Lydson),
    154–5
*Does Every Child's Matter,
    Post-Blair?*, 82–4, 90–91,
    133–6
Does my Bump Look Big in This?
    (Johnson), 17
Doherty, ???, 53
Duckett, P., 172
Dugdale, R., 151

Economic and Social Research
    Council, 169
egalitarianism
    salience in relation to action
        and evaluation research,
        32–3
emancipation
    characteristics as resource for
        qualitative research, 53–4, *54*

salience in relation to action and evaluation research, 32–3

emancipatory research
challenges within disability studies, 94–5

embodiment
as feature of 'lifeworlds', 9

Emmison, M., 183–4

empowerment, stakeholder
as feature of PAR, 24

enquiry, narrative
characteristics and centrality of, 130–33
evaluation of, 136–40, *139*
see also types e.g. narrative interviews

epistemology
as 'problem' for qualitative research, 209–10
contribution of disability to understanding of, 47–9, *48*
contribution of feminism to understanding of, 46–7
definition, 48
role as defining feature of phenomenology, 10–11

equipment
salience as practicality of interview process, 96

essences
as element of phenomenology, 5

ethics
as 'problem' for qualitative research, 216–18
challenges of within interview process, 95–6
critiquing of as focus of psychology research history, 167–71
role in observation process, 67
salience as element of report writing, 201–4
salience as feature of AR, 29–30
see also codes, ethical

ethnographic research
approaches to uses of senses in, 186–8
case study of, 82–4
characteristics and methods employed, 77–80

issues and considerations facing, 81–2

ethnography
characteristics and history of, 75–7

Eva (case study)
use of repertory grid analysis, 109–11, *110*

evaluation
relationship with action research, 30–31

evaluation research
salience of egalitarianism and emancipation, 32–3
salience of utility, 31–2

Every Child Matters (2004), 82, 91

experiences, personal
importance in phenomenology, 16

experiences, subjective
as element of phenomenology, 5–6

exploration, conversational
role and process as element of repertory grid analysis, 108–9

Fanon, F., 18, 82
Fay, D., 44–5
feelings, observer
salience and stereotypes of, 71
Feld, S., 188
feminism
and inequality, 41–3
as challenge to interview process, 92–4
as reaction and resistance to theories of disability, 45–6
as reaction and resistance to theories of gender, 44–5
contribution to understanding epistemology, ontology and methodology, 46–7
importance of viewpoint for qualitative research, 39–40
limitations of approach in qualitative research, 50–51
Féré, C., 151
Ferguson, P., 49
Ferrero, G., 152, 155
Fido, R., 132

findings, research
importance of addressing in report writing, 205–6
Finkelstein, V., 49
Finlay, L., 12–13
Fletcher, R., 154
Flowers, P., 15
flexibility
need for in overcoming research 'problems,' 218–20
Fontana, A., 92
Foucault, M., 145–6
Fransella, F., 103
Freeman, R., 3–4, 5
Freud, S., 63
Frey, J., 92
Furedi, F., 113

Gall, F., 150
Garofalo, J., 155
gatekeepers
as consideration for ethnographic research, 81
Gaventa, J., 28
gender
feminism and CDS as reactions to theories of, 44–5
Giorgi, G., 5
Glaser, B., 82
Glassner, B., 95
goals
salience as feature of AR, 29
Goffman, E., 66, 170
Gombrich, E., 183
Goodley, D., 43, 53, 77
Goodson, I., 90
Goodwin, D., 81
Greenberg Adair, E., 79
grids, repertory
characteristics and potential, 103–4
process of generating, 105–9, *106, 108*
research process of negotiating, 104–5
strengths and weaknesses, 112–13
see also analysis, repertory grid
groups, focus
as ethnographic research method, 79
Guba, E., 7

guidelines, ethics
    salience as element of report
        writing, 202

Hammersley, M., 77–8, 84
Hardt, M., 129
Harri-Augstein, E., 105
Hartnett, S., 182
Hearing Voices Network, 16
Heidegger, M., 5
Helsby, G., 31–2
Henriques, J., 51, 52
Hepburn, A., 91, 97
Hesse-Biber, S., 189
Higher Education Funding
    Council for England,
    165
history (historical analysis)
    salience in field of psychology,
        143–7
    see also forms e.g. analysis,
        discourse
Holland, J., 47
Homo criminalis see 'Criminal
    Man'
Howes, D., 181
Huberman, A., 167
Hull, J., 184
humanism, radical
    approach to theories of
        disability, 49
Husserl, E., 5, 8, 14

image, qualitative research
    salience of upholding viable,
        218–20
inequality
    as starting point for qualitative
        research, 41–4
information technologies (IT)
    as ethnographic research
        method, 80
    see also specific e.g. internet
internet
    as ethnographic research
        method, 80
interpretations
    as 'problem' for qualitative
        research, 215–16
    salience in relation to action
        and evaluation research,
        30–31

interpretations, research
    of observation of queueing
        processes, 70–71
interpretive phenomenological
    analysis (IPA), 15–16
interpretivism
    approach to theories of
        disability, 49
intersubjectivity
    as feature of 'lifeworlds', 9
interviews
    challenges posed as
        methodology, 90–96
    characteristics and origins,
        78–9, 88–9
    practicalities of process, 96–7
    see also analysis, interview
    see also type e.g. narrative
        interviews; semi-structured
        interviews; structured
        interviews; unstructured
        interviews
introduction, report
    salience as element of report
        writing, 197–8
IPA (interpretive
    phenomenological analysis),
    15–16
IT (information technologies)
    as ethnographic research
        method, 80
    see also specific e.g. internet

Janesick, V., 189
Jarviluoma, H., 50
Johnson, S., 17
Jowett, M., 44, 47
Jukes, The (Dugdale), 151
Jung, K., 41

Kagan, C., 23–4, 113
Karniel-Miller, O., 40, 42
Katz, J., 15
Kellock, A., 185
Kelly, G., 100–103, 111, 113
Kessler, S., 65
King, N., 12, 13, 15
Kitsuse, J., 137
Kitzinger, S., 40
Klein, M., 119, 123, 124, 125
Kothari, U., 189
Kozinets, R., 80

Krebs, H., 144
Kuhn, A., 185
Kvale, S., 91, 95, 96

Lacan, J., 119–20, 123, 124–5
Lafrance, M., 39, 40, 42, 50, 52
Lambroso, C., 147, 148, 149, 151,
    152, 153–4, 155
Lammer, C., 187
Lamont, P., 145
Lane, F., 156
Langdridge, D., 8, 12, 16, 17
Langer, E., 73
Langness, L., 49, 53, 130–31
language
    consideration of as element
        of research reports,
        194–6
    salience in psycho-historical
        discourse analysis, 153–4
Lash, S., 138
Latané, B., 63
Law, L., 187
Lawthom, R., 53
Leavy, P., 189
Lee, E., 18
legitimacy
    as 'problem' for qualitative
        research, 211–14
Levine, H., 49, 53, 130–31
Lewin, K., 22–3, 30
Lexis (case study)
    use of repertory grid analysis,
        109–11, 110
'lifeworlds'
    as element of phenomenology,
        5–6
    definition and features, 9
Lincoln, Y., 7, 81, 179, 180
Linton, S., 45, 131
Lohmann, K., 144
Lopez, K., 14
L'uomo delinquente (Lombroso),
    149
Lydson, G. F., 154–5

McAlister, S., 41–2, 45, 47, 50, 51
McDougall, W., 145
McLaughlin, J., 137–8
Macrae, R., 112
Malinowski, B., 76
Mantegazza, P., 152

mapping, qualitative research theories of, 48–9, *48*
Marshall, C., 64
Mason, J., 212, 213
Mastain, L., 14
Maudsley, H., 149
May, T., 46–7
Mayhew, H., 149–50
Measuring Disablement in Society project, 54
media (multimedia)
   as ethnographic research method, 80
   significance of as tool for qualitative research, 174–5
   see also specific e.g. technologies, information
Merleau-Ponty, M., 5
methodology and methodologies
   case for future decolonising of in psychology, 171–3
   contribution of disability to understanding of, 47–9, *48*
   contribution of feminism to understanding of, 46–7
   definition, 48
   mixing of as 'problem' for qualitative research, 211–13
   role as defining feature of phenomenology, 13–15
   salience of pluralism of in AR, 26
   see also elements and processes e.g. ethics; writing, research
   see also tools and specific e.g. grids, repertory; interviews; observation; participants and participation
Michalko, R., 7–8, 8–9, 11, 184
Miles, M., 167
Milgram, S., 166
Miller, J., 95
Minuchin, S., 65
models and theories
   as consideration for ethnographic research, 81–2
   gender resistances, 44–5
   paradigms of qualitative research, 6–7
   personal construct theory, 100–103
   qualitative research mapping, 48–9, *48*

Mohanty, C., 16
Moore, P., 188
Morgan, G., 6, 47–8
Morris, J., 78, 83
Morrison, W., 151
Moulding, M., 42–3, 45
Murphy, E., 167–8
My Gypsy Childhood (Freeman), 3

Nader, L., 169–70, 173
narrative interviews
   characteristics and case study, 133–6
   evaluation of form, 136–40, *139*
narratives
   as approach to interview analysis, 90
   topicality of, 129
narratives, creative, 131–2
narratives, critical analysis (CNA), 17
narratives, historical, 132–3
notes, research
   role in observation process, 67
   see also reports, research
Negotiator, The (film), 120–22
Negri, A., 129
Neill, G., 41–2, 45, 47, 50, 51
Nutbrown, C., 47–8

Oakley, A., 40, 44, 93
objects, psychological
   role in history discourse analysis, 147–8
observation
   case study of, 69–71
   characteristics and examples, 64–6
   process of, 66–9
   role in psychological research, 63
   strengths and weaknesses as research method, 71–3
observation, participant
   features as element of ethnographic research, 77–8
Ochs, E., 134
O'Leary, Z., 39, 47, 50, 52–3
Olkin, R., 133
ontology
   contribution of disability to understanding of, 47–9, *48*

   contribution of feminism to understanding of, 46–7
   definition, 47–8
   role as defining feature of phenomenology, 11–12
openness
   need for in overcoming qualitative research 'problems,' 218–20
Origin of Species (Darwin), 150–51
O'Toole, G., 44, 47, 130
Ottolenghi, S., 156
overuse
   as challenge to interview process, 91
ownership
   characteristics as element of qualitative research, 52–3

PAR (participatory action research), 24–5
paradigms
   of contemporary qualitative research, 6–7
Parker, I., 183
participants and participation
   access to as consideration for ethnographic research, 81
   characteristics as element of qualitative research, 53–4, *54*
   see also anonymity, participant; observation, participant; vulnerability, participant; well-being, participant
participatory action research (PAR), 24–5
participatory rural appraisal (PRA), 80
partnerships, collaborative
   salience as feature of AR, 27–8
pastoralism
   salience as element of analysis of power, 156
patriarchy
   salience as element of analysis of power, 155
Pawson, R., 30, 32
Pelias, R., 189
personal construct theory (PCT)
   characteristics and history, 100–103

see also elements e.g. grids, repertory
phenomenology
defining and mapping of, 7–10
definition and characteristics, 4–6
future directions, 17–18
see also analysis, interpretive phenomenology
see also core concerns e.g. subjectivity
see also research elements impacted e.g. epistemology; methodology and methodologies; ontology; positionality
photography
approach to alternatives and uses in social research, 184–5
Piaget, J., 63
pictures
approach to alternatives and uses in social research, 183–4
Pink, S., 186–7
Polkinghorne, D., 90
Pope, M., 103
positionality
as challenge to interview process, 91–2
role as defining feature of phenomenology, 12–13
Potter, J., 91, 97, 173
Potts, M., 132
power
as challenge within interview process, 93–4
as 'problem' for qualitative research, 218
salience in psycho-historical discourse analysis, 154–7
prefigurative action research (PreAR), 23–4
Price, J., 51
Prins, E., 26
priorities
need to enunciate in qualitative research, 218–20
salience as feature of AR, 28
Prisoners and Paupers (Boies), 148
problems, quantitative research
examples of, 208–18
salience of overcoming, 218–20

properties, emergent
salience as feature of AR, 25
psychological research
critiquing as focus of history of, 167–71
historical development, 165–7
role of observation, 63
see also elements e.g. analysis, psychosocial; ethics
psychology
history of qualitative research in, 165–7
salience of historical analysis within, 143–7
see also objects, psychological
see also elements for consideration e.g. ethics; methods and methodology

quality
salience as feature of AR, 28–9
queueing
case study of observation of, 69–71
Quinlan, E., 26

Ramazanoglu, C., 44, 47
Ramcharan, P., 168
realism
as approach to interview analysis, 90
reality, researcher
as feature of phenomenology, 9
Reason, P., 64, 205–6
Reavey, P., 184
reduction, phenomenological
as element of phenomenological analysis, 5
Reeve, D., 132–3
references
salience as element of report writing, 201
reflexivity
as 'problem' for qualitative research, 216
salience as element of report writing, 200–201
salience as feature of AR, 26–7
Reid, C., 27, 29
reports, research
considerations of language and style, 194–6

importance of research findings in, 205–6
role and characteristics of observational, 67–8
salience of ethics and values as elements, 201–5
structure of, 196–201
see also notes, research
see also stages e.g. writing, research
representations, visual
approach to alternatives and uses in social ethnography, 183–6
research, qualitative
context of emerging approaches to, 179–80
defining and mapping phenomenology as approach to, 7–10
need to enunciate practices, 218–20
neglected and 'problem' areas, 208–18
overcoming qualitative versus quantitative divide, 173–4
paradigms of contemporary, 7
position of phenomenology within, 6–7, 6
salience and limitations of feminism as approach, 39–40, 50–51
salience of critical disability sitpoint, 40–41
salience of overcoming 'problems' and image of, 218–20
see also interpretations, research
see also concepts and elements e.g. epistemology; methodology and methodologies; ontology; ownership; participants and participation; subjectivity; 'voice'; writing, research
see also subjects and drivers e.g. inequality; sciences, social
see also tools e.g. media
see also types e.g. action research; emancipatory

research; ethnographic
    research; evaluation research;
    participatory action
    research; psychological
    research
Rhodes, J., 15
Richards, G., 145
Richardson, L., 182
Ricouer, P., 15
risks
    salience as feature of AR, 28
Rogers, C., 5
Rose, G., 92
Rose, N., 145
Roseman, M., 187
Rosenhan, D., 170
Rossman, G., 64
Rowan, J., 64, 205–6
Roxberg, A., 12, 13

Salmon, A., 42, 44, 52
Salmon, P., 105, 112
Sapsford, R., 206
Sarbin, T., 137
Satre, J-P., 5, 18
Saunders, M., 31–2
Savin, H., 201, 204
sciences, social
    alternatives and uses of
        research visual
        representations in, 183–6
    case study of engaging with
        subject wording, 182–3
    emerging qualitative research
        representations in, 180–82
    see also particular e.g.
        psychology
Scott-Hill, M., 137
selection
    as 'problem' for qualitative
        research, 214–15
semi-structured interviews, 89–90
senses, the
    uses in social ethnography,
        186–8
Serres, M., 181
Shepherd, 205
Sherry, M., 45, 46
Shildrick, M., 51
Silverman, D., 90, 95, 189
Slavoj, Z., 149
Smail, D., 113

Smith, J., 5, 12, 15, 17
Smith, L., 32, 171
Smith, P., 131, 132, 137, 183–4
Smits, P., 31
Sociological Initiatives
    Foundation, 29
Sparkes, A., 131, 132, 137
spatiality
    as feature of 'lifeworlds', 9
Stainton-Rogers, W., 113, 175
stakeholders
    empowerment of as feature of
        PAR, 24
Stanford Prison Experiment, 204
Stanley, L., 39, 44, 52
status and value
    as consideration for
        ethnographic research, 81
    as feature of AR, 28–9
    salience as element of report
        writing, 204–5
Stenner, P., 146, 147
Stephenson, N., 42–3, 47, 50–51
Stevenson, R. L., 151
Stocker, R., 29
Stoker, B., 151
Stoppard, J., 39, 40, 42, 50, 52
storytelling
    as approach to interview
        analysis, 90
    topicality of, 129
    see also enquiry, narrative
Strange Case of Doctor Jekyll and
    Mr Hyde, The (Stevenson),
    151
Strauss, A., 82
structuralism, radical
    approach to theories of
        disability, 49
structured interviews, 89–90
studies, critical disability (CDS)
    as reaction and resistance to
        theories of disability,
        45–6
    as reaction and resistances to
        theories of gender, 44–5
    challenges of by emancipatory
        research, 94–5
    limitations of approach in
        qualitative research, 51–2
    salience of sitpoint for
        qualitative research, 40–41

studies, pilot
    role in observation process, 66
styles, writing
    considerations of as element of
        research reports, 194–6
subjectivity
    as feature of PAR, 24
    characteristics as resource
        for qualitative research,
        52–4, 54
    definition and features of
        individual, 9
    importance in phenomenology,
        16
    salience as feature of AR, 26–7

TAB (Temporarily Able Bodied)
    (concept), 43
Tarde, G., 153
Taylor, S., 7, 51–2
techniques, criminology
    salience in psycho-historical
        discourse analysis, 152–3
technologies, information
    as ethnographic research
        method, 80
    see also specific e.g. internet
Tedlock, B., 76
temporality
    as feature of 'lifeworlds', 9
Temporarily Able Bodied (TAB)
    (concept), 43
text, humane
    narrative interviews as, 138
themes
    salience in psycho-historical
        discourse analysis, 148–9
theories and models see models
    and theories
Thomas, C., 46
Thomas, L., 105
Thome, B., 11, 15
Thompson, B., 112
Thomson, G., 41
Thomson, J., 148–9, 155
Tilley, N., 30, 32
Time Machine, The (Wells), 151
Tindall, A., 103, 112
Titchkosky, T., 84, 180
titles
    salience as element of report
        structures, 196–7

transcription
    salience as practicality of
        interview process, 96–7
Travers, M., 47
trust
    salience as feature of AR, 29–30

unstructured interviews, 89–90
Ussher, J., 42
utility
    importance in evaluation and
        AR, 31–2

Valkenburg, B., 29–30
value and status
    as consideration for
        ethnographic research, 81
    as feature of AR, 28–9
    salience as element of report
        writing, 204–5
Van Manen, M., 11
Villella, G., 148–9
Vlachou, A., 76–7

'voice'
    as challenge to interview
        process, 94
    characteristics as element of
        qualitative research, 52–3
vulnerability, participant
    salience as feature of AR, 29

Walker, B., 102
Walker, M., 38, 44, 45, 52
Walker, R., 138
Watts, J., 40, 42–3, 47, 50–51, 52
Weatherell, M., 173
Webb, E., 65
Weber, M., 156
Weiss, C., 30, 31
well-being, participant
    salience as feature of AR, 29
Wells, H. G., 151
Wertz, F., 14, 18
Westmarland, M., 39, 44
Wilde, O., 151
Wilkinson, S., 44, 200, 201

Williams, F., 131
Willig, C., 7, 8, 10, 14, 39, 112, 196
Willis, D., 14
Wilson, A., 133
Winter, D., 102
Wise, L., 39, 44, 52
words
    uses and alternatives in social
        science research, 182–3
World Wide Web
    as ethnographic research
        method, 80
Wright Mills, C., 41, 130
Wrightson, K., 187–8
writing, research
    role and characteristics of
        observational, 67–8
    see also output e.g. reports,
        research
Wundt, W., 166

Zarb, G., 53
Zimbardo, P., 201